CARDIO KIDNEY METABOLIC MEDICINE 2026

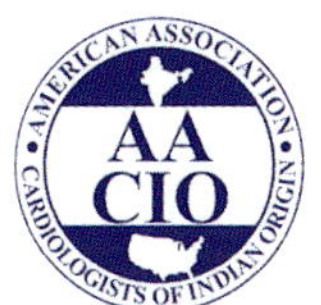

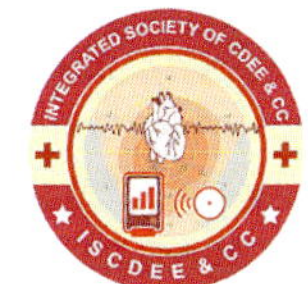

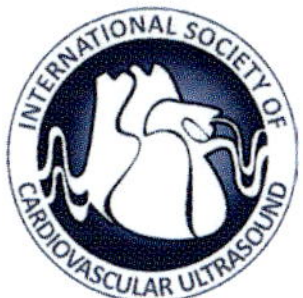

CARDIO KIDNEY METABOLIC MEDICINE 2026

Editor-in-Chief

PC Manoria
MD DM FACC FESC FCAPSC FICC FICP
Director
Department of Cardiology
Manoria Heart and Critical Care Hospital, Bhopal
Former Professor and Head
Department of Cardiology
Gandhi Medical College
Bhopal, Madhya Pradesh, India
Past Chairman, Hypertension Council
Asian Pacific Society of Cardiology
Past Vice President, SAARC Cardiac Society
Past President, CSI, API, ICC, IFUMB, HSI, IACM, GSI
Past Dean, ICP, ICMU

Forewords

Peter EH Schwarz
Prakash Deedwania
YS Chandrashekhar
Navin C Nanda

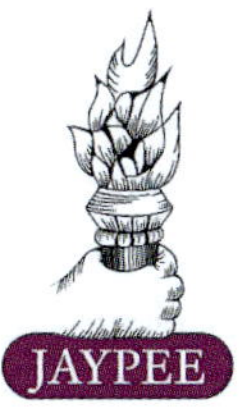

JAYPEE BROTHERS MEDICAL PUBLISHERS
The Health Sciences Publisher
New Delhi | London

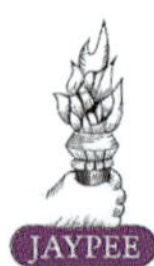

Jaypee Brothers Medical Publishers (P) Ltd

Headquarters
EMCA House, 23/23-B
Ansari Road, Daryaganj
New Delhi 110 002, India
Landline: +91-11-23272143, +91-11-23272703
+91-11-23282021, +91-11-23245672
e-mail: jaypee@jaypeebrothers.com

Corporate Office
4838/24, Ansari Road, Daryaganj
New Delhi 110 002, India
Phone: +91-11-43574357
Fax: +91-11-43574314
e-mail: jaypee@jaypeebrothers.com

Overseas Office
JP Medical Ltd
83 Victoria Street, London
SW1H 0HW (UK)
Phone: +44-20 3170 8910
e-mail: info@jpmedpub.com

EU GPSR Authorised Representative
Logos Europe, 9 rue Nicolas Poussin
17000, La Rochelle, France
Phone: +33 (0) 6 67 93 73 78
e-mail: contact@logoseurope.eu

Website: www.jaypeebrothers.com
Website: www.jaypeedigital.com

Inquiries for bulk sales may be solicited at: jaypee@jaypeebrothers.com

Cardio Kidney Metabolic Medicine 2026

First Edition: **2026**

ISBN: 978-93-7202-435-7

Printed at: Samrat Offset Pvt. Ltd.

Contributors

Akshat Banga MBBS
Resident (MD)
Department of Internal Medicine
Mount Auburn Hospital
Cambridge, MA, USA

Alok Modi MD (Med)
Consultant
Department of Diabetology
Kevalya Hospital
Mumbai, Maharashtra, India

Anuj Maheshwari
MD FICP FIACM FIMSA FRSSDI FACP (USA) FACE (USA) FRCP (London, Edinburgh)
Diabetologist and Metabolic Physician
Department of Medicine
Hind Institute of Medical Sciences
Lucknow, Uttar Pradesh, India

Ashok L Kirpalani
MD (Internal Medicine), MNAMS (Nephrology)
Professor Emeritus
Department of Nephrology
Bombay Hospital Institute of Medical Sciences
Mumbai, Maharashtra, India

Avani Verma MBBS
Junior Resident PGY3 (MD)
Department of Dermatology, Venereology and Leprosy
Mahatma Gandhi Medical College and Hospital
Jaipur, Rajasthan, India

Banshi Saboo MD PhD
Chairman and Chief Diabetologist
Dia Care, Diabetes Care and Hormone Clinic
Ahmedabad, Gujarat, India

Brij Mohan Makkar
MD FIAMS FICP FRCP (Glasg, Edin) FACP (USA) FACE (USA) FRSSDI
Senior Diabetologist and Obesity Specialist
Dr Makkar's Diabetes and Obesity Centre
New Delhi, India

Dilip A Kirpalani
MD DM (Nephrology)
Assistant Professor
Department of Nephrology
Bombay Hospital Institute of Medical Sciences
Mumbai, Maharashtra, India

Elmutaz Abdalla Mekki Kanani MS (General Surgery)
Specialist (General Surgery)
Fellow, Upper GI, Bariatric and Metabolic Surgery
Laparo Obeso Centre (LOC Healthcare LLP)
Pune, Maharashtra, India

Hardik K Shah
MD (Internal Medicine), DNB (Nephrology)
Associate Professor
Department of Nephrology
Bombay Hospital Institute of Medical Sciences
Mumbai, Maharashtra, India

Harish Ranjani PhD CDE
Senior Scientist and Head
Department of Preventive and Digital Health Research
Madras Diabetes Research Foundation and Dr Mohan's Diabetes Specialities Centre
Chennai, Tamil Nadu, India

Hemant Phatale
DM (Endocrine)
Senior Endocrinologist
Samrat Endocrine Institute of Diabetes, Obesity and Thyroid
Chhatrapati Sambhaji Nagar, Maharashtra, India

Kanishka Manikandan
MBBS
Medical Graduate
Government Medical College and Hospital
Coimbatore, Tamil Nadu, India

Mala Dharmalingam
MD DM (AIIMS) FDiab FAMS FACE (US)
Consultant Endocrinologist
Bangalore Endocrinology and Diabetes Research Centre
Bengaluru, Karnataka, India

Manish Kumar Verma MD
Additional Professor
Department of Physiology
Dr Ram Manohar Lohia Institute of Medical Sciences
Lucknow, Uttar Pradesh, India

Manisha Arora
MD (Internal Medicine)
Consultant
Department of Internal Medicine
CK Birla Hospital
New Delhi, India

Mohamed Thajudeen MD
Senior Medical Officer
Clinical Research
Twin Health
Chennai, Tamil Nadu, India

Narsingh Verma MD
Principal
Hind Institute of Medical Sciences
Sitapur, Uttar Pradesh, India

Navin C Nanda
MD DSc (Hon) DSc (Med) (Hon) FACC FAHA FASE FISCU (D)
Distinguished Professor of Medicine and Cardiovascular Disease
University of Alabama at Birmingham
Birmingham, Alabama, USA
President, International Society of Cardiovascular Ultrasound

Neeta Deshpande
MD (Medicine) FRCP (Edinburgh) PG ENDO (London) ASBP Cert Obesity (USA)
Diabetologist and Bariatric Physician
Belgaum Diabetes Center
Belagavi, Karnataka, India

Nitin Patankar MD (Medicine)
Consultant (Diabetes and Obesity)
Adi Arogyam Suman Ramesh Tulsiani Hospital
Thane, Maharashtra, India

Pankaj Manoria
MD DM FACC FESC FSCAI
Chief Interventional Cardiologist
Manoria Heart and Critical Care Hospital
Bhopal, Madhya Pradesh, India

PC Manoria
MD DM FACC FESC FCAPSC FICC FICP
Director
Department of Cardiology
Manoria Heart and Critical Care Hospital, Bhopal
Former Professor and Head
Department of Cardiology
Gandhi Medical College
Bhopal, Madhya Pradesh, India
Past Chairman, Hypertension Council
Asian Pacific Society of Cardiology
Past Vice President, SAARC Cardiac Society
Past President, CSI, API, ICC, IFUMB, HSI, IACM, GSI
Past Dean, ICP, ICMU

Piyush Manoria
MD DM (Gastroenetrology)
Gastroenterologist
Manoria Heart and Critical Care Hospital
Bhopal, Madhya Pradesh, India

Prakash Deedwania MD
Professor
Department of Cardiovascular Medicine
University of California San Francisco
Fresno, CA, USA

Pramod Kumar Thyparambil Aravindakshan MSc MPhil PhD
Scientist
Research Operations and Diabetes Complications
Madras Diabetes Research Foundation
ICMR—Collaborating Centre of Excellence
Chennai, Tamil Nadu, India

Priti Phatale MBBS DCH
Pediatrician and Childhood and Adolescent Obesity Specialist
Samrat Endocrine Institute of Diabetes, Obesity and Thyroid
Chhatrapati Sambhaji Nagar
Maharashtra, India

Radha Deshpande
MD (General Medicine)
Senior Resident
Department of Medicine
MGM Medical College and Hospital
Navi Mumbai, Maharashtra, India

Rajeev Gupta
MD PhD
Chairman
Preventive Cardiology and Medicine
Eternal Heart Care Centre and Research Institute
Jaipur, Rajasthan, India

Rajesh Rajput
MD DM (Endocrinology) FRCP (Edin) FACE (USA) FICP FIACM FISH FIMSA FRSSDI
Director
Division of Endocrinology and Diabetes
Medanta—the Medicity
Gurugram, Haryana, India

Rakesh M Parikh
MBBS FCPS (Med) Dip Diabetology
Consultant
Department of Diabetology
CKS Hospital
Jaipur, Rajasthan, India

Ranjit Mohan Anjana
MD PhD FRCP
President and Managing Director
Madras Diabetes Research Foundation and Dr Mohan's Diabetes Specialties Centre
Chennai, Tamil Nadu, India

Sagar Phatale
MBBS
General Physician
Family Health Clinic
Chhatrapati Sambhaji Nagar
Maharashtra, India

Saifullah Syed MD
Internal Medicine Resident
Indiana University School of Medicine
Indianapolis, Indiana, USA

Sana M Sahigara
Renal Nutritionist BSc, Dip Nutrition and Dietetics
Dietician
Kidney and Blood Pressure Clinic
Indian Cancer Society Medical Centre
Mumbai, Maharashtra, India

Sharma Nitika
MSc Foods Nutrition and Dietetics
Project Manager
Department of Digital and Preventive Health Research
Madras Diabetes Research Foundation and Dr Mohan's Diabetes Specialties Centre
Chennai, Tamil Nadu, India

Shashank S Shah
MS FAIS FICS FIAGES FALS
Senior Consultant and General, Laparoscopic, Bariatric and Metabolic Surgeon
Director and Head
Laparo Obeso Centre
(LOC Healthcare LLP)
Pune, Maharashtra, India

Shivam Verma MD DNB
Assistant Professor
Department of Physiology
Dr Ram Manohar Lohia Institute of Medical Sciences
Lucknow, Uttar Pradesh, India

Siddhant Rajput MD (Medicine)
Student (DM)
Department of Nephrology
Nizam's Institute of Medical Sciences (NIMS)
Hyderabad, Telangana, India

Somyata Somendra
MD DM Cardiology
Consultant Cardiology
Eternal Hospital
Jaipur, Rajasthan, India

Subhajyoti Ghosh
MD PhD (Diabetes)
Consultant Physician and Diabetologist
Apollo Clinic
Dibrugarh, Assam, India

Vineet Sankhla
MD DM Cardiology
Cardiologist
Palmerston North Hospital
New Zealand

Viswanathan Mohan
MD FRCP PhD DSc FNASc FASc FAMS FNA FACE FTWAS MACP FRSE
Chairman
Department of Diabetology
Madras Diabetes Research Foundation
(ICMR-Collaborating Centre of Excellence)
Dr Mohan's Diabetes Specialties Centre
(IDF Centre of Excellence in Diabetes Care)
Chennai, Tamil Nadu, India

Yaser Ahmad MD
Internal Medicine Resident
University of Alabama at Birmingham
Birmingham, Alabama, USA

Foreword

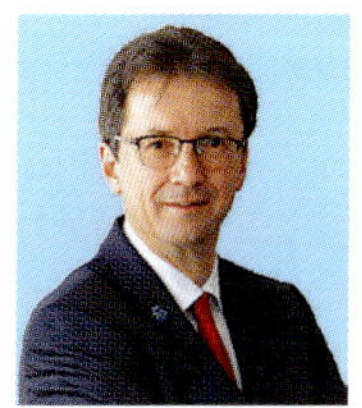

As President of the International Diabetes Federation (IDF), it is a great pleasure and honor to write the foreword to this timely and forward-looking book *Cardio Kidney Metabolic Medicine 2026*.

We are living through a global epidemic of obesity, type 2 diabetes, hypertension, chronic kidney disease, and heart failure—conditions that do not occur in isolation but are deeply interconnected and mutually reinforcing. This volume brings these links consequently together: From obesity and sarcopenic obesity, to metabolic dysfunction-associated steatotic liver disease (MASLD), heart failure and CKD, and on to pharmacotherapy with SGLT2-inhibitors and new antihypertensive agents. It reflects a modern understanding that prevention, early diagnosis, and comprehensive care must all be organized around the *entire* cardio-kidney metabolic continuum.

I am particularly encouraged by the clear focus on the future of diabetes care. Chapters on Continuous Glucose Monitoring, Digital Twins, Artificial Intelligence, and Digital Diabetes Care illustrate how rapidly our toolbox is expanding—and how crucial it is that we use these innovations to close, not widen, existing gaps in care. For clinicians, researchers, nurses, educators, and policymakers, this book offers both an up-to-date overview and many very practical insights that can be translated into better everyday care for people living with or at high risk of diabetes.

At IDF, we are convinced that no single profession, discipline, or country can solve the cardiometabolic challenge alone. The broad and distinguished group of authors assembled here—spanning obesity, pediatrics, cardiology, nephrology, diabetology, pharmacotherapy and digital health—embodies exactly the kind of multidisciplinary collaboration we need. Their combined expertise makes this book a rich resource for anyone committed to improving outcomes across the life course.

I warmly congratulate the editors and contributors on this important achievement. I am confident that this book will inspire its readers to think more integratively, act more proactively, and advocate more powerfully for people at risk of, or living with, diabetes and related conditions. May it support you in your daily work and motivate us all to move faster toward a world where prevention, remission where possible, and high-quality, person-centered care are a reality for everyone.

Peter EH Schwarz

Prof. Dr med. habil, MBA

Department for Prevention and Care of Diabetes

Faculty of Medicine Carl Gustav Carus

Technische Universität Dresden, Dresden, Germany

Paul Langerhans Institute Dresden, Helmholtz Zentrum München

University Hospital and Faculty of Medicine, TU Dresden, Dresden, Germany

German Center for Diabetes Research (DZD e.V.), Neuherberg, Germany

President

International Diabetes Federation (IDF), Brussels, Belgium

Foreword

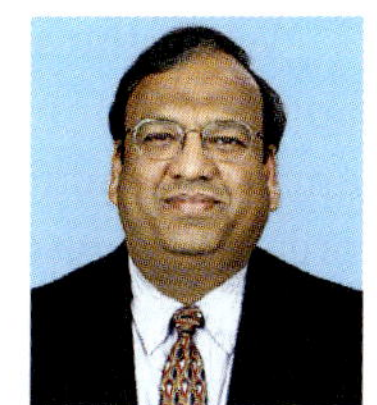

The recent recognition of cardio-kidney metabolic syndrome in an American Heart Association Presidential Advisory marked a defining moment in contemporary medicine as it emphasizes the ever-increasing public health burden of obesity and diabetes globally. For decades, diabetes, cardiovascular disease, obesity, metabolic disorders, and chronic kidney disease have been defined as distinct clinical entities. However, the advances in epidemiology, pathophysiology, and therapeutic strategies have now revealed a far more integrated reality that these conditions form a biologically interconnected continuum driven by shared mechanisms and reciprocal progression. It is now well recognized that there are overlapping mechanisms like inflammation, insulin resistance, endothelial dysfunction, and neurohormonal activation that link obesity, diabetes, metabolic abnormalities, cardiovascular disorders, and even hepatic dysfunction. This paradigm shift is reshaping how we conceptualize these chronic disorders, use various therapeutic strategies, and deliver care.

This book titled, *Cardio Kidney Metabolic Medicine 2026* by Dr PC Manoria comes at a time of remarkable scientific progress and therapeutic advances in this field. The book makes a timely and meaningful contribution by evolving science into clinical perspective. It promotes a unified approach to patient management and highlights the need for early identification and interventions to prevent target end-organ damage.

The foundational chapters on obesity, diabetes, and insulin resistance establish the biological and clinical substrate upon which CKM disease develops. Obesity is appropriately recognized as a chronic, biologically driven disorder that serves as a major upstream determinant of insulin resistance, metabolic dysfunction, inflammation, hypertension, and cardiometabolic risk. Diabetes is described not merely as a disorder of hyperglycemia, but as a systemic disease with profound cardiovascular and renal consequences. Subsequent chapters build upon this foundation by examining the multisystem consequences of these disorders, including heart failure, atherosclerotic cardiovascular disease, chronic kidney disease, and MASLD. This progression reinforces the concept that CKM represents a continuum beginning early in the course of metabolic dysfunction and advances silently before the onset overt clinical events.

A major strength of this book lies in its comprehensive and contemporary discussion of newer therapeutic agents, particularly sodium-glucose cotransporter inhibitors (SGLTis) and glucagon-like peptide-1 receptor agonists (GLP-1Ras). These chapters highlight a paradigm shift in treatment strategy—from the glucocentric management to organ—protective, disease-modifying therapy. The evidence presented demonstrates that SGLT confers far more than glucose control by showing robust cardiovascular and renal protection, including dramatic reduction in heart failure hospitalization and slowing the progression of CKD benefits that extend well beyond those demonstrated with glycemic control. Similarly, GLP-1RAs have been shown to favorably influence various components of CKM though weight reduction, improvement in insulin resistance, reduction in major CV events, and emerging benefits in MASLD.

Taken together various chapters in this book bridge the gap between complex medical science and clear understanding by providing links between pathophysiology and clinical consequences, offering the readers a cohesive, evidence-based framework for the holistic management of CKM disorders. Furthermore, the chapters not only explain how these conditions develop but also provide guidance as to how practical and simple lifestyle choices, integrated medical care, and informed decision making can dramatically reduce risk and improve quality of life.

While the statistics and epidemiologic data surrounding CKM, diabetes, CKD, and heart disease appear alarming, the message of this book is ultimately one of hope. With education, commitment, and timely action emphasizing early identification and appropriate therapeutic intervention to prevent organ damage we can change the course of these diseases and protect both heart and overall well-being.

I am confident that this book will serve as a trusted guide by providing an authoritative roadmap to manage the rapidly growing global public heath challenge with CKM disorders.

Prakash Deedwania
MD FACC FAHA FASH FHFSA FESC
Professor of Medicine
UCSF School of Medicine
San Francisco, California, USA

Foreword

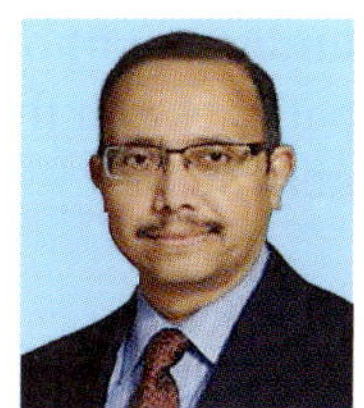

Medicine is evolving rapidly, and one major welcome development is that we are moving away from identifying and treating individual disease entities (e.g., obesity, diabetes, or hypertension) to addressing the patient more holistically—seeing the patient as a whole entity rather than addressing one disease at a time in a siloed manner. One area where we are currently witnessing this massive paradigm shift is in the *Cardiovascular-Kidney-Metabolic (CKM) syndrome*, a syndromic complex that simultaneously involves several seemingly disparate systems, together—obesity, metabolic dysregulation, kidney dysfunction, and adverse effects in the cardiovascular system. The problem is huge, for example, nearly 90% of the US population displays at least one component of CKM. The situation is far worse in the developing world and is likely to get worse very rapidly.

It is now known that current strategies, that treat each of these individual components separately, often by distinctly separate cardiovascular, renal, and metabolic medicine specialties, are grossly inadequate. On the other hand, there is new evidence that CKM is reversible in its early stages; recognizing and addressing all these multisystem connections, in a coordinated and evidence-based manner, can improve outcomes significantly.

Unfortunately, CKM is massively under-recognized and even worse, most patients are suboptimally treated. A major reason seems to be the lack of adequate understanding of what CKM really is, knowing how to detect it, and confusion about how best to treat this highly reversible condition.

This excellent book, *Cardio Kidney Metabolic Medicine 2026,* edited by Dr PC Manoria and colleagues thus arrives at a critical juncture while also filling a dire need—providing evidence based, easily implementable, practical knowledge about CKM—with comprehensive information for both the experts as well as for the less expert clinicians managing this complex and highly prevalent condition. It serves as a definitive road map for clinicians navigating multisystem pathology, covering everything that is important from the looming threat of obesity across the life spectrum, pathogenetic concepts including chronic inflammation and insulin resistance, role of biomarkers, new data in management of diabetes and hypertension, recent information on newer drugs like SGLT2 inhibitors and GLP/GIP agonists, and then leads into recognition, prevention, and treatment of major organ-specific syndromes like heart failure, MASLD, and CKD.

What makes this book particularly timely is its futuristic perspective. It does not just address current best practices but also gives the reader a glimpse of what is coming into newer therapies, wearable-monitoring devices, and the possibly transformative role of artificial intelligence and digital twin technology in personalized care.

As someone who regularly sees a lot of patients with this syndrome and as well having seen the devastating impact of delayed and fragmented care first-hand, I believe this textbook is more than a reference—it is a call for evidence-driven, integrated care model and shows you how to incorporate that into your practice. It provides practitioners with practical tools to act at the reversible stage of CKM, holistically addressing each of the components of CKM, long before they cause irreversible damage.

I greatly enjoyed reading and learning from this book, and I invite you to delve deeply into it to understand holistic, patient-centered care in CKM and thus improve the lives of the hundreds of patients with this condition that you see now and will undoubtedly be seeing even much more in the near future.

YS Chandrashekhar
MD FACC
Professor of Medicine
University of Minnesota
Minneapolis, Minnesota, USA
Editor-in-Chief, JACC Cardiovascular Imaging

Foreword

I am most pleased and honored to write this foreword for the book *Cardio Kidney Metabolic Medicine 2026*, which is edited by none other than Dr (Professor) PC Manoria. He has been hosting the remarkably successful World Congress on the afore-mentioned subject regularly.

I have had the privilege of knowing and interacting with Dr PC Manoria for several decades. He is one of the most illustrious cardiologists in India who has conducted several international Conferences and Congresses in India on various aspects of cardiology (including echocardiography) and metabolic diseases for the past several years.

The contents of this book consist of 20 chapters listed under the headings of introduction, obesity, diabetes reversal/remission, continuous glucose monitoring (CGM), hypertension, metabolic dysfunction-associated steatotic liver disease (MASLD), heart failure, chronic kidney disease (CKD), pharmacotherapy, and future of diabetes. All the chapters in the book are written by experts in their field and consist of most current updates in each subject. Our group's contribution is on noninvasive assessment of epicardial adipose tissue and its impact on cardiometabolic risk.

The book will be useful to a wide audience of all physicians and paramedical personnel, especially cardiologists, endocrinologists, and internal medicine practitioners. My heartfelt appreciation and congratulations to Professor PC Manoria and all contributors for their hard work in publishing this very important and most timely book.

Navin C Nanda
MD DSc (Hon) DSc (Med) (Hon) FACC FAHA FASE FISCU (D)
Distinguished Professor of Medicine and Cardiovascular Disease
University of Alabama at Birmingham
Birmingham, Alabama, USA
President, International Society of Cardiovascular Ultrasound

Preface

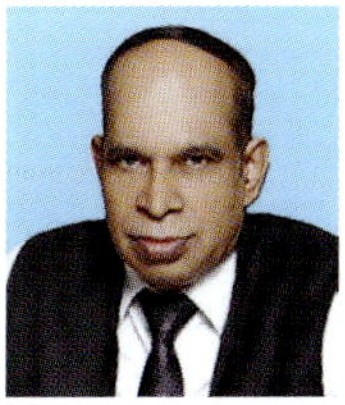

In the rapidly evolving landscape of Cardiovascular Kidney Metabolic Medicine, 2026 marks a pivotal year of convergence. Cardiovascular-kidney-metabolic (CKM) syndrome represents a unified framework to understand the interconnected bidirectional cascade that challenges traditional siloed care.

This book, *Cardio Kidney Metabolic Medicine 2026*, distills the year's most impactful evidence in terms of obesity, diabetes, hypertension, metabolic dysfunction-associated steatotic liver disease (MASLD), heart failure, and CKD. A section is also devoted to future of diabetes.

Our goal is practical, equipping clinicians, researchers, and trainees with actionable strategies to mitigate CKM progression, optimize guideline-directed therapies, and pioneer personalized interventions.

As global burdens rise with CKD affecting 850 million worldwide and cardiometabolic deaths projected at 25 million by 2030, this volume underscores urgency and opportunity. We invite you to explore these frontiers, fostering a unified response to the CKM epidemic.

PC Manoria

Preface

Contents

SECTION 6: MASLD

SECTION 7: HEART FAILURE

SECTION 8: CHRONIC KIDNEY DISEASE

SECTION 9: PHARMACOTHERAPY

SECTION 10: FUTURE OF DIABETES

SECTION 1

Introduction

CHAPTER 1

Cardio–kidney–metabolic Medicine: The Necessity for Adopting Globally

PC Manoria

ABSTRACT

The need for cardiovascular–kidney–metabolic (CKM) syndrome stems from recognizing that heart disease, kidney disease, and metabolic issues (like diabetes and obesity) are not separate problems but interconnected conditions, often starting with unhealthy lifestyles and excess fat, leading to severe multi-organ failure, if untreated. This framework promotes an integrated, holistic approach to early detection, risk reduction, and coordinated treatment (lifestyle and new drugs) for better outcomes, preventing severe complications such as heart failure, stroke, and kidney failure.

Keywords: Cardiovascular–kidney–metabolic syndrome, cardiometabolic risk, chronic kidney disease, metabolic syndrome, lifestyle modification

INTRODUCTION

Cardiovascular-kidney-metabolic (CKM) medicine focuses on the widespread adoption of an integrated care framework to address the interconnected nature of these diseases, implementation barriers, and the use of novel therapeutics. CKM medicine represents a paradigm-shifting framework that unifies the battle against cardiovascular (CV), kidney, and metabolic epidemics, poised to save millions amid their explosive global surge. CMK poses alarming global crisis with over 1.5 billion people grapple with CKM risks, fueling 45% of worldwide mortality-equivalent to a major city vanishing daily. Stage 4 extremes ravage 1 in 4 adults, with low-resource hotspots like India facing three times higher CKD escalation, devouring $500B+ in avoidable costs yearly. Siloed care and training deficits block progress, despite guidelines [American Heart Association (AHA)/Kidney Disease: Improving Global Outcomes (KDIGO)] blueprints proving 60% risk slashing via sodium-glucose cotransporter 2 inhibitors (SGLT2i)/glucagon-like peptide-1 receptor agonist (GLP-1 RA) combos. Stigma and inequities sideline 70% of at-risk populations in low- and middle-income countries (LMICs), demanding bold steps.

CKM medicine integrates management of CV, kidney, and metabolic disorders, which share common pathways like inflammation and insulin resistance. Global adoption is crucial due to their synergistic risks, affecting over 1 billion people worldwide and driving 40% of global deaths.

CKM syndrome stages patients from 0 (no risks) to 4 (extreme risk), with Stage 3+ prevalent in 20–30% of adults in high-income nations. In low-resource areas such as India, undiagnosed cases exacerbate CKD progression to end-stage renal disease, costing billions annually. Integrated screening could prevent 50% of events through SGLT2 inhibitors and GLP-1 agonists.

EVOLUTION OF THE CONCEPT: FROM CARDIORENAL TO CARDIOVASCULAR–KIDNEY–METABOLIC SYNDROME

The concept builds upon earlier frameworks:

- *Metabolic syndrome:* Focused on CV risk, clustering hypertension, dyslipidemia, hyperglycemia, and abdominal obesity.

- *Cardiorenal syndromes:* Classified (types 1–5) the bidirectional heart-kidney interactions in acute and chronic settings. CKM syndrome expands these by integrating metabolic dysfunction as a central, driving component that initiates and accelerates both cardiac and renal injury, creating a vicious and self-perpetuating cycle.

PATHOPHYSIOLOGICAL PILLARS OF CARDIOVASCULAR–KIDNEY–METABOLIC SYNDROME

The interconnection is driven by overlapping mechanisms:

- *Insulin resistance and hyperglycemia:* Chronic hyperglycemia and insulin resistance promote advanced glycation end-product (AGE) formation, oxidative stress, and endothelial dysfunction, damaging both the glomerular filtration barrier and coronary vasculature.
- *Chronic low-grade inflammation and immune dysregulation:* Adipose tissue, especially visceral fat, acts as an endocrine organ secreting proinflammatory adipokines (e.g., leptin and resistin) and cytokines [e.g., tumor necrosis factor-α (TNF-α) and interkeukin-6 (IL-6)]. This systemic inflammation accelerates atherosclerosis, promotes renal fibrosis, and worsens insulin resistance.
- *Neurohormonal activation renin-angiotensin-aldosterone system (RAAS) and sympathetic nervous system (SNS):* Overactivity of the RAAS and the SNS is a final common pathway. It drives hypertension, sodium retention, myocardial fibrosis, and progressive glomerulosclerosis.
- *Endothelial dysfunction and microvascular disease:* A hallmark of CKM syndrome, leading to impaired vasodilation, a prothrombotic state, and capillary rarefaction, affecting the heart, kidneys, and other organs.
- *Hemodynamic and fluid overload:* Kidney dysfunction leads to sodium/water retention, increasing preload and afterload, precipitating or worsening heart failure [especially heart failure with preserved ejection fraction (HFpEF)]. Conversely, reduced cardiac output in heart failure decreases renal perfusion, exacerbating chronic kidney disease (CKD).

CLINICAL STAGING AND RISK STRATIFICATION

A proposed staging system adapted from the AHA[1] facilitates risk assessment and guides preventive actions:

- *Stage 0 (At risk):* No CKM risk factors. *Focus:* Healthy lifestyle.
- *Stage 1 (Excess adiposity):* Overweight/obesity, or dysfunctional adipose tissue (e.g., elevated waist circumference). *Focus:* Weight management.
- *Stage 2 (Metabolic risk factors):* Includes type 2 diabetes mellitus (T2DM), hypertension, hypertriglyceridemia, and metabolic syndrome. *Focus:* Risk factor control.
- *Stage 3 (Subclinical CKM):* Evidence of end-organ damage without symptoms: e.g., high CV risk (by calculators), left ventricular (LV) hypertrophy, albuminuria (≥30 mg/g), estimated glomerular filtration rate (eGFR) 30–59 mL/min/1.73 m^2. *Focus:* Disease-modifying therapies.
- *Stage 4 (Clinical CKM):* Symptomatic disease: Cardiovascular disease (CVD) (heart failure, coronary artery disease, atrial fibrillation, and stroke), CKD (eGFR <30), or both. Subclassified by kidney function (a–d). *Focus:* Multidisciplinary specialty care.

KEY CURRENT ISSUES AND FOCUS AREAS IN 2025

- *Integrated care and breaking down silos:* A primary issue is moving away from traditional, organ-specific "siloed" care models (e.g., separate cardiologists, nephrologists, and care pathways is essential to improve the prognosis and quality of life for a vast population of patients globally. Embracing this holistic paradigm is the next critical step in combating interconnected noncommunicable diseases.

REFERENCES

1. Ndumele CE, Janani R, Chow SL, Neeland IJ, Tuttle KR, Khan SS, et al. Cardiovascular-kidney-metabolic health: a presidential advisory from the American Heart Association. Circulation. 2023;148:1606-35.
2. Rumrill SM, Shlipak MG. The new cardiovascular-kidney-metabolic (CKM) syndrome: an opportunity for CKD detection and treatment in primary care. Am J Kidney Dis. 2025;85(4) 399-402.
3. Singh A, Kesani H, Verma S, Saleh TM, Rai M. Cardio-renal metabolic syndrome: an integrated approach to prevention and management. Cureus. 2025;17(10):e94134.

SECTION 2

Obesity

CHAPTER 2

Obesity: A Looming Cardiometabolic Threat

Brij Mohan Makkar, Manisha Arora, Alok Modi

ABSTRACT

Obesity is now a major global and national health challenge, with rapidly increasing prevalence in India across all age groups. It is a chronic, progressive, and relapsing disease driven by genetic, metabolic, environmental, and behavioral factors rather than lifestyle imbalance alone. Asian Indians are particularly vulnerable due to higher body fat and central adiposity at lower body mass index (BMI) levels, leading to early cardiometabolic complications.

Assessment of obesity should extend beyond BMI to include measures of central adiposity such as waist circumference and waist-to-height ratio. Comprehensive evaluation using the 5A's framework and Edmonton Obesity Staging System (EOSS) enables risk-based management. Treatment requires individualized strategies including lifestyle modification, pharmacotherapy, bariatric surgery, and long-term follow-up. Emerging therapies, precision medicine, and digital health tools are reshaping modern obesity care toward sustained metabolic health improvement.

Keywords: Cardiometabolic risk, EOSS, obesity management, pharmacotherapy.

INTRODUCTION: THE EVOLVING LANDSCAPE OF OBESITY

Obesity, once considered a disease of high-income countries, has rapidly become a global pandemic, with low- and middle-income countries now experiencing the largest increases. In India, a country facing a double burden of malnutrition, obesity rates are rising across all age groups, contributing to premature mortality from noncommunicable diseases (NCDs) such as diabetes, cardiovascular disease, and cancer. Projections for 2025 and beyond suggest that this largely silent health crisis will continue to escalate, placing substantial strain on the Indian healthcare system.[1-3]

DEFINING OBESITY

Obesity is a complex and chronic disease characterized by abnormal or excessive body fat accumulation that increases health risk. It is no longer viewed simply as a consequence of lifestyle choices or a basic energy imbalance; rather, it reflects an interplay of genetic susceptibility, environmental exposures, and behavioral determinants that drive onset and persistence. Importantly, obesity is progressive and relapsing, warranting comprehensive and sustained medical management comparable to other chronic diseases. Beyond its physical phenotype, obesity is commonly associated with low-grade systemic inflammation and metabolic dysfunction, which together increase the risk of multiple comorbidities, particularly cardiovascular and endocrine disorders.[4-6]

PREVALENCE IN INDIA AND GLOBALLY

Global adult obesity has more than doubled since 1990, while adolescent obesity has quadrupled.

By 2022, approximately one in eight people worldwide were living with obesity, and by 2030, the global costs of overweight and obesity are predicted to reach US$3 trillion per year.[1,2]

Prevalence in India

Recent data from the National Family Health Survey-5 (NFHS-5) indicate that nearly 24% of women and 22.9% of men in India are classified as overweight or obese, representing a significant increase compared with 2015–2016. Projections are more concerning: a recent Lancet analysis estimates that nearly one-third of the Indian population may be obese by 2050 and forecasts that India could have the second-highest number of overweight and obese individuals globally, with approximately 450 million affected.[4,6]

- *Children and adolescents:* The percentage of overweight children under 5 years of age increased from 2.1 to 3.4% between 2015–2016 and 2019–2021. The World Obesity Atlas 2022 estimates that by 2030, 10.81% of children aged 5–9 years and 6.23% of those aged 10–19 years in India will be obese.[4,5]

PATHOPHYSIOLOGY OF OBESITY[7-10]

Obesity is initiated by sustained positive energy balance, but its clinical consequences extend well beyond caloric excess. It is best understood as an endocrine and inflammatory disorder driven by adipose tissue dysfunction, resulting in integrated metabolic and vascular injury.[8,10]

- *Adipose tissue as an endocrine organ:* Adipose tissue is an active endocrine organ that releases hormones, cytokines, and signaling molecules (adipokines). In health, adipokines such as adiponectin support insulin sensitivity and exert anti-inflammatory effects. In obesity, this profile shifts toward inflammation, with increased secretion of leptin and proinflammatory mediators [e.g., tumor necrosis factor-α (TNF-α)] and reduced adiponectin. This imbalance is central to insulin resistance and chronic low-grade inflammation.[8]
- *Insulin resistance and β-cell dysfunction:* Hypertrophic adipocytes release excess free fatty acids, impairing insulin signaling in skeletal muscle and liver and promoting insulin resistance. The pancreas initially compensates through hyperinsulinemia, but persistent metabolic stress eventually leads to β-cell dysfunction and failure, driving progression to type 2 diabetes mellitus (T2DM).[8]
- *Chronic inflammation:* Visceral adipose tissue becomes infiltrated with macrophages and other immune cells that amplify cytokine release [e.g., interleukin-6 (IL-6) and TNF-α]. This sustained low-grade inflammatory state promotes endothelial dysfunction, accelerates atherosclerosis, and further worsens insulin resistance.[8,10]
- *The "South Asian Phenotype":* Many Asian Indians demonstrate a propensity for central (abdominal) adiposity and higher body fat percentage at lower or even "normal" body mass index (BMI) (normal weight obesity). This phenotype is characterized by increased visceral fat, which is metabolically active and proinflammatory, explaining why cardiometabolic complications—particularly T2DM and cardiovascular disease—often occur at lower BMI thresholds than in Western populations.[7,9]

Unique Cardiometabolic Risks in Asian Indians

Asian Indians commonly display a "normal weight obesity" (NWO) phenotype—normal BMI but higher body fat percentage, particularly central (abdominal) adiposity. This visceral fat excess, even in the absence of high BMI, is strongly associated with cardiometabolic dysfunction. Abdominal obesity has been linked to substantially higher risk of T2DM, hypertension, and atherosclerotic cardiovascular disease (ASCVD), partly driven by a characteristic atherogenic dyslipidemic profile.[9,10]

MEASURES OF OBESITY

Body weight and BMI are convenient screening tools, but they do not capture fat distribution or distinguish fat mass from lean mass. Central (android) adiposity—especially visceral fat—is more metabolically active and proinflammatory, and is, therefore, more strongly associated with insulin resistance, dyslipidemia, chronic inflammation, and adverse cardiovascular outcomes than total fat mass alone. Accordingly, obesity assessment should prioritize measures of central adiposity and, where feasible, body composition, to improve risk stratification beyond BMI.[10]

TRADITIONAL ANTHROPOMETRIC MEASURES OF OBESITY

Body Mass Index (Fig. 1)

Body mass index is a calculated measure of body weight relative to height, serving as a widely used screening tool for macronutritional status. It is calculated as an individual's weight in kilograms divided by the square of their height in meters (kg/m^2).

For adults aged 20 years and older, the World Health Organization (WHO) and Centers for

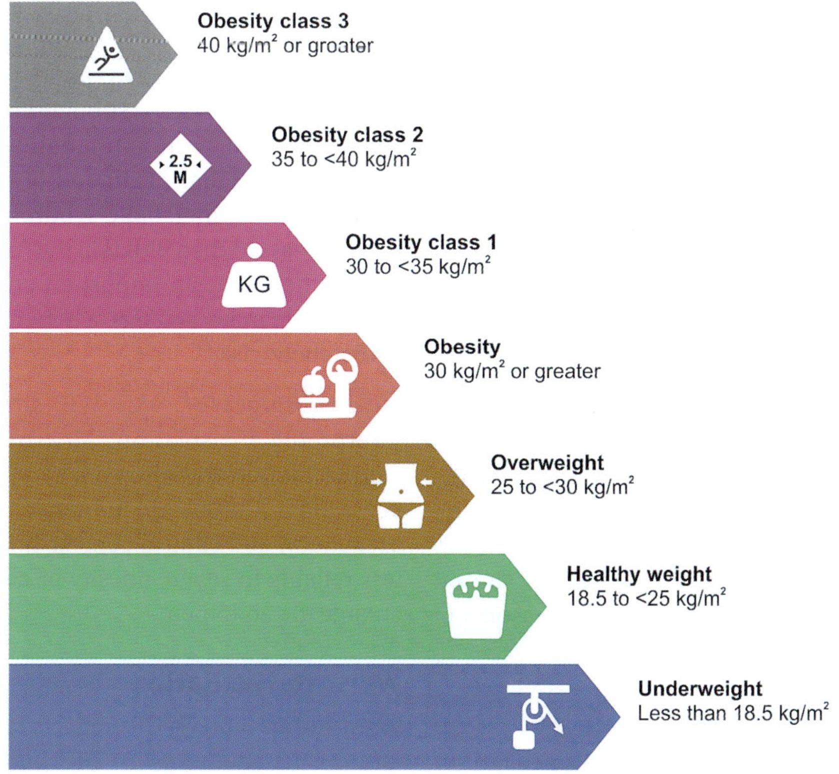

Fig. 1: Body mass index (BMI) classification pyramid.

Disease Control and Prevention (CDC) classify BMI categories as follows:

- *Underweight:* Less than 18.5 kg/m^2
    - *Healthy weight:* 18.5 to <25 kg/m^2
    - *Overweight:* 25 to <30 kg/m^2 (also referred to as preobesity)
    - *Obesity:* 30 kg/m^2 or greater.

Obesity is further subdivided into *Class 1 (30 to <35 kg/m^2), Class 2 (35 to <40 kg/m^2), and Class 3 (Severe obesity, ≥40 kg/m^2).* For children and adolescents (2–19 years), different age- and sex-specific cutoff points are used, often based on percentiles (e.g., ≥95th percentile for obesity).

Because the Asian Indians have higher body fat percentage even at lower level, lower cutoffs of BMI (normal 18.0–23.0 kg/m^2, overweight 23.0–24.9 kg/m^2, and obesity >25.0 kg/m^2) and waist circumference (WC) (<80 cm for women and <90 cm for men) are recommended for defining overweight and obesity in south Asian Indians.[11]

Advantages of BMI: BMI is simple, rapid, inexpensive, and feasible in routine practice and population surveys. It is useful for epidemiologic surveillance and for tracking weight change over time in adults. Extreme BMI values also correlate with higher likelihood of clinically significant undernutrition or severe obesity-related disease.

Disadvantages of BMI: BMI is an imprecise proxy for adiposity because it does not distinguish fat from lean mass and cannot identify fat distribution. It may misclassify muscular individuals as overweight and overlook excess body fat in people with low muscle mass. Crucially, BMI fails to detect central/visceral adiposity, thereby underestimating cardiometabolic risk in "normal-BMI" individuals. Hence, BMI should be interpreted with complementary measures of central adiposity and clinical risk.[10]

Waist Circumference

Waist circumference is a practical measure of central (abdominal) adiposity and correlates strongly with visceral fat and cardiometabolic risk. It should be measured at the midpoint between the lower rib margin and the iliac crest at the end of normal expiration with the patient standing, using a standardized technique; 2–3 readings can be taken and averaged for accuracy.

Risk Thresholds (WHO, NICE, Heart and Stroke Canada)

- Increased risk:
    - *Males:* >94 cm (37 inches)
    - *Females:* >80 cm (31.5 inches)
- Substantially increased risk (or "substantially increased risk"/"greatly increased risk"):
    - *Males:* >102 cm (40 inches)
    - *Females:* >88 cm (35 inches)

WHO also categorizes risk for women as normal (<80 cm), increased (80–88 cm), or substantially increased (>88 cm).

Advantages of WC: WC is a simple and low-cost marker of central adiposity and correlates closely with visceral fat, which is strongly linked to insulin resistance and cardiometabolic risk. A high WC predicts higher likelihood of hypertension, T2DM, ASCVD, metabolic syndrome, and some cancers—even when BMI is in the "normal" range. WC is, therefore, an important complement to BMI and, in many settings, a better discriminator of metabolic risk.[10]

Disadvantages of WC: WC should not be interpreted in isolation. Measurements vary with technique and observer, so standardization is essential. Cutoffs are influenced by ethnicity, pregnancy, and clinical context, and WC may be less reliable in severe obesity or conditions that enlarge the abdomen.

Waist-to-Hip Ratio

Waist-to-hip ratio (WHR) reflects fat distribution and is calculated as *waist circumference divided by hip circumference (W/H).* Waist is measured at the narrowest point or standardized midpoint, and hips at the widest circumference.

WHO/National Institute of Diabetes and Digestive and Kidney Diseases (NIDDK) abdominal obesity thresholds:

- *Males:* Above 0.90 (WHO), or ≥1.0 (NIDDK)
- *Females:* Above 0.85 (WHO), or ≥0.8 (NIDDK)

A ratio higher than 1.0 for either sex signifies a much higher chance of health problems.

Risk levels (for BMI < 35 kg/m^2, both sexes, all ethnicities, including muscular adults):

- *<0.4–0.49:* Healthy (not increased health risks)
- *0.5–0.59:* Increased central adiposity (increased health risks)—"Take care"
- *≥0.6:* High central adiposity (further increased health risks)—"Take action".

A WHtR cutoff of 0.5 is generally accepted as a universal cutoff for central obesity in children (aged ≥6 years) and adults across different sex and ethnic groups.

Advantages of WHR: WHR is a rapid indicator of fat distribution ("apple" vs. "pear") and correlates with visceral adiposity. In some populations—particularly older adults—it may predict cardiometabolic outcomes and mortality better than BMI, and it can be useful where lean mass varies substantially (e.g., sarcopenia).[10]

Disadvantages of WHR: WHR can be harder to interpret at very high BMI and may rise due to either increased abdominal fat or reduced hip/gluteal muscle mass. Measurement technique and body-shape variation can affect reproducibility, and some evidence suggests WHtR may outperform WHR for cardiovascular risk screening.

Waist-to-Height Ratio

Waist-to-height ratio (WHtR) is calculated as *waist circumference divided by height* (same units). NICE recommends a simple screening threshold: *waist < half of height (WHtR < 0.5)* for adults.[12]

Advantages of WHtR: The WHtR is a simple and low-cost marker of central adiposity that, in multiple systematic reviews and meta-analyses, performs better than BMI and often better than WC in predicting early cardiometabolic risk (T2DM, hypertension, and cardiovascular disease). By adjusting waist for height, WHtR reduces misclassification in very short or tall individuals. A practical "universal" threshold (*WHtR < 0.5*) applies to adults and children ≥6 years, supporting clear screening and public-health messaging: *keep waist circumference less than half of height.*[12]

Disadvantages of WHtR: WHtR is not recommended for routine use in children <6 years due to limited validation and greater age-dependence. Its accuracy depends on standardized waist measurement, and some populations may benefit from sex- or ethnicity-specific cutoffs to optimize sensitivity and specificity.[12]

Neck Circumference

Neck circumference (NC) is an inexpensive and noninvasive measure of upper-body subcutaneous fat. It is measured at mid-neck (just below the laryngeal prominence in men) and correlates with BMI and waist-based indices. NC is quick to perform and may be particularly useful when waist measures are impractical (e.g., severe obesity, pregnancy, and limited mobility). Higher NC has been associated with adverse metabolic markers, including dysglycemia, blood pressure elevation, triglyceride/HDL abnormalities, and insulin resistance, suggesting potential value as an adjunct screening tool.

Disadvantages of NC: While various studies have determined NC cutoffs for diagnosing obesity or metabolic syndrome in different populations (e.g., Nigerian, Brazilian, and Turkish children), there is no widely accepted universal standard, and cutoffs can be influenced by cultural and ethnic variables. Examples include:

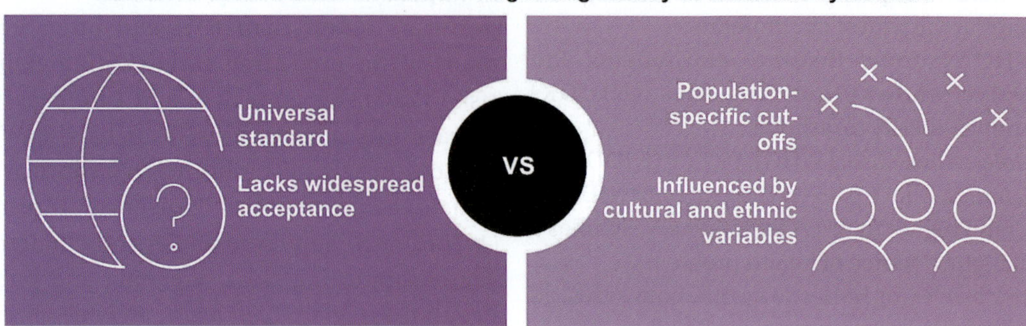

Fig. 2: Neck circumference cutoffs.

- *Males:* 44.0 cm (Nigeria), 42 cm (Brazil), and 37 cm (nondiabetic).
- *Females:* 40 cm (Nigeria), 36 cm (Brazil), and 33 cm (metabolic syndrome).
- *Children (6–10 years):* 27.9 cm for boys and 26.9 cm for girls for overweight/obesity.

While it reflects upper body adiposity, NC does not directly quantify visceral fat in the same way as abdominal measures like WC or WHtR. Although studies show associations, more direct comparisons between NC, and other anthropometric measures are needed to solidify its role in standard guidelines and practices **(Fig. 2)**.

EMERGING ANTHROPOMETRIC INDICES FOR ADVANCED OBESITY ASSESSMENT

Newer indices—such as the visceral adiposity index (VAI), a body shape index (ABSI), conicity index (CI), fat mass index (FMI), and the fat mass/fat-free mass (FM/FFM) ratio—aim to refine obesity assessment beyond BMI and simple waist measures. These tools better reflect fat distribution, body composition, and metabolic risk, and may improve diagnostic and prognostic precision when traditional anthropometry is insufficient.

Advanced Body Composition Analysis Techniques

When more precise assessment is required, body composition can be quantified using advanced methods:

- *Dual-energy X-ray absorptiometry (DEXA/DXA):* Provides accurate estimates of fat mass, lean mass, and bone mineral density with minimal radiation.
- *Bioelectrical impedance analysis (BIA):* Low-cost and noninvasive, but accuracy is affected by hydration status and may be less reliable in severe obesity or fluid overload.
- *Air displacement plethysmography (ADP):* Noninvasive method for estimating body volume and density without radiation.
- *CT/MRI:* Most accurate for distinguishing visceral from subcutaneous fat and assessing tissue-level composition, but limited by cost and availability.

Overall, these techniques—and newer anthropometric indices—should be viewed as *complements* to BMI and waist measures, supporting a *multimetric assessment* for more accurate risk stratification when clinically indicated.

5As OF OBESITY MANAGEMENT

Key principles of obesity care include:

- Obesity is progressive and relapsing; it requires long-term management like diabetes or hypertension.
- Success should be judged by health improvement, not only scale weight; even modest loss can yield meaningful metabolic benefit.
- Identify and address root causes and barriers (biological, psychological, and socioeconomic), including low basal metabolic rate, overeating, and physical inactivity.
- "Success" is individualized—prevention of further gain, improved quality of life and energy, ~5% weight loss, maintenance of best achievable weight, or improved overall health.
- Targets should be realistic and sustainable; the "best weight" a patient can maintain may be more appropriate than an idealized weight.[6]

1. Ask: Initiating Patient-centered Conversations

The first step is to *ask permission* to discuss weight, as this topic is sensitive and often associated with stigma. A respectful and nonjudgmental approach builds trust and improves engagement (e.g., "Would it be okay if we discussed your weight and its impact on your health?"). Clinicians should actively minimize weight bias by using *person-first language,* avoiding blame, and applying motivational interviewing skills (open-ended questions, empathy, affirmation, and reflective listening). The patient's response also provides insight into readiness for change; if they are not ready, offering resources and revisiting later maintains a therapeutic relationship without coercion.[6]

2. Assess: Comprehensive Patient Evaluation

"Assess" involves a *holistic evaluation* beyond BMI—understanding the patient's trajectory, drivers of weight gain, barriers to change, and obesity-related complications. This includes detailed history, physical examination, standardized anthropometry, dietary and activity assessment, relevant laboratory testing, and screening for comorbidities and psychosocial contributors to ensure individualized, and complication-focused management.[6]

Medical History and Physical Examination

A focused history should document the patient's usual weight trajectory and recent change, as rapid gain can suggest endocrine or metabolic contributors. Core elements include dietary pattern (portion size, energy-dense foods, and binge/emotional eating), physical activity/sedentary time, sleep, alcohol/tobacco, prior medical/surgical illness (including mental health), current medications (including weight-promoting drugs), and family history of obesity, diabetes, dyslipidemia, and premature cardiovascular disease.[6]

Examination should assess general health and function, vital signs (especially blood pressure), and clinical markers of metabolic risk or complications. This includes features of dyslipidemia (e.g., xanthelasma/xanthomas), skin findings (e.g., acanthosis and intertrigo), neuropathic signs in those with diabetes risk, and an overall functional assessment (mobility and activities of daily living), supplemented by targeted systemic evaluation.[6]

Anthropometric Measurements: Beyond Body Mass Index

BMI remains a practical screening tool, but it does not distinguish fat from lean mass and cannot

Patient evaluation ranges from simple to complex assessments

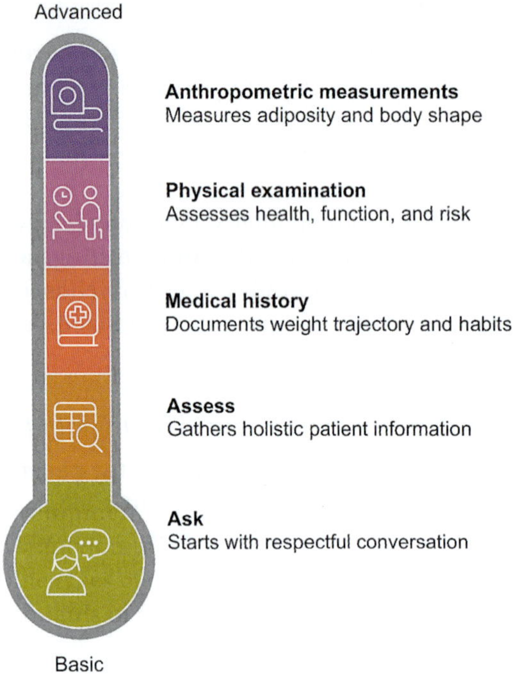

Advanced

Anthropometric measurements
Measures adiposity and body shape

Physical examination
Assesses health, function, and risk

Medical history
Documents weight trajectory and habits

Assess
Gathers holistic patient information

Ask
Starts with respectful conversation

Basic

Fig. 3: Multilevel assessment in obesity care.

capture fat distribution. Therefore, assessment should incorporate measures of central adiposity and body shape—*WC, WHtR, WHR, NC*—and, where relevant, composite indices such as *ABSI, conicity index (CI), visceral adiposity index (VAI), fat mass index (FMI), and FM/FFM ratio.* This approach improves risk stratification by prioritizing visceral adiposity and metabolic risk rather than body size alone[10] **(Fig. 3)**.

Comorbidities and Adiposity-related Complications

Assessment should identify and grade obesity-related conditions, commonly including T2DM, hypertension, dyslipidemia, ASCVD, obstructive sleep apnea, fatty liver disease, osteoarthritis, and obesity-associated cancers. Baseline investigations typically include glucose metrics, lipid profile, and liver enzymes, guided by clinical context.[6]

Psychosocial Factors: The 4M Framework

A comprehensive evaluation should also address drivers and barriers using the *4M framework*:

1. *Mechanical:* Mobility limitations, osteoarthritis, and functional impairment.
2. *Metabolic:* Insulin resistance, endocrine causes, dyslipidemia, hypertension, and diabetes.
3. *Mental:* Depression, anxiety, eating disorders, and stress-related overeating.
4. *Social milieu:* Socioeconomic constraints, food environment, cultural norms, and social support and triggers.

This structured assessment supports individualized and sustainable treatment planning. Incorporating psychosocial and environmental determinants is essential because they often *drive weight gain and impede treatment,* rather than merely coexisting with obesity. For example, chronic stress can promote emotional eating, while unsafe or inaccessible environments can limit physical activity and reduce adherence. Consequently, effective obesity care must extend beyond diet and medications to a *holistic and multidisciplinary approach,* often involving collaboration with mental health professionals, social support services, and community resources to improve sustainability.[6]

Disease Severity Staging: Edmonton Obesity Staging System

The EOSS stages obesity severity based on *medical, psychological, and functional impact,* providing a more clinically meaningful assessment than BMI alone. Because EOSS better predicts health risk and mortality than BMI, it is useful for *risk stratification and treatment intensity*—from preventive counseling in Stage 0 to intensive multidisciplinary care, including pharmacotherapy and/or surgery, in Stages 3–4[13] **(Table 1)**.

TABLE 1: Edmonton obesity staging system (EOSS) stages and clinical implications.

EOSS stage	*Description*	*Clinical implications*
Stage 0	No apparent obesity-related risk factors, physical symptoms, or functional limitations	Focus on prevention and maintaining healthy lifestyle; no immediate need for weight management intervention
Stage 1	Presence of obesity-related risk factors (e.g., prehypertension and impaired glucose tolerance) but no established disease or functional limitations	Increased risk of future complications. Lifestyle interventions and close monitoring are indicated
Stage 2	Established obesity-related diseases (e.g., type 2 diabetes mellitus, hypertension, sleep apnea, moderate functional limitations, and mild–moderate psychological issues)	Requires active management of comorbidities and weight. Lifestyle changes, pharmacotherapy, or surgical options may be considered
Stage 3	Significant obesity-related complications impacting daily life (e.g., severe uncontrolled diabetes, severe heart disease, significant functional limitations, and severe psychological issues)	Intensive, multidisciplinary intervention often required, including pharmacotherapy and/or bariatric surgery. Focus on improving quality of life and managing severe complications
Stage 4	End-stage complications, severe disabilities, or life-threatening conditions directly attributable to obesity (e.g., end-stage organ failure, and severe debilitating osteoarthritis)	Complex, specialized care with a focus on palliative measures and maximizing remaining function

3. Advise: Evidence-based Treatment Strategies

After comprehensive assessment, "Advise" focuses on clear, evidence-based recommendations tailored to the patient's risk profile and goals. Counseling should link obesity to specific health risks and emphasize achievable benefits of treatment. Even *modest weight loss (~5%)* can produce clinically meaningful improvements in blood pressure, lipid parameters, and glycemic risk, reinforcing motivation through measurable health gains rather than scale weight alone.[13]

Personalized Lifestyle Modifications

Lifestyle therapy remains the foundation and should be individualized for feasibility and sustainability:[14]

- *Nutrition:* Medical nutrition therapy (MNT), ideally delivered by a trained dietitian, should be preference-sensitive, flexible, and oriented toward long-term adherence rather than restrictive short-term diets.[14]
- *Physical activity:* Regular aerobic activity (typically *30–60 minutes most days,* moderate–vigorous intensity) supports fat loss, improves cardiometabolic markers, and aids weight maintenance.[14]
- *Sleep and stress:* Optimizing sleep and stress regulation improves adherence and reduces behavioral drivers of weight gain.[14]
- *Psychological interventions:* When indicated, structured therapies such as *CBT* or *ACT* can address emotional eating and other behavioral contributors.[14]

Pharmacotherapy Options: Current Guidelines and Emerging Therapies

Because lifestyle intervention alone often yields *modest and difficult-to-maintain* weight loss, pharmacotherapy is now a core component of obesity treatment—used *alongside* lifestyle measures as part of chronic disease management. Medication choice should be individualized based on comorbidities, expected efficacy,

TABLE 2: Overview of pharmacological interventions for obesity management.

Medication class/drug	*Mechanism of action*	*Key indications/criteria*	*Goals of therapy*
GLP-1 receptor agonists (e.g., liraglutide and semaglutide)[14,15]	Mimics natural incretin hormones, enhancing glucose-dependent insulin secretion, slowing gastric emptying, and promoting satiety	BMI ≥ 30 kg/m^2 or BMI ≥27 kg/m^2 with obesity-related complications. Specific subpopulations: atherosclerotic cardiovascular disease, heart failure with preserved ejection fraction, metabolic dysfunction-associated steatohepatitis, prediabetes, type 2 diabetes mellitus, obstructive sleep apnea	Clinically, meaningful weight loss, improvement in obesity-related health complications, sustained weight loss and maintenance, prevention of weight regain
Dual GIP/GLP-1 receptor agonists (e.g., tirzepatide)[16]	Activates both glucose-dependent insulinotropic polypeptide (GIP) and glucagon-like peptide-1 (GLP-1) receptors	Similar to GLP-1 receptor agonists (RAs), with potential for greater efficacy	Enhanced weight loss and metabolic improvements, especially in type 2 diabetes mellitus
Naltrexone/Bupropion (combination tablet)	Naltrexone targets opioid receptors involved in reward pathways; Bupropion affects dopamine and norepinephrine, reducing appetite and cravings	BMI ≥ 30 kg/m^2 or BMI ≥ 27 kg/m^2 with obesity-related complications	Weight loss, reduction in cravings and appetite
Orlistat	Pancreatic lipase inhibitor, reducing dietary fat absorption	BMI ≥ 30 kg/m^2 or BMI ≥ 27 kg/m^2 with obesity-related complications	Modest weight loss and prevention of weight regain

(BMI: body mass index)

adverse effects, route and dosing frequency, drug interactions, cost, and patient's preferences, with long-term use considered when benefits outweigh risks[6] **(Table 2)**.

Surgical Interventions: Criteria and Types

Metabolic/bariatric surgery is indicated for selected patients with severe obesity or obesity-related complications. Common criteria include *BMI ≥ 40 kg/m², BMI ≥ 35–40 kg/m² with comorbidities, or BMI ≥ 30 kg/m² with poorly controlled T2DM.* Procedure selection—most commonly *sleeve gastrectomy, Roux-en-Y gastric bypass, or biliopancreatic diversion ± duodenal switch*—should be individualized through shared decision-making, balancing risk profile, comorbidity burden, and patient's preference.[17-19]

4. Agree: Collaborative Goal Setting and Shared Plan

"Agree" centers on shared decision-making and realistic goal setting. Targets should be *patient-valued* and health-focused (e.g., functional capacity, glycemic control, and BP reduction), not only weight-centric. A practical action plan should address identified drivers (mechanical, metabolic, mental, and social milieu) and translate them into *SMART goals* (specific, measurable, achievable, relevant, and time-bound), improving adherence and long-term sustainability.[6,20]

5. Assist: Ongoing Support and Follow-up

"Assist" emphasizes obesity as a chronic disease requiring longitudinal support. Follow-up should address barriers, prevent relapse, and adapt the plan over time. Effective care often requires a *team-based model,* integrating dietetic support, behavioral/psychological interventions, and specialist/surgical input when indicated. Structured monitoring and reinforcement of progress—clinical and functional—improves engagement and maintenance.[6,20]

PRECISION MEDICINE: TAILORING TREATMENT TO THE INDIVIDUAL

Obesity is heterogeneous; therefore, precision approaches aim to match therapy to underlying drivers and patient's phenotype rather than applying uniform recommendations. Phenotype-guided strategies (e.g., appetite dysregulation, emotional eating, and low energy expenditure) may improve outcomes by aligning behavioral and pharmacologic choices with dominant mechanisms. Genomic and advanced physiological phenotyping can further refine risk prediction and treatment selection, though implementation remains resource-dependent.[20]

ROLE OF ARTIFICIAL INTELLIGENCE AND DIGITAL TOOLS

Artificial intelligence-enabled models and digital platforms may support precision care by integrating multimodal data (clinical, behavioral, and wearable metrics) to improve risk stratification, personalize coaching, and optimize follow-up. Wearables and mHealth tools can facilitate real-time monitoring of activity and sleep and support behavior change at scale.

EVOLVING LANDSCAPE OF PHARMACOTHERAPY

Obesity pharmacotherapy is rapidly advancing with incretin-based agents and multiagonists achieving substantial and sustained weight loss. The pipeline includes *dual and triple agonists* and combination approaches aimed at improved efficacy and tolerability. Beyond incretins, newer mechanisms seek to improve *body composition* (fat loss with lean mass preservation) and expand options for patients with varied metabolic profiles.[15-17]

ADVANCES IN DRUG DELIVERY

Development is also focused on more convenient delivery (e.g., *oral agents* and less frequent injections/infusions) and targeted systems to improve adherence and potentially reduce adverse effects. Overall, these innovations reinforce obesity management as long-term, multimodal, and increasingly individualized.

CONCLUSION

Obesity should be managed as a chronic disease requiring long-term, patient-centered care. BMI alone is insufficient for risk assessment, particularly in Asian Indians, where central adiposity drives cardiometabolic risk. Clinical evaluation must integrate anthropometric measures, comorbidity assessment, and functional staging. Management should focus on realistic health goals using lifestyle therapy, medications, and surgery when indicated. Advances in incretin therapies, precision medicine, and digital monitoring are transforming obesity treatment toward individualized and sustainable care.

REFERENCES

1. NCD Risk Factor Collaboration (NCD-RisC). Worldwide trends in underweight and obesity from 1990 to 2022: a pooled analysis of 3663 population-representative studies with 222 million children, adolescents, and adults. Lancet. 2024;403(10431):1027-50.
2. GBD 2021 Adult BMI Collaborators. Global, regional, and national prevalence of adult overweight and obesity, 1990–2021, with forecasts to 2050: a forecasting study for the Global Burden of Disease Study 2021. Lancet. 2025;405(10481):813-38.
3. Sørensen TIA. Forecasting the global obesity epidemic through 2050. Lancet. 2025;405(10481):756-7.
4. Jacob JJ. Tackling the rising tide: understanding the prevalence of childhood obesity in India. Indian J Endocrinol Metab. 2024;28(2):101-3.
5. Zhang X, Li Y, Wang L, Reilly JJ, Ma J. Global prevalence of overweight and obesity in children and adolescents: a systematic review and meta-analysis. JAMA Pediatr. 2024;178(8):800-13.
6. Madhu SV, Srivastava A, Bhatt SP, Gulati S, Gupta R, Kalra S, et al. ESI clinical practice guidelines for the evaluation and management of obesity in India. Indian J Endocrinol Metab. 2022;26(4):295-318.
7. WHO Expert Consultation. Appropriate body-mass index for Asian populations and its implications for policy and intervention strategies. Lancet. 2004;363(9403):157-63.
8. Misra A, Khurana L. Obesity and the metabolic syndrome in developing countries. J Clin Endocrinol Metab. 2008;93(11 Suppl 1):S9-S30.
9. Misra A, Vikram NK. Insulin resistance syndrome (metabolic syndrome) and obesity in Asian Indians: evidence and implications. Nutrition. 2004;20(5):482-91.
10. Després JP. Body fat distribution and risk of cardiovascular disease: an update. Circulation. 2012;126(10):1301-13.
11. Misra A, Chowbey P, Makkar BM, Vikram NK, Wasir JS, Chadha D, et al. Consensus Statement for Diagnosis of Obesity, Abdominal Obesity and the Metabolic Syndrome for Asian Indians and Recommendations for Physical Activity, Medical and Surgical Management. J Assoc Physicians India. 2009;57:163-70.
12. Ashwell M, Gunn P, Gibson S. Waist-to-height ratio is a better screening tool than waist circumference and BMI for adult cardiometabolic risk factors: systematic review and meta-analysis. Obes Rev. 2012;13(3):275-86.
13. Sharma AM, Kushner RF. A proposed clinical staging system for obesity. Int J Obes (Lond). 2009;33(3):289-95.
14. Wadden TA, Tronieri JS, Butryn ML. Lifestyle modification approaches for the treatment of obesity in adults. Am Psychol. 2020;75(2):235-51.
15. Wilding JPH, Batterham RL, Calanna S, Davies M, Van Gaal LF, Lingvay I, et al. Once-weekly semaglutide in adults with overweight or obesity. N Engl J Med. 2021;384(11):989-1002.
16. Rubino D, Abrahamsson N, Davies M, Hesse D, Greenway FL, Jensen C, et al. Effect of continued weekly subcutaneous semaglutide vs placebo on weight loss maintenance in adults with overweight or obesity: the STEP 4 randomized clinical trial. JAMA. 2021;325(14):1414-25.
17. Jastreboff AM, Aronne LJ, Ahmad NN, Wharton S, Connery L, Alves B, et al. Tirzepatide once weekly for the treatment of obesity. N Engl J Med. 2022;387(3):205-16.
18. Sjöström L, Narbro K, Sjöström CD, Karason K, Larsson B, Wedel H, et al. Effects of bariatric surgery on mortality in Swedish obese subjects. N Engl J Med. 2007;357(8):741-52.
19. Rubino F, Nathan DM, Eckel RH, Schauer PR, Alberti KGMM, Zimmet PZ, et al. Metabolic surgery in the treatment algorithm for type 2 diabetes: a joint statement by international diabetes organizations. Diabetes Care. 2016;39(6):861-77.
20. Acosta A, Streett S, Kroh MD, Cheskin LJ, Saunders KH, Kurian M, et al. White Paper AGA: POWER—Practice Guide on Obesity and Weight Management, Education, and Resources. Clin Gastroenterol Hepatol. 2017;15(4):631-49.e10.

CHAPTER 3

Childhood Obesity: Current Concepts

Priti Phatale, Hemant Phatale, Sagar Phatale

ABSTRACT

Childhood obesity is an increasing global public health challenge. The rising trend is particularly concerning in low- and middle-income countries (LMICs), such as India, where early prevention is crucial.

Childhood obesity is a chronic, multifactorial disease influenced by genetic, environmental, behavioral, and socioeconomic factors. Obese children are at higher risk of early cardiometabolic, hepatic, orthopedic, and psychosocial complications and frequently remain obese into adulthood. Diagnosis is based on age- and sex-specific body mass index (BMI) percentiles, along with assessment of central adiposity and associated comorbidities. Management requires early identification, family-centered lifestyle modification, behavioral interventions, pharmacotherapy when indicated, and bariatric surgery in selected adolescents.

Decisive prevention—encompassing early screening, school-based interventions, and robust public health policies—is the most essential and impactful strategy to reverse the exponential surge in childhood obesity and its subsequent burden of noncommunicable diseases (NCDs).

Keywords: Childhood obesity, body mass index, cardiometabolic risk, comorbidities, lifestyle modification, prevention, noncommunicable diseases.

INTRODUCTION

Childhood obesity is a serious global public health challenge. The global prevalence of this condition has reached alarming levels. The World Health Organization (WHO) estimates that in 2024, 35 million children under 5 years were overweight, with almost half residing in Asia. >390 million children and adolescents aged 5–19 years were overweight globally, including 160 million with obesity, in 2022. This represents a quadrupling of the percentage of obese children and adolescents in this age group, rising from 2% in 1990 to 8% in 2022.[1]

The prevalence of obesity is rising fastest in low- and middle-income countries (LMICs), where early prevention is not just crucial, but urgent. The etiology of childhood obesity is complex and multifactorial, involving an interplay of biological, behavioral, environmental, and sociocultural factors. Overweight and obese children are likely to stay obese into adulthood and are more likely to develop noncommunicable diseases (NCDs) such as diabetes and cardiovascular diseases at a younger age. Childhood obesity, a preventable risk factor, significantly contributes to the rising burden of NCDs.[2] In addition, childhood obesity is a risk factor for cardiometabolic and psychosocial comorbidities, including hypertension, dyslipidemia, metabolic dysfunction-associated fatty liver disease (MAFLD), anxiety, and depression.

Once obesity develops, it poses significant challenges for the patient, their family, and society, as well as the nation. The goal of this review is to provide clinicians, healthcare professionals, and policymakers with a comprehensive overview of the current state of science and practice in combating childhood obesity.

DEFINITION AND DIAGNOSIS

The Obesity Medicine Association's definition of "Obesity is a chronic, relapsing, multifactorial, neurobehavioral disease wherein an increase in body fat that promotes adipose tissue dysfunction and abnormal fat mass physical forces, resulting in adverse metabolic, biomechanical, and psychosocial health consequences."[3]

The Lancet Diabetes and Endocrinology (2025) has further refined this definition, distinguishing between preclinical obesity and clinical obesity.

Preclinical obesity is defined as excess fat without current organ dysfunction or limitations in daily activities, but with an increased future health risk.

Clinical obesity, on the other hand, is a chronic systemic disease state directly caused by excess adiposity, which can lead to severe end-organ damage and potentially life-threatening complications such as heart attacks, strokes, and renal failure.[4]

Body mass index (BMI) is calculated as weight in kg/ height in m^2

$$\text{BMI} = \text{kg/m}^2$$

Age and sex-specific BMI percentile charts are used to classify both children and adolescents with high BMI.

For children <2 years of age: According to WHO growth standards, obesity in children under 5 years is defined as weight-for-recumbent length at or above the 97.7th percentile.[5]

- *For children and adolescents aged 2–20 years* ***(Table 1)***.[6]

The rising prevalence of severe obesity in adolescents is a significant public health concern requiring urgent attention.

In the Indian context, the Indian Academy of Pediatric growth charts for children aged 5–18 years utilize adult-equivalent BMI cut-offs, taking into account the specific characteristics of Asian children. An adult-equivalent BMI of 23 is considered overweight, and a BMI of 27 is considered obese.[7]

TABLE 1: Clinical thresholds for pediatric overweight and obesity classifications.

Category	*Body mass index (BMI) for age percentile*
Overweight	BMI ≥85th percentile but <95th percentile
Obese	BMI ≥95th percentile
Severe obesity	BMI ≥120% of the 95th percentile or ≥35 kg/m^2, whichever is lower, based on age and sex.

LIMITATIONS OF BODY MASS INDEX

For diagnosing childhood obesity, BMI is an inherently limited tool.

- It measures excess *weight*, not excess *body fat*, and fails to distinguish between muscle and fat mass.
- It cannot identify harmful visceral fat distribution, often misses up to 25% of children with excess adiposity (low sensitivity), and requires complex age- and sex-specific percentiles due to rapid growth.

Age- and sex-specific waist circumference reference curves have been established for Indian children, as the Indian ethnicity is prone to central obesity.

A waist circumference at or above the 70th percentile is used as a cut-off to screen for the risk of metabolic syndrome.[8]

EPIDEMIOLOGY

If current trends persist without intervention, the global prevalence and the number of young people (aged 5–19 years) with overweight or obesity are projected to increase from 22% (430 million) in 2016 to 39% (770 million) by 2035. Obesity Atlas 2024 projects an annual growth rate of 4.1% in adults with high BMI compared to 6.2%

for children with high BMI from 2020 to 2035. It indicates that childhood obesity is increasing at a faster rate than adult obesity, underscoring the urgency of addressing this issue.[9]

This rising trend is particularly worrying in LMICs, where early prevention is crucial. In India, a meta-analysis of 21 studies conducted from 2003 to 2023, encompassing data from 186,901 children, revealed a pooled prevalence of childhood obesity of 8.4% and a prevalence of 12.4% for childhood overweight.[10]

DRIVERS OF THE OBESITY EPIDEMIC IN INDIA

- *The nutritional transition:* Traditional Indian diets, rich in fiber and whole grains, are being replaced by energy-dense diets high in saturated fats, refined sugars, and salt. Increased consumption of processed foods, sugar-sweetened beverages, and fast food is the primary driver.
- *The sedentary shift:* The replacement of active play with screen time (television, smartphones, and gaming), increased academic pressure, and urban designs that lack safe recreational spaces all contribute to a sedentary lifestyle.
- The "Thin-fat" Indian phenotype is a critical driver: Research shows that for a given BMI; individuals of Indian ethnicity possess a significantly higher body fat percentage and lower muscle mass compared to other ethnic groups. This unique predisposition to central adiposity increases the risk of metabolic complications, such as insulin resistance, even at lower BMI thresholds. Overweight and obese children are likely to stay obese into adulthood and are more likely to develop NCDs such as diabetes and cardiovascular diseases at a younger age. The majority of these children, with an increasing NCD burden, will reside in middle-income countries, where most cases will remain undetected and untreated.

The risk of developing obesity-related NCDs is estimated by both the age of onset and the duration of obesity.

PATHOPHYSIOLOGY OF PEDIATRIC OBESITY

The energy imbalance and metabolic dysregulation in pediatric obesity are driven by a complex interplay of genetic, environmental, and behavioral factors.

Imbalance: The Core Drivers

The global rise in obesity is primarily attributed to a persistent energy imbalance, which is fueled by an *obesogenic environment* that promotes excessive caloric intake and reduces caloric expenditure.

Metabolic and Hormonal Dysregulation

The body's regulatory systems are significantly altered in pediatric obesity, leading to various metabolic complications:

- *Genetic predisposition*: Children are at a greater risk if they have a family history of obesity, indicating inherited genetic predispositions affecting metabolism, appetite regulation, and fat storage. Specific genes, like the fat mass and obesity-associated gene (*FTO*) and the melanocortin four receptor gene (*MC4R*), are linked to energy regulation and satiety.
- *Hormonal alterations*: Irregular or insufficient sleep can lead to altered hormonal regulation of hunger and satiety, specifically impacting *ghrelin* (hunger hormone) and *leptin* (satiety hormone) levels.
- *Central adiposity and insulin resistance*: The accumulation of visceral fat (central adiposity) is especially relevant in the *"Thin-fat" Indian phenotype*, where individuals, even at lower BMI values, have a higher body fat percentage

and lower muscle mass. This unique predisposition increases the risk of:

- Hyperinsulinism and *insulin resistance.*
- Prediabetes and type 2 diabetes mellitus.
- Metabolic syndrome.
- *MAFLD*
- Dyslipidemia (an atherogenic profile with elevated triglycerides and low high-density lipoprotein cholesterol (HDL-C).

NEUROENDOCRINE REGULATION OF APPETITE

Appetite is regulated by a complex neuroendocrine system, which involves the interaction of hormones and genetic elements to manage energy balance, the sensation of hunger, and the feeling of fullness (satiety).

Key Hormones

Insufficient or irregular sleep is associated with changes in the levels of two key hormones:

- *Ghrelin:* This is the hormone that stimulates hunger.
- *Leptin:* This is the hormone that signals satiety (fullness).

Genetic Pathways

Genetic predispositions affecting metabolism, appetite regulation, and fat storage also play a role.

- *Leptin-melanocortin neural pathway:* Single gene mutations within this pathway are often the cause of rare, severe forms of early-onset obesity (monogenic obesity), leading to severe, early-onset obesity and hyperphagia (excessive eating).
- *Specific genes* linked to energy regulation and satiety include the fat mass and *FTO* and the *MC4R* gene.
- *Endocrine obesity:* Hormonal imbalances can result in endocrine obesity, which is often clinically distinguished by impaired linear growth or short stature.

ETIOLOGY: A MULTIFACTORIAL CHRONIC DISEASE

The etiology of childhood obesity is complex and multifactorial, involving an interplay of biological, behavioral, environmental, and sociocultural factors.[11]

These include genetics, epigenetics, alterations in the gut microbiome, and intrauterine influences.

Genetic and Epigenetic Factors

Children with a family history of obesity are at greater risk due to inherited genetic predispositions affecting metabolism, appetite regulation, and fat storage. Specific genes, such as the *FTO* gene and the *MC4R* gene, have been linked to obesity through their effects on energy regulation and satiety.[12]

Obesity may be polygenic or monogenic.

- *Polygenic obesity:* A common condition of variable severity and late onset, influenced by the modest contribution of hundreds of genetic variants in combination with significant environmental factors. *Example:* Exogenous obesity.
- *Monogenic obesity:* A rare, severe form of early-onset obesity caused by a single gene mutation, often within the leptin-melanocortin neural pathway, leading to severe, early-onset obesity and hyperphagia.

Examples: Mutations in genes such as the leptin (*LEP*) gene, leptin receptor (*LEPR*) gene, and the *MC4R* gene.[13]

Epigenetics

Common manifestations of epigenetics in childhood obesity include:

- Small for gestational age due to poor gestational weight gain.

- Large for gestational age (associated with mothers with preconception BMIs at or above 30 kg/m^2, excessive gestational weight gain, or gestational diabetes mellitus (GDM).[14]

SYNDROMIC OBESITY

Occurs as part of a wider genetic syndrome that includes dysmorphic features, intellectual disability, and other organ system abnormalities

Syndromic forms of obesity include Prader–Willi syndrome (PWS), Alstrom syndrome, Bardet–Biedl syndrome, and Cohen syndrome, among others.

ENDOCRINE OBESITY

Results from hormonal imbalances. The clinical hallmark that distinguishes it from other forms is short stature or impaired linear growth. Conditions include:

- Hypothyroidism
- Growth hormone (GH) deficiency
- GH resistance
- Leptin deficiency or resistance to leptin action
- Glucocorticoid excess (Cushing syndrome)

Complex Interplay of Environmental, Psychosocial, and Behavioral Factors

The global escalation of obesity and related metabolic disorders is driven mainly by an obesogenic environment.

These include:

- Easy access to inexpensive, high-calorie, and ultraprocessed foods.
- Built environments that discourage physical activity.
- Emotional stress, depression, and low self-esteem may lead to overeating or binge eating behaviors.
- Parental modelling of unhealthy behaviors (e.g., poor diet and sedentary lifestyle) has a direct influence on children's habits.

Dietary Habits

- High consumption of energy-dense, nutrient-poor foods (e.g., processed snacks, sugary beverages, and fast food) contributes to excessive caloric intake.
- Skipping breakfast, frequent snacking, and consuming oversized portions are associated with an increased risk of obesity.
- In infancy, early introduction of sugary foods and inappropriate feeding practices may set the stage for lifelong unhealthy eating habits.

Physical Inactivity

- Sedentary lifestyles, characterized by reduced physical activity and increased screen time (including smartphones, TV, and video games), are significant contributors to energy imbalance.
- The lack of structured physical education in schools and reduced opportunities for outdoor play.

Socioeconomic and Environmental Factors

Children with lower socioeconomic status (SES) often face additional challenges like limited access to nutritious foods, food insecurity, and disparities in healthcare accessibility and quality that contribute to the risk of obesity.

High consumption of energy-dense, nutrient-poor foods (e.g., processed snacks, sugary beverages, and fast food) contributes to excessive caloric intake.

Skipping breakfast, frequent snacking, and consuming oversized portions are associated with an increased risk of obesity.

In infancy, early introduction of sugary foods and inappropriate feeding practices may set the stage for lifelong unhealthy eating habits.

Sleep Patterns

Irregular or insufficient sleep has been linked to altered hormonal regulation of hunger and satiety, i.e., ghrelin and leptin, respectively.[15]

Medications

Certain medications (e.g., corticosteroids, some antidepressants, or antipsychotics) may contribute to weight gain in children and adolescents.

For about >90% of cases are idiopathic; <10% are associated with genetic or hormonal causes.[16]

CRITICAL PERIODS RELEVANT TO OBESITY RISK

There appear to be at least three critical periods for the development of *childhood obesity*. These include the following: Fetal life; the period of *adiposity* rebound between ages 4 and 6 years, in which BMI, after a rise in infancy and subsequent decline, begins to increase again; and finally, the period of adolescence.[17]

HEALTH CONSEQUENCES AND COMORBIDITIES

Childhood obesity is associated with a higher chance of premature death and disability in adulthood. Alarmingly, 55% of obese children remain obese in adolescence, and 80% persist into adulthood.[18] These overweight and obese children are more likely to develop NCDs such as diabetes and cardiovascular diseases at a younger age. Obese children and adolescents suffer from both short-term and long-term health consequences.

Cardiovascular and Endocrine Complications

Obesity during childhood and adolescence is associated with several cardiovascular and endocrine complications:

- Hyperinsulinism and insulin resistance
- Prediabetes and type 2 diabetes mellitus
- Hypertension
- Dyslipidemia
- Metabolic syndrome
- Polycystic ovary syndrome (PCOS)

Central adiposity in adolescents, characterized by an android or abdominal fat distribution, is more strongly associated with cardiovascular risk factors than the peripheral (gynoid or gluteal pattern) of fat deposition.

Prediabetes and Type 2 Diabetes Mellitus

According to a nationally representative study, the prevalence of prediabetes/diabetes was 12.3% and 8.4% among adolescent boys and girls, respectively, in India.[19]

Hypertension

In children <13 years of age, the definition of hypertension remains ≥95th percentile for age, sex, and height on ≥3 occasions. However, for adolescents ≥13 years of age, hypertension is now defined as blood pressure (BP) ≥ 130/80, regardless of age, sex, or height.[20]

A systematic review of a total of 64 studies published in The Indian Journal of Pediatrics in 2021 by Goyal et al., reported that obese Indian children and adolescents had a significantly higher prevalence of hypertension (29%) compared to normal-weight children (7%).[21]

Dyslipidemia

The prevalence and patterns of dyslipidemia were evaluated among overweight and obese children aged 2–18 years residing in a tribal region. Dyslipidemia was identified in 63.6% of the study population. The most common dyslipidemia pattern observed was the combined low HDL-C and elevated triglyceride levels, observed in 32.5% (n = 49) of participants. Among overweight children, isolated low HDL-C was the most common lipid abnormality (32.3%, n = 19), whereas among obese children, the predominant pattern was combined low HDL-C with elevated triglycerides (42.3%, n = 39).[22]

Polycystic Ovary Syndrome

- PCOS is a common condition, affecting approximately 10% of women of reproductive age and 3–11% of teenage patients.[23]
- This syndrome can lead to various complications and frequently coexists with other health issues. Research is increasingly focusing on the association between PCOS and conditions, such as metabolic syndrome, hypertension, obesity, insulin resistance, type 2 diabetes, and MAFLD.

Liver and Gallbladder

Metabolically-dysfunction-associated fatty liver disease, formerly known as nonalcoholic fatty liver disease (NAFLD), is a significant complication observed in children with obesity. MAFLD is characterized by excessive accumulation of fat in hepatocytes in the absence of secondary causes, such as alcohol consumption or other liver diseases. MAFLD is defined by the presence of hepatic steatosis in individuals with metabolic dysfunction, namely obesity, type 2 diabetes mellitus, or at least two metabolic risk factors, such as:

- Elevated waist circumference
- Hypertension
- Low HDL-cholesterol
- Hypertriglyceridemia
- Prediabetes
- Homeostasis model assessment of insulin resistance (HOMA-IR)
- Elevated high-sensitivity C-reactive protein (CRP) levels[24]

The pathogenesis is closely linked to insulin resistance, adipose tissue dysfunction, increased hepatic lipogenesis, chronic fibrosis, and long-term cardiovascular and metabolic complications. If left untreated, MAFLD can progress to nonalcoholic steatohepatitis (NASH), fibrosis, and long-term cardiovascular and metabolic complications, making early identification and intervention essential in children with obesity.

Psychosocial Consequences

Obese children and adolescents frequently experience social stigmatization, bullying, low self-esteem, anxiety, depression, and eating disorders.[25]

Orthopedic Disorders

Children with obesity are more prone to numerous orthopedic disorders, including:

- Genu valgus deformity
- Slipped capital femoral epiphysis
- Blount disease

DIAGNOSIS

Obesity management starts with determining whether the obesity is exogenous or endogenous. If history and physical examination reveal abnormalities, additional evaluations based on the findings are necessary. For attenuated growth velocity, an endocrine evaluation is required, including thyroid function test (TSH) and free thyroxine (FT4), GH levels, cortisol levels, and other relevant hormones to rule out conditions such as hypothyroidism, GH deficiency, or Cushing's syndrome.

For children with early-onset, severe, or syndromic obesity, a genetic evaluation is needed.

In cases of central nervous system (CNS) injury or hypothalamic obesity, we need to reevaluate pituitary function and consider hormone therapy. If the patient is on antipsychotic medications, a review of drug therapy options is required.

A detailed family history may assist in identifying genetic risk factors and guiding further diagnostic evaluation **(Flowchart 1)**.

Flowchart 1: Clinical indicators and metabolic markers for cardiovascular health assessment.[26,27]

BMI ≥85th percentile

History and physical examination

Abnormal

Additional evaluations based on findings

Antipsychotic drug use

Normal

Evaluate for obesity comorbidities

Attenuated growth velocity

Neuro-developmental abnormalities or severe hyperphagia

CNS injury

Reevaluate drug therapy/ choice

Present

Initiate lifestyle changes and specific treatment of comorbidity

Absent

Initiate lifestyle changes

Continued weight gain >6 months

Weight loss/ stabilization

Endocrine evaluation

Genetic evaluation

Hypothalamic obesity

Consider pharmacotherapy and/or surgery

Maintain support for lifestyle changes and comorbidity treatment

Continued weight gain

Reevaluate pituitary function and/or hormone therapy

Data supporting use of these interventions are limited to pubertal individuals

Is there developmental delay?

Yes

Karyotype; DNA methylation studies

Positive

Prader–Willi syndrome

Negative

Is there evidence of retinal dystrophy, photophobia, or nystagmus?

Positive

Bardet–Biedl syndrome
Alstroms syndrome
Tub deficiency

Negative

Albrights hereditary Osteodystrophy
BDNF, TrkB, SIM1 deficiency

Negative

Measure leptin, insulin*, and proinsulin*

Positive

Congenital leptin deficiency
PCSK1 deficiency

Negative

Molecular genetic studies

Leptin/leptin receptor deficiency
POMC deficiency
MC4R deficiency
SH2B1 deficiency
KSR2 deficiency

(BMI: body mass index; bp: blood pressure; DBP: diastolic blood pressure; HDL-C: high-density lipoprotein cholesterol; LDL-C: low-density lipoprotein cholesterol; SBP: systolic blood pressure; TC/HDL-C: total cholesterol to high-density lipoprotein ratio; VLDL-C: very low-density lipoprotein cholesterol)

*Measure insulin and proinsulin in patients with clinical features of PCSK1 deficiency.

MANAGEMENT

Obesity is a chronic, relapsing, and multifactorial disease that necessitates a lifelong, multidisciplinary management approach, as endorsed by the WHO, the American Academy of Pediatrics (AAP), and the Endocrine Society.

Clinical Management

In managing childhood obesity, it's essential to establish both family and clinical goals.

Family Goals

Obesity management should begin with family counseling. Obesity is increasingly recognized and managed as a complex chronic disease driven by multiple physiological, genetic, behavioral, and environmental factors. Acknowledging it as a disease is part of a modern, non-stigmatizing approach to treatment.

Clinical Goals

Involve altering body composition: The focus is on decreasing central body adiposity (visceral fat), as this more accurately reflects metabolic risk, and to progress toward a normal body composition for the child's age and gender.

- Improving cardiometabolic health: Achieving a 5–10% body weight reduction can significantly enhance obesity-related comorbidities, such as dyslipidemia and insulin resistance.[28]
- Personalized obesity interventions must account for genetic determinants and characteristic behavioral traits—particularly hyperphagia—to optimize treatment outcomes.
- *Enhancing quality of life*: To improve the child's physical, social, and psychological well-being.

These goals can be achieved by:

An early personalized and tailored intervention for obesity management through a multidisciplinary team approach, along with screening for comorbidities, is required.

Effective treatment strategies must address the complex interplay of genetic, behavioral, environmental, and metabolic determinants of obesity.

Comprehensive family counseling should ensure that interventions do not adversely affect the child's growth and development.

The core components of obesity management encompass sustained lifestyle modifications that focus on dietary optimization, increased physical activity, and behavioral interventions. These components not only aid in weight reduction but also enhance overall metabolic health.

A focused review of systems is crucial for evaluating related comorbidities:

Obtain a sleep history, including symptoms of snoring, daytime somnolence, nocturnal enuresis, morning headaches, and inattention, to evaluate for obstructive sleep apnea (OSA).

- Monitor for symptoms of depression and conduct annual evaluation for depression for adolescents 12 years and older.
- Among female adolescents with obesity, evaluate for menstrual irregularities and signs of hyperandrogenism (e.g., hirsutism and acne) to assess risk for PCOS.
- Perform a physical examination (e.g., internal hip rotation in growing children and gait) and musculoskeletal review of systems as part of their evaluation for obesity related orthopedic comorbidity.

In cases of comorbidities, appropriate management and/or specialist referrals should be provided whenever necessary.

"The 2023 AAP Clinical Practice Guideline advocates for a proactive and structured approach to management".

THE STEPPED-CARE MODEL

Management should be delivered in a tiered fashion, progressively intensifying the intervention based on the child's age, degree of obesity, comorbidities, and response to initial treatments.[29]

- *Step 1:* For all children with overweight or obesity, foundational management and motivational interviewing, core education on nutrition, physical activity, and sleep are essential.
- *Step 2:* Intensive health behavior and lifestyle treatment (IHBLT). According to the 2023 AAP Clinical Practice Guideline, IHBLT should be family-based and multicomponent, incorporating nutrition, physical activity, and behavioral change support, and should be delivered with sufficient intensity to achieve clinically meaningful outcomes.[29]

  Intensive health behavior and lifestyle treatment is the most effective evidence-based nonpharmacologic treatment for childhood obesity, recommended for children aged 6 years and older.

  It involves a multidisciplinary team and consists of ≥26 hours of face-to-face, family-based, multicomponent counselling over a 3–12-month period, an intensity level supported by rigorous evidence reviews.[29]
- *Step 3:* Adjunctive therapies—when IHBLT for children with more severe obesity proves unsuccessful, pharmacotherapy may be used as an adjunct to IHBLT.

Pharmacotherapy

Antiobesity medications are **(Table 2)**:

Early Growth Hormone Intervention in Prader–Willi Syndrome

Growth hormone therapy significantly prevents severe obesity in PWS by increasing lean body mass and reducing fat mass, effectively modifying the condition's natural history. Clinical data show that starting therapy in infancy—ideally before two years of age—leads to a more optimal body composition and lower BMI-SDS compared to starting later.[31]

TABLE 2: Pharmacological interventions and clinical efficacy in pediatric obesity management.

Name of the drug	*Mechanism of action*	*Recommended age group*
Semaglutide	• Glucagon-like peptide-1 (GLP-1) receptor agonist • Clinical trials demonstrated a mean change in BMI of –16.1% compared to +0.6% with placebo +0.6% with placebo.[30]	Adolescents aged >12 years
Liraglutide	GLP-1 receptor agonist	Adolescents aged >12 years
Orlistat	Lipase inhibitor	Adolescents aged >12 years
Phentermine-topiramate[29]	Suppresses appetite and helps you feel fuller	Adolescents aged >16 years in some regions[29]

Metabolic and Bariatric Surgery

Metabolic and bariatric surgery is indicated in adolescents with severe obesity, defined as a BMI ≥ 120% of the 95th percentile in the presence of significant comorbidities, or a BMI exceeding 140% of the 95th percentile, irrespective of comorbidity status.[32]

This approach has shown substantial and sustained weight loss, as well as improvement or resolution of comorbidities.

PREVENTIVE STRATEGIES

Addressing an exponential rise in childhood and adolescent obesity requires a multipronged and collaborative approach involving individuals, families, schools, healthcare professionals, and policymakers.

- *School-based interventions:* Schools are the best platforms for promoting healthy behaviors through structured physical education, healthy canteen options, and health education curricula.

- *Policy interventions:* Government policies can play a crucial role in combating the obesity epidemic. These may include regulations on the marketing of unhealthy foods and beverages to children, implementation of clear front-of-pack food labelling, and investment in public infrastructure that promotes physical activity (e.g., parks and safe walking paths)
- *Early screening and management:* Pediatricians and other pediatric healthcare providers (PHCPs) should measure height and weight, calculate BMI, and assess BMI percentile using age- and sex-specific Centers for Disease Control (CDC) growth charts at least annually for all children aged 2–18 years to screen for overweight, obesity, and severe obesity for early identification and intervention.
- *Breastfeeding:* Mounting evidence indicates that exclusive breastfeeding in the first 6 months of life may have longer-term benefits of reducing the risk of being overweight and obesity in childhood and adolescence.
- *Future research:* Continued research is necessary to gain a deeper understanding of the complex interplay of factors contributing to obesity and to develop culturally relevant and effective interventions.

CONCLUSION

Childhood and adolescent obesity is a significant and growing public health concern. Childhood obesity is a complex, multifactorial disease that requires a comprehensive and individualized approach for management. Early intervention, a focus on long-term health outcomes, and family involvement are crucial elements in the successful management of childhood obesity. As research in this field continues to evolve, it is essential for healthcare providers to stay informed about the latest evidence-based strategies and to work collaboratively with families to implement effective prevention and treatment programs. A concerted effort from all sectors of society is imperative to reverse this alarming trend and ensure a healthier future for the next generation.

REFERENCES

1. World Health Organization. Obesity and overweight. Geneva: World Health Organization; 2025.
2. World Health Organization. Noncommunicable diseases: Childhood overweight and obesity. Geneva: World Health Organization; 2025.
3. Obesity Medicine Association. Obesity medicine association 2020 obesity Algorithm. [Online] Available from https://obesitymedicine.org/resources/obesity-algorithm/ [Last accessed March, 2026].
4. The Lancet Diabetes Endocrinology. Childhood obesity: prioritising a healthy start. Lancet Diabetes Endocrinol. 2025;13(7):537.
5. WHO Child Growth Standards based on length/height, weight, and age. Acta Paediatr Suppl. 2006;450:76-85.
6. Styne DM, Arslanian SA, Connor EL, Farooqi IS, Murad MH, Silverstein JH, et al. Pediatric obesity-assessment, treatment, and prevention: an Endocrine Society clinical practice guideline. J Clin Endocrinol Metab. 2017;102(3):709-57.
7. Indian Academy of Pediatrics Growth Charts Committee; Khadilkar V, Yadav S, Agrawal KK, Tamboli S, Banerjee M, et al. Revised IAP growth charts for height, weight, and body mass index for 5- to 18-year-old Indian children. Indian Pediatr. 2015;52(1):47-55.
8. Khadilkar A, Ekbote V, Chiplonkar S, Khadilkar V, Kajale N, Kulkarni S, et al. Waist circumference percentiles in 2-18-year-old Indian children. J Pediatr. 2014;164(6):1358-62.
9. World Obesity Federation. World Obesity Atlas 2024: No area of the world is unaffected by the consequences of obesity. [Online] Available from https://www.worldobesity.org/news/world-obesity-atlas-2024 [Last accessed March, 2026].
10. Singh S, Awasthi S, Kapoor V, Mishra P. Childhood obesity in India: a two-decade meta-analysis of

prevalence and socioeconomic correlates. Clin Epidemiol Glob Health. 2023;23:101390.
11. Daley AF, Balasundaram P. Obesity in Pediatric Patients. In: Treasure Island (FL): StatPearls Publishing; 2026.
12. Loos RJF, Bouchard C. Obesity—is it a genetic disorder? J Intern Med. 2003;254(5):401-25.
13. Loos RJF, Yeo GSH. The genetics of obesity: from discovery to biology. Nat Rev Genet. 2022;23(2):120-33.
14. Dalrymple KV, El-Heis S, Godfrey KM. Maternal weight and gestational diabetes impacts on child health. Curr Opin Clin Nutr Metab Care. 2022;25(3):203-8.
15. Miller AL, Lumeng JC, LeBourgeois MK. Sleep patterns and obesity in childhood. Curr Opin Endocrinol Diabetes Obes. 2015;22(1):41-7.
16. medscape.com. Pediatrics: General Medicine. [Online] Available from https://reference.medscape.com/guide/pediatrics-general [Last accessed March, 2026].
17. Dietz WH. Critical periods in childhood for the development of obesity. Am J Clin Nutr. 1994;59(5):955-9.
18. Simmonds M, Llewellyn A, Owen CG, Woolacott N. Predicting adult obesity from childhood obesity: a systematic review and meta-analysis. Obes Rev. 2016;17(2):95-107.
19. Kumar P, Srivastava S, Mishra PS, Mooss ETK. Prevalence of pre-diabetes/type 2 diabetes among adolescents (10-19 years) and its association with different measures of overweight/obesity in India: a gendered perspective. BMC Endocr Disord. 2021;21(1):146.
20. Batisky D. Screening for pediatric hypertension: How many readings are enough? J Clin Hypertens (Greenwich). 2019;21(9):1358-9.
21. Meena J, Singh M, Agarwal A, Chauhan A, Jaiswal N. Prevalence of hypertension among children and adolescents in India: a systematic review and meta-analysis. Indian J Pediatr. 2021;88(11):1107-14.
22. Dyslipidemia Among Overweight and Obese Children in Jharkhand: A Hospital-Based Study. Indian Pediatrics. 2023;60(8):641-3.
23. Jakubowska-Kowal K, Skrzyńska K, Gawlik-Starzyk A. Treatment and complications of PCOS in adolescents - what's new in 2023? Front Endocrinol (Lausanne). 2024;15:1436952.
24. Boccatonda A, Andreetto L, D'Ardes D, Cocco G, Rossi I, Vicari S, et al. From NAFLD to MAFLD: definition, pathophysiological basis and cardiovascular implications. Biomedicines. 2023;11(3):883.
25. www.mayoclinic.org. (2025). Childhood obesity. [Online] Available from https://www.mayoclinic [Last accessed March, 2026].
26. August GP, Caprio S, Fennoy I, Freemark M, Kaufman FR, Lustig RH, et al. Prevention and treatment of pediatric obesity: an Endocrine Society clinical practice guideline based on expert opinion. J Clin Endocrinol Metab. 2008;93(12):4576-99.
27. Farooqi SOR, O'Rahilly S. Genetic obesity syndromes. In: Grant S, ed. The Genetics of Obesity. New York, NY: Springer; 2104. pp. 23-32.
28. Ryan DH, Yockey SR. Weight loss and improvement in comorbidity: differences at 5%, 10%, 15%, and over. Curr Obes Rep. 2017;6(2):187-94.
29. Hampl SE, Hassink SG, Skinner AC, Armstrong SC, Barlow SE, Bolling CF, et al. Clinical practice guideline for the evaluation and treatment of children and adolescents with obesity. Pediatrics. 2023;151(2):e2022060640.
30. Weghuber D, Barrett T, Barrientos-Pérez M, Gies I, Hosszú E, Jeppesen OK, et al. Once-weekly semaglutide in adolescents with obesity. N Engl J Med. 2022;387(24):2245-57.
31. Wolfgram PM, Carrel AL, Allen DB. Long-term effects of recombinant human growth hormone therapy in children with Prader-Willi syndrome. Curr Opin Pediatr. 2013;25(4):509-14. doi: 10.1097/MOP.0b013e328362c7a2. PMID: 23782572; PMCID: PMC4396180.
32. Pratt JSA, Browne A, Browne NT, Brethauer S, Cuda S, Furbish A, et al. ASMBS pediatric metabolic and bariatric surgery guidelines, 2018. Surg Obes Relat Dis. 2018;14(7):882-901.

Sarcopenic Obesity: An Overlooked but High-risk Syndrome

Neeta Deshpande, Nitin Patankar, Radha Deshpande

ABSTRACT

Sarcopenic obesity (SO) is an increasingly recognized but underdiagnosed condition characterized by the coexistence of sarcopenia—low muscle mass, strength, and function—and obesity. The interaction between these two conditions creates a synergistic pathophysiological burden, leading to greater adverse health outcomes than either disorder alone. Chronic low-grade inflammation, insulin resistance, oxidative stress, and mitochondrial dysfunction form the central mechanisms driving SO, with hormonal dysregulation, ectopic fat deposition, and gut microbiota alterations further contributing. Epidemiological evidence indicates that SO prevalence rises with age but can also manifest in younger individuals with obesity or metabolic disease. Clinically, SO is associated with impaired functional capacity, frailty, falls, fractures, type 2 diabetes, cardiovascular disease, and higher all-cause mortality. Diagnosis requires combined assessment of sarcopenia and obesity, using methods such as handgrip strength, gait speed, dual-energy X-ray absorptiometry (DXA), or bioelectrical impedance analysis (BIA). Currently, management relies on multimodal interventions including resistance and aerobic exercise, protein-optimized nutrition, moderate caloric restriction, and in select cases, bariatric surgery or emerging pharmacological agents. Early recognition and targeted strategies are essential to reduce morbidity, mortality, and healthcare burden associated with SO.

Keywords: Sarcopenic obesity, sarcopenia, obesity, muscle mass, muscle strength, inflammation, insulin resistance, oxidative stress

INTRODUCTION

Sarcopenic obesity (SO) is an emerging concept characterized by the simultaneous presence of two complex medical states—(1) Sarcopenia and (2) obesity. This combination, a condition of excessive adipose tissue, and reduced skeletal muscle mass and function, is SO.[1] The coexistence of both conditions contributes to compounded, synergistic health risks, functional decline, and increased mortality, particularly in aging populations but not exclusive to them. Apart from lower muscle mass, in sarcopenia, muscle function is compromised too. Although multiple factors have been known to be determinants of sarcopenia, age is one of the predominant factors.[2] As a natural process of aging, every year, the fat mass increases, and the skeletal muscle mass starts to dip. But other determinants may predominate such that sarcopenia can supervene even at younger age. Obesity itself is an independent determinant of muscle loss, owing to its propensity to cause inflammation.[3] This can lead to oxidative stress, which in turn can lead to lowering of skeletal muscle mass. Therefore, obesity and sarcopenia have a bidirectional relationship.

Again, aging brings with it a slew of metabolic disorders, that can act as predisposing factors for SO. For example, type 2 diabetes mellitus (T2DM). Just like obesity, T2DM and sarcopenia also have a bidirectional relationship. The common determinants between obesity and T2DM in causation of sarcopenia seem to be inflammation, oxidative stress, and insulin resistance (IR). Normal cellular function is impaired, at the level of the skeletal muscle, leading to sarcopenia. As skeletal muscle is one of the important targets of insulin action, sarcopenia in turn leads to worsen glucose control.

PATHOPHYSIOLOGY AND ETIOLOGY

The pathophysiology of SO is a complex and multifactorial process, primarily driven by a detrimental interplay between excess adipose tissue and declining skeletal muscle mass and function.[4] This creates a "vicious cycle" where obesity and sarcopenia synergistically enhance each other, leading to worse health outcomes than either condition alone.[5] The primary mechanisms involved include chronic low-grade inflammation, IR, oxidative stress, hormonal changes, and myocellular dysfunction.

CORE MECHANISMS: INFLAMMATION, INSULIN RESISTANCE, AND OXIDATIVE STRESS

A central feature in the etiopathogenesis of SO is a state of chronic, low-grade systemic inflammation.[4] In obesity, white adipose tissue expands and becomes dysfunctional, leading to infiltration of immune cells such as macrophages, which shift to a proinflammatory M1 phenotype. These cells secrete a range of proinflammatory cytokines and adipokines, including tumor necrosis factor alpha (TNF-α), interleukin 6 (IL-6), IL-1β, and monocyte chemoattractant protein 1 (MCP-1), while reducing the secretion of anti-inflammatory adiponectin.

These inflammatory mediators also enter the systemic circulation and exert damaging effects on skeletal muscle.

In skeletal muscle, elevated levels of TNF-α and IL-6 are negatively associated with muscle mass and strength. They promote muscle atrophy by upregulating protein degradation pathways, such as the ubiquitin-proteasome system, and inducing apoptosis (programmed cell death) of myocytes.[6] Increased levels of IL-6 and C-reactive protein (CRP) are associated with a twofold to threefold increased risk of significant muscle strength loss.[7]

Insulin resistance is considered a primary cause and a core pathophysiological factor of SO. The inflammatory state driven by obesity is a major contributor to IR.[8]

- At the molecular level, the accumulation of lipids within muscle cells, known as intramyocellular lipids (IMCL)—including metabolites such as ceramides and diacylglycerol (DAG)—disrupts insulin signaling. These lipids activate kinases such as protein kinase C (PKCθ), which interfere with insulin receptor substrate 1 (IRS-1) and prevent the translocation of glucose transporter 4 (GLUT4) to the cell surface. This severely impairs glucose uptake by the muscle.[9]
- The resulting IR leads to "anabolic resistance", where the muscle's ability to synthesize new protein in response to stimuli like amino acids is blunted.[10] Insulin normally activates the mTORC1 protein complex, a key regulator of muscle protein synthesis; in an insulin-resistant state, this process is impaired. Simultaneously, IR promotes protein breakdown by activating the FoxO family of transcription factors.[11]

The combination of inflammation and dysfunctional metabolism leads to oxidative stress, characterized by an overproduction of reactive oxygen species (ROS). This stress is exacerbated by mitochondrial dysfunction and a deficiency in endogenous antioxidants such as glutathione (GSH). ROS can damage cellular components, including mitochondrial DNA and proteins, which reduces adenosine triphosphate (ATP) synthesis, activates apoptotic pathways, and promotes cellular senescence, all contributing to muscle loss.

MYOCELLULAR AND MITOCHONDRIAL MECHANISMS

The muscle tissue itself undergoes significant changes in SO.

- *Myosteatosis and lipotoxicity:* A key feature is *myosteatosis*, the infiltration of fat into and between muscle fibers [intermuscular adipose tissue (IMAT)] and within the muscle cells themselves (IMCL). This ectopic fat deposition is not just a storage issue but actively contributes to "lipotoxicity", further driving inflammation, IR, and mitochondrial dysfunction within the myocyte.
- *Mitochondrial dysfunction:* Mitochondria are central to the pathology of SO. In SO, there is often a reduction in both the number and volume of mitochondria. Their function is impaired due to the overload of fatty acids, which leads to incomplete β-oxidation, increased ROS production, and reduced energy (ATP) generation. There is also evidence for impaired mitochondrial quality control, with excessive mitochondrial fission and declining mitophagy (the process of clearing damaged mitochondria), which further compromises muscle performance.
- *Muscle fiber and stem cell alterations:* The accelerated muscle loss in SO is characterized by an imbalance between protein synthesis and breakdown. It specifically involves the atrophy of type II muscle fibers, which are larger and generate force more rapidly. Furthermore, the function and number of muscle stem cells, known as satellite cells, are diminished, which impairs the muscle's ability to repair and regenerate.

ENDOCRINE AND SIGNALING DYSREGULATION

Hormonal and signaling imbalances are critical drivers of SO.

- *Sex hormones:* Aging leads to a natural decline in anabolic hormones. Decreased *testosterone* in men and *estrogen* in women remove their protective effects on muscle mass and protein synthesis. Obesity worsens this by increasing the activity of the aromatase enzyme in fat tissue, which converts testosterone to estradiol.
- *Dysregulated adipokines and myokines:*
  - *Adipokines:* Although circulating levels of the adipokine leptin are often increased in SO, muscle tissue appears to be resistant to its anabolic effects. Similarly, levels of adiponectin, which is normally anti-inflammatory and improves insulin sensitivity, are reduced or its action is blunted.[12]
  - *Myokines:* Secretions from muscle also contribute to the pathology. Myostatin, a myokine that inhibits muscle growth, is often elevated, while irisin, which is positively associated with muscle mass, is decreased.
- *Key signaling pathways:* Proinflammatory signals, particularly TNF-α, lead to the activation of the nuclear factor-κB (NF-κB) transcription factor, a central regulator of muscle wasting.[13] The cellular energy sensor AMP-activated protein kinase (AMPK) also becomes dysregulated, affecting mitochondrial health and substrate metabolism.

THE GUT MICROBIOTA PERSPECTIVE

Emerging evidence suggests that the gut microbiota plays a role in the etiology of SO.

- *Dysbiosis and "inflammaging":* Both aging and obesity are associated with dysbiosis, an unhealthy alteration in the composition of gut microbes.[14] This dysbiosis contributes to systemic inflammation (termed "inflammaging") by increasing intestinal permeability.

This "leaky gut" allows bacterial components to enter the bloodstream, triggering an inflammatory response that exacerbates IR.

- *Altered metabolite production:* A dysbiotic gut produces fewer beneficial metabolites, such as short-chain fatty acids (SCFAs), which are important for maintaining gut barrier integrity and reducing inflammation.

EPIDEMIOLOGY

The incidence of SO is rapidly increasing, driven by the dual global health challenges of an aging population and the obesity epidemic. However, its exact prevalence is difficult to establish due to the lack of a universally accepted definition and standardized diagnostic criteria.[15] A meta-analysis found a global prevalence of approximately 11% in adults aged 60 and older. The prevalence increases dramatically with age. For example, the Dutch Lifelines cohort study reported a prevalence of 16.7% in the 80–89 years age group.[16] SO can also be observed in middle-aged and even younger obese individuals, often in the presence of chronic illnesses or following rapid changes in body weight. Epidemiological evidence consistently demonstrates that SO is a more severe condition that confers a poorer prognosis than either sarcopenia or obesity alone, due to a synergistic negative effect on health. SO is associated with a significantly higher risk of all-cause mortality.[17]

CLINICAL CONSEQUENCES

Functional Decline

The combination of excess fat mass and low muscle mass and strength in SO leads to significant functional impairment and a loss of independence. This complex condition carries a twofold to threefold greater risk of functional impairment compared to either sarcopenia or obesity alone. Individuals with SO often experience difficulties with physical function, such as walking, rising from a chair, and climbing stairs. This decline is a strong predictor of future disability, particularly in performing activities of daily living. The condition is also associated with frailty, gait limitations, and an increased risk of falls and fractures. Consequently, SO has a significant negative impact on health-related quality of life (HRQoL), with studies showing that patients with SO report a poorer quality of life compared to those with obesity alone.[18]

Metabolic Risk

Insulin resistance is considered a primary cause and a core pathophysiological feature of SO. The pathogenesis is multifactorial, but inflammatory mediators and IR play a key role. SO is strongly associated with an increased risk of developing T2DM.[19] The relationship appears to be bidirectional, with chronic inflammation connecting the two conditions. Furthermore, the IR seen in the adipose tissue, skeletal muscle, and liver of individuals with SO is a primary characteristic of nonalcoholic fatty liver disease (NAFLD), as SO compromises insulin signaling in hepatocytes, leading to increased fat production and reduced fat breakdown in the liver.[20]

Cardiovascular Risk

The SO is associated with an increased risk of cardiovascular disease (CVD) and its related risk factors, such as hypertension. Atherosclerosis is considered a primary pathological contributor to CVD in SO patients, driven by chronic low-grade inflammation and IR. Proinflammatory cytokines, including TNF-α and IL-6, secreted from adipose and muscle tissue can directly damage the vascular endothelium, which in turn worsens IR and accelerates the progression of atherosclerosis.[3] This is supported by studies showing an independent correlation between SO and coronary artery calcification, a marker of advanced atherosclerosis. The relationship between SO and CVD is mutually causative; preexisting CVD can contribute to the development of SO by causing exercise intolerance, disrupting blood flow to muscles, and impairing mitochondrial function, which promotes muscle atrophy.

Mortality

Sarcopenic obesity is a strong predictor of all-cause mortality. The combination of obesity and sarcopenia has a synergistic effect, leading to a higher mortality risk than either condition alone. Multiple prospective studies and a meta-analysis have confirmed this association.[21,22]

DIAGNOSIS

As a subclinical disease, SO lacks a universally accepted set of diagnostic criteria, which means its identification is based on diagnosing its two distinct components—(1) sarcopenia and (2) obesity.

Assessment of Sarcopenia

The diagnosis of sarcopenia typically involves evaluating three key parameters—(1) low muscle mass, (2) diminished muscle strength, and (3) poor physical performance. Various working groups have put forth different criteria, but a common diagnostic pathway begins with screening at-risk patients with questionnaires such as the SARC-F, which assesses a person's ability to perform daily activities. A positive screen is followed by quantitative and functional testing for confirmation.

Diagnostic Benchmarks for Sarcopenia (EWGSOP 2019)[23] *(Table 1)*

The quantity of muscle can be measured using several techniques.

- *Dual-energy X-ray absorptiometry (DXA):* This is often considered a reference method for measuring muscle and fat mass. DXA uses two X-ray photons to distinguish between bone, fat, and lean tissues. It is a quick procedure with minimal radiation exposure, but its precision can be compromised in individuals with a high Body Mass Index (BMI), and variations in software can make test comparisons challenging.
- *Bioelectrical impedance analysis (BIA):* BIA is an accessible, inexpensive, and portable method that estimates body composition by measuring electrical conductivity. Its accuracy can be influenced by the patient's hydration level, and it may overestimate lean mass and underestimate fat mass in individuals with a BMI over 34 kg/m^2.

TABLE 1: EWGSOP 2019 diagnostic benchmarks for sarcopenia.

Parameters	*Assessment method*	*Threshold (men)*	*Threshold (women)*
Muscle strength	Handgrip dynamometry	<27 kg	<16 kg
	Time to rise from a chair (5 reps)	>15 seconds	>15 seconds
Muscle mass	Appendicular skeletal muscle mass	<20 kg	<15 kg
	Muscle mass index (ASM/height^2)	<7.0 kg/m^2	<5.5 kg/m^2
Physical performance	Gait speed (usual walking pace)	<0.8 m/s	<0.8 m/s
	Short physical performance battery	≤8 points	≤8 points
	Timed get-up-and-go test	≥20 seconds	≥20 seconds
	400 m walk	>6 minutes or incomplete	>6 minutes or incomplete

- *Computed tomography/magnetic resonance imaging (CT/MRI):* These high-resolution imaging tools can precisely measure muscle mass, differentiate between various types of fat and lean tissue, and quantify fat infiltration within the muscle, a condition known as myosteatosis. However, their use is limited by high costs, lack of portability, and radiation exposure in the case of CT.

Assessment of Obesity

The World Health Organization (WHO) defines obesity as an "abnormal or excessive fat accumulation that poses a health risk".

- *Challenges:* BMI alone misclassifies many.
  - The most common tool for diagnosing obesity is the BMI, with a value of ≥30 kg/m^2 typically indicating obesity. This value is ≥23 kg/m^2 for the Indian population.
  - However, BMI is not considered a reliable standalone measure of body fat because it fails to capture variations in body composition. Individuals of different ethnicities can have substantially different body fat percentages at an identical BMI.
  - Additionally, using BMI in older adults can be problematic due to age-related changes such as a decrease in height, which can inflate the BMI value even if body weight is stable.
- *BMI, waist circumference, and body fat percentage:*
  - To improve accuracy, waist circumference is frequently measured alongside BMI. It is important to recognize that cut-off points for waist circumference also differ among ethnic groups.
  - Given the limitations of indirect measures, the direct assessment of body fat percentage is viewed as a more dependable method for diagnosing SO. Techniques such as DXA, BIA, CT, and MRI are used for this purpose.

MANAGEMENT STRATEGIES

Currently, there are no approved drug therapies specifically for SO; therefore, treatment is centered on a multimodal approach that integrates lifestyle modifications, nutritional therapy, and in some cases, bariatric surgery or emerging pharmacological interventions. The primary therapeutic goal is the preservation of muscle strength and function, with a secondary objective of achieving weight loss that specifically targets fat mass, not muscle.[24]

Lifestyle Interventions

Lifestyle changes, particularly caloric restriction (CR) and physical exercise, are considered the cornerstone of treatment for SO.

- *Physical exercise:* Exercise is regarded as the most effective single intervention for sarcopenia, as it can restore mitochondrial function and reduce inflammatory responses.[25]
  - *Resistance training* is viewed as the most effective type of exercise for inducing muscle hypertrophy, improving muscle strength, and enhancing physical performance in older adults.[26]
  - *Aerobic exercise* is particularly useful for managing obesity and improves cardiovascular health, IR, and muscle capacity.[27]
  - A combination of resistance and aerobic exercise appears to be the most beneficial strategy, leading to greater improvements in physical function and quality of life than either modality alone.[28]
- *Nutritional therapy:* Dietary management is crucial for supporting muscle health while promoting fat loss.
  - *CR:* While CR is a standard treatment for obesity, very-low-calorie diets should be avoided in SO as they can worsen muscle and bone loss.[29] A moderate CR with a weight loss goal of <5–8% of initial body

weight is recommended. Combining a calorie-restricted diet with exercise is synergistic, preserving lean mass while improving muscle function.[30]

- *Protein intake:* Higher protein intake is necessary to overcome the "anabolic resistance" of aging and prevent muscle loss during weight reduction.[31] Recommendations support 1.0–1.2 g/kg of body weight per day for older adults, increasing to 1.2–1.5 g/kg for those with chronic illness.
- *Protein quality and specific nutrients:* Proteins of high biological value, particularly those rich in the amino acid leucine (e.g., whey protein), are more effective at stimulating muscle protein synthesis.[32] Supplements containing whey protein, leucine, and vitamin D have been shown to be an effective strategy.[33] Other nutrients such as beta-hydroxy-methyl-butyrate (HMB), creatine, and omega-3 fatty acids may also offer benefits.

- *Bariatric surgery:* Bariatric surgery is an effective treatment for morbid obesity, but its role in SO is still being evaluated. While surgery leads to significant fat loss, it can also cause a substantial loss of muscle mass (over 15% in some patients), which is associated with poorer metabolic outcomes.[34] The prevalence of sarcopenia may significantly increase after surgery, highlighting the need for careful preoperative assessment of muscle mass.
- *Pharmacological and emerging therapies:* While no specific drugs are approved for SO, several pathways are under investigation.

Hormonal and Anabolic Therapies

- Testosterone replacement may be used in men to restore androgen balance, though its use in older adults is limited by cardiovascular risks.[35] The data on its impact remain conflicting.
- Selective androgen receptor modulators (SARMs) offer a more targeted approach by activating receptors primarily in muscle and bone, potentially providing more benefit than testosterone.[36]
- *Myostatin inhibitors*, such as the monoclonal antibody bimagrumab, block negative regulators of muscle growth and have been shown to increase muscle mass.[37]
- Other agents such as glucagon-like peptide 1 (GLP-1) receptor agonists and the ghrelin agonist anamorelin are also being considered for their beneficial effects on body composition and lean mass.[38]

Metabolic and Antioxidant Agents

- *AMPK agonists* like resveratrol and metformin can improve mitochondrial function and protein synthesis, though metformin has shown mixed results, potentially blunting the benefits of exercise in older adults.[39]
- *Antioxidants* may help counteract the oxidative stress underlying SO. Supplementing with glycine and N-acetylcysteine (GlyNAC) is a promising approach to correct GSH deficiency, which improves muscle function and reduces oxidative stress.[40]
- *Vitamin D* deficiency is linked to SO, but evidence for the effectiveness of supplementation on muscle strength has been inconsistent.[41]

CONCLUSION

Sarcopenic obesity is underrecognized yet high-risk. SO is a growing health problem that often goes undiagnosed due to a lack of consensus on diagnostic criteria. This condition poses a greater risk for severe adverse outcomes—including disability, CVD, and increased mortality—than either sarcopenia or obesity alone. The synergistic negative effects make it a critical public health challenge, particularly in aging populations.

Identifying and treating it requires a dual focus on fat and muscle. Effective management must simultaneously target the reduction of fat mass while preserving or enhancing muscle mass and function. The cornerstone of treatment is a multimodal lifestyle intervention combining nutritional therapy and physical exercise. This approach typically includes moderate CR, a high-protein diet to counteract muscle loss, and a combination of resistance and aerobic exercises to improve both muscle strength and metabolic health.

Early diagnosis and tailored interventions may reduce morbidity, mortality, and healthcare burden. Timely identification of SO is crucial for mitigating its severe health consequences. Establishing standardized diagnostic criteria is essential for both clinical practice and research. Tailored, multimodal interventions centered on diet and exercise can improve physical function, enhance quality of life, and ultimately reduce the high risk of morbidity and mortality associated with the condition, thereby lessening the significant burden on healthcare systems.

REFERENCES

1. Barazzoni R, Bischoff S, Boirie Y, Busetto L, Cederholm T, Dicker D, et al. Sarcopenic obesity: time to meet the challenge. Obes Facts. 2018;11(4):294-305.
2. Makizako H. Frailty and sarcopenia as a geriatric syndrome in community-dwelling older adults. Int J Environ Res Public Health. 2019;16(20): 4013.
3. Hong SH, Choi KM. Sarcopenic obesity, insulin resistance, and their implications in cardiovascular and metabolic consequences. Int J Mol Sci. 2020;21(2):494.
4. Karaağaç Y. Sarcopenic obesity, pathogenesis, and treatment with a focus on exercise and protein intake. J Mind Med Sci. 2023;10(2): 237-46.
5. Rolland Y, Lauwers-Cances V, Cristini C, Van Kan GA, Janssen I, Morley JE, et al. Difficulties with physical function associated with obesity, sarcopenia, and sarcopenic-obesity in community-dwelling elderly women: the EPIDOS Study. Am J Clin Nutr. 2009;89(6):1895-900.
6. Kob R, Bollheimer LC, Bertsch T, Fellner C, Djukic M, Sieber CC, et al. Sarcopenic obesity: molecular clues to a better understanding of its pathogenesis? Biogerontology. 2015;16(1):15-29.
7. Wang J, Leung KS, Chow SK, Cheung WH. Inflammation and age-associated skeletal muscle deterioration (sarcopaenia). J Orthop Translat. 2017;10:94-101.
8. Gusmao-Sena MH, Curvello-Silva K, Barreto-Medeiros JM, Da-Cunha-Daltro CH. Association between sarcopenic obesity and cardiovascular risk: Where are we? Nutr Hosp. 2016;33:592.
9. Wei S, Nguyen TT, Zhang Y, Ryu D, Gariani K. Sarcopenic obesity: epidemiology, pathophysiology, cardiovascular disease, mortality, and management. Front Endocrinol (Lausanne). 2023;14:1185221.
10. Wilkinson DJ, Piasecki M, Atherton PJ. The age-related loss of skeletal muscle mass and function: measurement and physiology of muscle fibre atrophy and muscle fibre loss in humans. Ageing Res Rev. 2018;47:123-32.
11. Lecker SH, Goldberg AL, Mitch WE. Protein degradation by the ubiquitin-proteasome pathway in normal and disease states. J Am Soc Nephrol. 2006;17:1807-19.
12. Sabaratnam R, Skov V, Paulsen SK, Juhl S, Kruse R, Hansen T, et al. A signature of exaggerated adipose tissue dysfunction in type 2 diabetes is linked to low plasma adiponectin and increased transcriptional activation of proteasomal degradation in muscle. Cells. 2022;11;2005.
13. Vaughan S, Jat PS. Deciphering the role of nuclear factor-kappaB in cellular senescence. Aging (Albany NY). 2011;3:913-9.
14. Livshits G, Kalinkovich A. Inflammaging as a common ground for the development and maintenance of sarcopenia, obesity, cardiomyopathy and dysbiosis. Ageing Res Rev. 2019;56:100980.
15. El Ghoch M, Calugi S, Grave RD. Sarcopenic Obesity: definition, health consequences and clinical management. Open Nutr J. 2018; 12(1):70-3.

16. Wagenaar CA, Dekker LH, Navis GJ. Prevalence of sarcopenic obesity and sarcopenic overweight in the general population: the lifelines cohort study. Clin Nutr. 2021;40:4422-9.
17. Stenholm S, Harris TB, Rantanen T, Visser M, Kritchevsky SB, Ferrucci L. Sarcopenic obesity-definition, etiology and consequences. Int J Obes. 2008;11(6):693-700.
18. Itani L, Kreidieh D, El Masri D, Tannir H, El Ghoch M. The impact of sarcopenic obesity on health-related quality of life in treatment-seeking patients with obesity. Curr Diabetes Rev. 2020;16:1-7.
19. Lim HS, Park YH, Suh K, Yoo MH, Park HK, Kim HJ, et al. Association between Sarcopenia, Sarcopenic Obesity, and Chronic Disease in Korean Elderly. J Bone Metab. 2018;25(3):187-93.
20. Donnelly KL, Smith CI, Schwarzenberg SJ, Jessurun J, Boldt MD, Parks EJ. Sources of fatty acids stored in liver and secreted via lipoproteins in patients with nonalcoholic fatty liver disease. J Clin Invest. 2005;115(5):1343-51.
21. Atkins JL, Whincup PH, Morris RW, Lennon LT, Papacosta O, Wannamethee SG. Sarcopenic obesity and risk of cardiovascular disease and mortality: a population-based cohort study of older men. J Am Geriatr Soc. 2014;62:253-60.
22. von Berens A, Obling SR, Nydahl M, Koochek A, Lissner L, Skoog I, et al. Sarcopenic obesity and associations with mortality in older women and men: a prospective observational study. BMC Geriatr. 2020;20:199.
23. Cruz-Jentoft AJ, Bahat G, Bauer J, Boirie Y, Bruyère O, Cederholm T, et al. Sarcopenia: revised European consensus on definition and diagnosis. Age Ageing. 2019;48:16-31.
24. Deutz NE, Bauer JM, Barazzoni R, Biolo G, Boirie Y, Bosy-Westphal A, et al. Protein intake and exercise for optimal muscle function with aging: recommendations from the ESPEN Expert Group. Clin Nutr. 2014;33(6):929-36.
25. Lo JH, U KP, Yiu T, Ong MT, Lee WY. Sarcopenia: Current treatments and new regenerative therapeutic approaches. J Orthop Translat. 2020;23:38-52.
26. Hsu KJ, Liao CD, Tsai MW, Chen CN. Effects of exercise and nutritional intervention on body composition, metabolic health, and physical performance in adults with sarcopenic obesity: a meta-analysis. Nutrients. 2019;11(9):2163.
27. Stensvold D, Viken H, Steinshamn SL, Dalen H, Stoylen A, Loennechen JP, et al. Effect of exercise training for five years on all cause mortality in older adults—the generation 100 study: randomised controlled trial. BMJ. 2020;371:m3485.
28. Villareal DT, Aguirre L, Gurney AB, Waters DL, Sinacore DR, Colombo E, et al. Aerobic or resistance exercise, or both, in dieting obese older adults. N Engl J Med. 2017;376:1943-55.
29. Batsis JA, Villareal DT. Sarcopenic obesity in older adults: aetiology, epidemiology and treatment strategies. Nat Rev Endocrinol. 2018;14:513-37.
30. Camajani E, Feraco A, Proietti S, Basciani S, Barrea L, Armani A, et al. Very low calorie ketogenic diet combined with physical interval training for preserving muscle mass during weight loss in sarcopenic obesity: a pilot study. Front Nutr. 2022;9:955024.
31. Breen L, Phillips SM. Skeletal muscle protein metabolism in the elderly: Interventions to counteract the 'anabolic resistance' of ageing. Nutr Metab (Lond). 2011;8:68.
32. Rooks D, Roubenoff R. Development of pharmacotherapies for the treatment of sarcopenia. J Frailty Aging. 2019;8:120-30.
33. Camajani E, Persichetti A, Watanabe M, Contini S, Vari M, Di Bernardo S, et al. Whey protein, L-leucine and vitamin d supplementation for preserving lean mass during a low-calorie diet in sarcopenic obese women. Nutrients. 2022;14(9):1884.
34. Vaurs C, Diméglio C, Charras L, Anduze Y, Chalret duRieu M, Ritz P. Determinants of changes in muscle mass after bariatric surgery. Diabetes Metab. 2015;41:416-21.
35. Bhasin S. Testosterone supplementation for aging-associated sarcopenia. J Gerontol A Biol Sci Med Sci. 2003;58:1002-8.
36. von Haehling S, Anker SD. Treatment of cachexia: an overview of recent developments. J Am Med Dir Assoc. 2014;15:866-72.
37. Lach-Trifilieff E, Minetti GC, Sheppard K, Ibebunjo C, Feige JN, Hartmann S, et al. An anti-body blocking activin type II receptors induces strong skeletal muscle hypertrophy and protects from atrophy. Mol Cell Biol. 2014;34:606-18.

38. Temel JS, Abernethy AP, Currow DC, Friend J, Duus EM, Yan Y, et al. Anamorelin in patients with non-small-cell lung cancer and cachexia (ROMANA 1 and ROMANA 2): results from two randomised, double-blind, phase 3 trials. Lancet Oncol. 2016;17:519-31.
39. Konopka AR, Laurin JL, Schoenberg HM, Reid JJ, Castor WM, Wolff CA, et al. Metformin inhibits mitochondrial adaptations to aerobic exercise training in older adults. Aging Cell. 2019;18:e12880.
40. Kumar P, Liu C, Suliburk J, Hsu JW, Muthupillai R, Jahoor F, et al. Supplementing glycine and N-acetylcysteine (GlyNAC) in older adults improves glutathione deficiency, oxidative stress, mitochondrial dysfunction, inflammation, physical function, and aging hallmarks: a randomized clinical trial. J Gerontol A Biol Sci Med Sci. 2022;78:75-89.
41. Kim MK, Baek KH, Song KH, Kang MI, Park CY, Lee WY, et al. Vitamin D deficiency is associated with sarcopenia in older Koreans, regardless of obesity: the fourth Korea national health and nutrition examination surveys (KNHANES IV) 2009. J Clin Endocrinol Metab. 2011;96: 3250-6.

CHAPTER 5

Epicardial Adipose Tissue: Clinical Biomarker of Cardiometabolic Risk

Kanishka Manikandan, Yaser Ahmad, Saifullah Syed, Navin C Nanda

ABSTRACT

This chapter discusses the clinical importance of assessing epicardial adipose tissue not only as a marker of cardiometabolic risk but also as a contributor to disease. Various noninvasive modalities used in its evaluation including echocardiography are also described together with their advantages and limitations.

Keywords: Epicardial adipose tissue, echocardiography, computed tomography, magnetic resonance imaging, cardiometabolic diseases.

INTRODUCTION

In the modern era of a rising trend in cardiovascular diseases, heart health is receiving the utmost attention. With evidence-based medicine at the forefront, everyone from primary care physicians to leading cardiologists is calculating various cardiovascular risk scores and often focus on parameters such as serum cholesterol levels, blood pressure, and hemoglobin A1C. However, another important, yet less well-known, marker of cardiometabolic risk is located anatomically over the heart itself—epicardial adipose tissue (EAT).[1]

Epicardial adipose tissue presents as a layer rich in fat l located between the outer surface of the myocardium and the visceral pericardium. It is therefore in direct contact with the myocardium and epicardial coronary arteries and is perfused through the same vascular network as the myocardium, positioning it as a key player in cardiac and metabolic regulation.[2]

Under physiological conditions, EAT plays protective roles by providing energy to the myocardium, offering thermal insulation, mechanically cushioning the heart, and secreting cardioprotective adipokines. However, in some metabolic states, EAT undergoes pathologic remodeling and releases harmful inflammatory and fibrosis-promoting cytokines and hence can serve as a clinical biomarker of cardiometabolic risk.[3-8]

This chapter will explore the functions, clinical implications, and various assessment methods of EAT. It will also address ongoing debates, controversies, and limitations, highlighting why EAT is increasingly regarded as a biomarker of cardiometabolic risk.

CURRENT IMAGING MODALITIES FOR EPICARDIAL ADIPOSE TISSUE ASSESSMENT (TABLE 1)

Various noninvasive imaging modalities have been employed to measure EAT, each with distinct advantages and limitations.

Two-dimensional Transthoracic Echocardiography

Epicardial adipose tissue thickness can be assessed noninvasively using two-dimensional transthoracic echocardiography (2DTTE), a widely used and cost-effective imaging modality. Standard parasternal long **(Fig. 1A)** and short axis **(Fig. 1B)** views allow for an accurate

TABLE 1: Imaging modalities for epicardial adipose tissue assessment.

Modality	*Technique*	*Advantages*	*Limitations*
2DTTE	Thickness of EAT on RV free wall	Widely available, cost-effective, and radiation free	Operator-dependent, limited spatial detail. Does not provide EAT volume
CT	Volumetric quantification (Reference range: *mean volume 68 ± 34 mL to 124 ± 50 mL*)[20]	High resolution, good reproducibility, can be done along with CAC scoring, potential for artificial intelligence-derived measurements[21]	Radiation exposure with risk of cancer. Contrast may be required. PCCT largely investigational
MRI	T1-weighted fat segmentation	Gold standard for soft tissue visualization, no radiation exposure	Expensive and time consuming

(2DTTE: two-dimensional transthoracic echocardiography; CAC: coronary artery calcium; CT: computed tomography scan; EAT: epicardial adipose tissue; MRI: cardiac magnetic resonance imaging; PCCT: photon-counting computed tomography; RV: right ventricular)

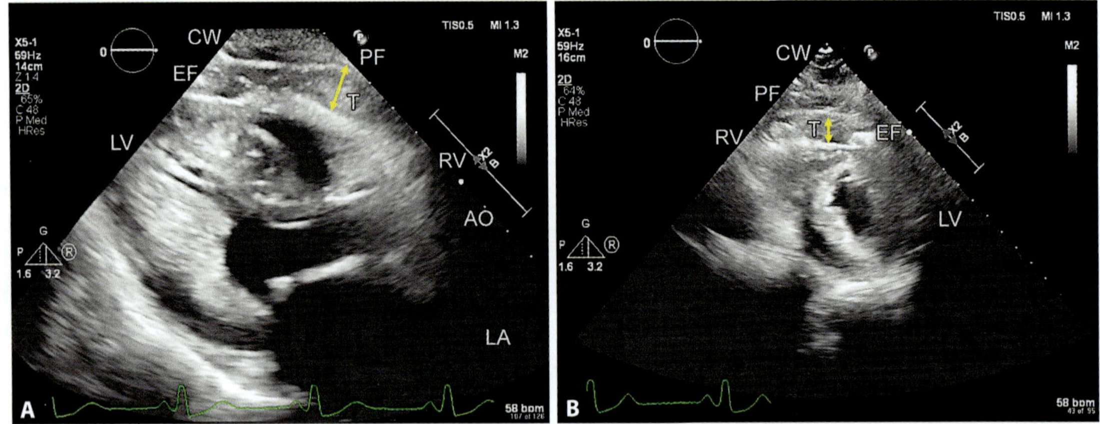

Figs. 1A and B: (A) Two-dimensional transthoracic echocardiographic assessment of epicardial adipose tissue (EF). Parasternal long axis view. Maximal thickness (T) of EF is 13 mm; (B) Two-dimensional transthoracic echocardiographic assessment of epicardial adipose tissue (EF). Maximal thickness (T) of EF is 13 mm. Parasternal short axis view. (AO: aorta; CW: chest wall; LA: left atrium; LV: left ventricle; PF: pericardial fat pad; RV: right ventricle)
Courtesy: Dr Navin C Nanda.

measurement of EAT thickness.[1] The maximum thickness of EAT is assessed perpendicularly along the right ventricular free wall. It typically presents as a predominantly echolucent or low echo dense region situated between the myocardium's outer surface and the visceral pericardium on imaging. Measurements are typically taken at end systole when the heart is contracted, as this phase often provides a clearer delineation of the EAT layer. In the literature, measurements have varied from 1 to 23 mm with maximum thickness >7 mm often considered as abnormal. However, there is no consensus on this. Measurements taken in end-diastole can be more consistent with computed tomography (CT) scans and magnetic resonance imaging (MRI). End-systolic measurements are larger than end-diastolic measurements.[9] To ensure accuracy, measurements are often taken over three cardiac cycles, and the average value is calculated.[1,9] Three-dimensional TTE may provide more reliable assessment of EAT than 2DTTE, but studies using this technique are lacking in the literature. EAT is distinguished echocardiographically from pericardial adipose tissue, which is identified as a hypoechoic space anterior to the EAT between the parietal and visceral layers of pericardium.[1] The paracardiac adipose tissue, on the other hand, is located outside the parietal pericardium **(Fig. 2)**.[10] In summary, due to its availability, low cost, and accuracy, 2DTTE serves as the preferred modality for routine EAT assessment.

Cardiac Computed Tomography Imaging

Computed tomography offers high-resolution, three-dimensional imaging, allowing for precise volumetric assessment of EAT. Following segmentation of epicardial fat, its volume is determined by aggregating the cross-sectional areas across all slices and multiplying by the slice thickness, yielding a precise volumetric measurement expressed in milliliters.[11]

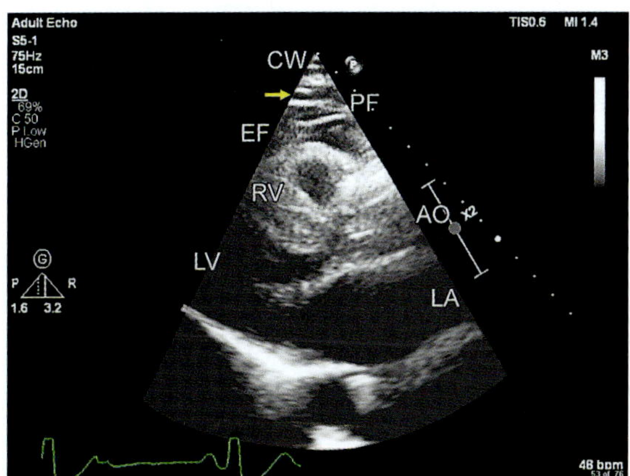

Fig. 2: Two-dimensional transthoracic echocardiographic assessment of epicardial adipose tissue (EF) in another patient. Parasternal short axis view. Arrow points to paracardiac fat.
(AO: aorta; CW: chest wall; LA: left atrium; LV: left ventricle; PF: pericardial fat pad; RV: right ventricle)
Courtesy: Dr Navin C Nanda.

It is particularly useful in individuals receiving coronary artery calcium (CAC) scoring or CT angiography. While CAC scoring measures calcified plaque burden within the coronary vessels, EAT volume provides additional information about noncalcified, metabolically active fat surrounding the coronary arteries.[12,13]

Studies indicate that combining EAT volume with CAC scores significantly enhances risk stratification for major adverse cardiovascular events. Elevated EAT volume independently correlates with increased risk beyond CAC scores alone. This suggests that EAT quantification can refine risk stratification, especially in patients with intermediate CAC scores.[14] Artificial intelligence (AI) models, trained on vast imaging datasets, can swiftly and accurately identify pericardial boundaries on CT and help quantify and segment EAT volume accurately, enhancing risk stratification for cardiovascular events.[15]

Photon-counting CT (PCCT) may offer more accurate volumetric EAT assessment with potentially lower radiation doses. Unlike conventional CT scanners, which measure the sum-total energy of X-ray photons collectively, PCCT employs advanced detectors that count individual X-ray photons while simultaneously measuring their precise energy levels. This approach provides more detailed and precise imaging, allowing for improved tissue characterization and material differentiation.[16] Research has shown that PCCT can accurately measure EAT attenuation and the fat attenuation index (FAI) at different energy levels, providing insights into pericoronary inflammation—a marker of cardiac risk.[17,18]

Cardiac Magnetic Resonance Imaging

Cardiac MRI enables precise volumetric quantification of EAT and additionally can assess myocardial inflammation, perfusion, and fat infiltration using advanced sequences such as T1/T2 mapping and fat suppression techniques. By transforming standard scans such as CTs and MRIs into rich datasets, radiomics helps delve deeper into tissue characteristics, providing a comprehensive profile of EAT's structural and compositional attributes **(Table 1)**.[19]

EPICARDIAL ADIPOSE TISSUE AS A MARKER OF CARDIOMETABOLIC RISK

Atherosclerosis

Coronary Artery Disease

Epicardial adipose tissue actively contributes to coronary artery disease (CAD) and acute coronary syndrome (ACS) by releasing inflammatory cytokines and adipokines that trigger vascular inflammation and contribute to cardiac remodeling. Increased EAT thickness by coronary CT angiography has been shown to be a valuable marker in predicting the presence of obstructive CAD.[22] In a 2025 cross-sectional study, Zhihong et al. compared 175 patients with ACS to non-ACS controls. Coronary CT angiography was used to quantify EAT. They revealed that patients with ACS not only had quantitatively larger volumes of EAT but also denser, more inflamed fat. Importantly, EAT density—reflecting inflammatory activity—was a stronger independent predictor of ACS than traditional risk factors, with an odds ratio of 6.94 and an area under the curve (AUC) of 0.859. These findings position EAT, particularly its density, as a potential biomarker for ACS risk assessment.[23] Similar findings have been demonstrated in a 2023 study, where 2DTTE-measured EAT thickness has been linked to greater CAD burden.[24]

Additionally, radiomic analysis of EAT has been utilized to differentiate between unstable angina and non-ST segment elevation myocardial infarction, demonstrating its potential in enhancing diagnostic accuracy of CAD.[25] The combined thickness of the intima and media layers of the carotid artery wall correlates strongly with an increased risk of myocardial infarction, stroke, and cardiovascular mortality. A cross-sectional study by Kocaman et al. involving 252 patients demonstrated a strong, positive correlation between EAT thickness measured using 2DTTE and carotid intima-media thickness. This potentiates EAT's role as a surrogate marker of early subclinical atherosclerosis.[26]

The EAT surrounding the epicardial coronary arteries is referred to as pericoronary adipose tissue. The inflammatory milieu created by dysfunctional EAT is linked with the progression of CAD.[27] Particularly, through paracrine effects, the EAT can induce and cause the progression of coronary plaques.[28] While traditionally atherosclerosis was thought to be initiated by intimal injury in an "inside-out" paradigm, the effects of perivascular inflammation on atherosclerosis has led to an "outside-in" approach.[29] In a study by Yu et al., patients suspected to have CAD underwent myocardial perfusion imaging along with CT to calculate CAC scoring and EAT volume. EAT volume correlated significantly with myocardial ischemia, suggesting its utility in primary or secondary prevention.[30]

Coronary Microcirculatory Disease

Epicardial adipose tissue thickness, as measured by 2DTTE, is also correlated with coronary microvascular dysfunction (CMD), likely due to local inflammatory properties of the EAT.[31] Patients at risk for CMD could benefit from EAT assessment.

Stroke

A 2021 meta-analysis by Rosa et al. demonstrated a significant association between increased EAT and stroke risk, independent of traditional cardiovascular risk factors. EAT was consistently elevated in stroke patients when measured by 2DTTE, CT, and MRI across multiple global cohorts. These results imply that EAT could act as an imaging-based indicator for identifying individuals at elevated stroke risk.[32] These results support expanding the role of EAT assessment beyond CAD to cerebrovascular risk evaluation.

Peripheral Artery Disease

Epicardial adipose tissue may serve as a panvascular biomarker, reflecting not only coronary atherosclerosis but also systemic vascular disease such as peripheral artery disease (PAD). A cross-sectional study of 54 patients undergoing CT coronary angiography found EAT volume positively correlated with total cholesterol and CAC scores, both proxies for systemic atherosclerosis, including PAD.[33] Roever et al. also proposed EAT as a potential PAD marker in adults aged 40–70. This systematic review clarified the association between EAT, metabolic syndrome, and PAD, with implications for early risk stratification and preventive strategies.[34]

Hypertension

A recent retrospective cohort study using MRI revealed that hypertensive individuals with left ventricular hypertrophy (LVH) exhibit significantly higher EAT volumes compared to those without LVH. Moreover, hypertensive patients as a whole show greater EAT accumulation than healthy controls. These observations underline EAT's role as both a marker and potential therapeutic target in the progression of hypertensive cardiovascular disease. Furthermore, imaging markers of myocardial fibrosis and strain abnormalities have been shown to mediate the relationship between increased EAT volume and ventricular remodeling, especially in hypertensive patients, suggesting that EAT promotes diffuse fibrosis and functional impairment in the heart muscle.[35]

Consistent findings have also been observed in a study by Eroglu et al., in which 2DTTE showed increased EAT thickness in patients with hypertension compared to normotensives, and was even higher in patients with uncontrolled hypertension.[36]

Type 2 Diabetes Mellitus

Epicardial adipose tissue emerges as a metabolic instigator in the evolution of type 2 diabetes mellitus (T2DM) by promoting insulin resistance, chronic inflammation, and myocardial dysfunction. A 2025 cross-sectional study by Tarabay et al. demonstrated that individuals with T2DM had substantially greater EAT thickness compared to nondiabetic controls using 2DTTE. Elevated EAT thickness was more strongly associated with left ventricular (LV) diastolic dysfunction in diabetic patients than in nondiabetic individuals, even in the absence of overt cardiovascular disease.[37] CT studies show that glucagon-like peptide-1 (GLP-1) receptor agonists such as semaglutide can reduce EAT thickness and modulate proinflammatory adipogenesis induction in T2DM patients.[38,39] These findings underscore EAT's potential as both a marker and mediator of cardiometabolic risk in T2DM patients.

Obesity

General

In obesity, adipocyte hypertrophy and inflammatory cell infiltration increase EAT size, releasing free fatty acids and cytokines that impair insulin signaling, promote oxidative stress, and induce lipotoxicity. Aitken-Buck et al. used 2DTTE to measure EAT thickness in obese and nonobese patients. Increased EAT thickness positively correlated with higher body mass index.[40] Therefore, EAT serves as both a driver and potential biomarker of the obese HFpEF phenotype.

Visceral Fat

Excess visceral adipose tissue (VAT) within the intra-abdominal cavity and organs in obesity is considered an additional factor for atherosclerosis.[41,42] In a study by Iacobellis et al., EAT thickness measured by 2DTTE was compared to traditional measurements of VAT such as waist circumference as well as MRI. They found that EAT thickness correlated well to both waist circumference and MRI-measured abdominal VAT, suggesting that 2DTTE assessment of EAT thickness could be a practical method of assessing VAT.[43] Additionally, the amount of EAT is directly correlated with general body adiposity.[5]

Myocardial Fat

Epicardial adipose tissue adipocytes may infiltrate into the myocardium.[44] Malavazos et al. found a correlation between measured EAT thickness using 2DTTE and myocardial fat volume using MRI spectroscopy. Increased myocardial fat is associated with T2DM.[45]

Kidney Function

The newly recognized entity of "cardiovascular-kidney-metabolic syndrome" reflects the shared impact of metabolic risk factors on the heart and kidney. Nakanishi et al. have noted a negative correlation between glomerular filtration rate (GFR) and EAT volume in patients undergoing CT for evaluation of CAD.[46] In patients with essential hypertension, Ozturk et al. found that those with microalbuminuria had significantly increased EAT thickness on 2DTTE, suggesting its potential as a marker of kidney damage.[47]

Steatotic Liver Disease

In a retrospective longitudinal study with over 11 years of follow-up, excess EAT and steatotic liver disease, both quantified by CT, were independently linked to a higher likelihood of developing albuminuria, an early marker of chronic kidney disease (CKD). The combination of both conditions conferred a markedly higher renal risk, reinforcing the value of EAT and hepatic fat quantification in early CKD risk stratification.[48]

Obstructive Sleep Apnea

Obstructive sleep apnea (OSA) is now widely acknowledged as a key cardiometabolic risk factor due to the recurrent episodes of hypoxia, sympathetic activation, and systemic inflammation that accelerate vascular dysfunction.[49] In this context, EAT has emerged as a potential link between OSA and cardiometabolic disease. A meta-analysis of nine studies comprising 1,178 participants demonstrated that patients with OSA have substantially increased EAT thickness compared to non-OSA controls. This increase in EAT was consistently observed through 2DTTE measurements, and the thickness appeared to rise in tandem with the severity of OSA, from mild to severe cases.[50] These observations underscore a potential connection between EAT accumulation and the advancement of OSA, supporting its role as a useful indicator of disease burden.

Left Ventricular Diastolic Dysfunction

Nakanishi et al. noted that as EAT volume by CT increased, LVDD by 2DTTE decreased in 100 patients they studied.[51] A similar relationship was seen by Takahari et al., who concluded that increased EAT volume resulted in increased LVDD, possibly due to the mechanical effect of EAT on LV because of its proximity.[52] Given the relationship between LVDD and heart failure, EAT may be helpful in risk stratification.

Heart Failure with Preserved Ejection Fraction

Heart Failure with Preserved Ejection Fraction Obesity Phenotype

A 2025 study found that individuals with obesity and diabetes exhibited increased MRI measured EAT volumes, which is connected to adverse changes in heart structure and function, highlighting its crucial influence in driving HFpEF in patients with obesity.[53] These findings indicate the potential of targeting EAT in developing personalized therapies for HFpEF.

Atrial Fibrillation in Heart Failure with Preserved Ejection Fraction

Epicardial adipose tissue contributes to atrial fibrillation (AF) pathogenesis by promoting atrial remodeling and fibrotic infiltration through the release of inflammatory and fibrotic mediators, which can affect the electrophysiological properties of myocytes.[54] In patients with HFpEF, AF often coexists due to shared underlying mechanisms.[55] Notably, emerging evidence highlights EAT-expressed genes are implicated in the overlapping pathophysiology of HFpEF and AF, positioning them as potential early diagnostic biomarkers. A 2025 study evaluated EAT thickness using 2DTTE in HFpEF patients and discovered notably higher values in those with AF, with a cut-off EAT of 7.5 mm.[55] These findings highlight EAT as a critical imaging biomarker in stratifying AF risk in HFpEF patients.

Lone Atrial Fibrillation

In a 2011 study, individuals undergoing radiofrequency ablation for AF were compared to age- and gender-matched controls undergoing CT screening for CAD with no history of AF. Total EAT volume using CT was significantly increased in the group with AF. Total EAT volume appears to predict AF recurrence after catheter ablation. Notably, this study also observed accumulation of EAT in the vicinity of the left atrium was tied to AF recurrence.[56]

Similarly, another study noted a relationship of EAT thickness between the left atrium and esophagus with AF using CT, highlighting the regional significance of EAT.[57]

Left Atrial Function During Exercise

Emerging evidence suggests EAT impairs cardiovascular performance during physical exertion. In a recent study, patients with higher EAT volume on cardiac CT showed significantly reduced LA emptying fraction and lower LA reservoir strain during exercise, indicating compromised atrial compliance under stress. These patients also demonstrated markedly lower peak oxygen consumption (VO_2 peak), highlighting a link between elevated EAT and diminished aerobic capacity.[58] These findings highlight excess EAT as a biomarker for impaired LA function and reduced exercise capacity.

Aortic Stenosis and Transcatheter Aortic Valve Replacement

Epicardial adipose tissue is gaining recognition as a key player in the progression of [aortic stenosis (AS)]. Growing evidence indicates that its accumulation may trigger or intensify inflammation, oxidative stress, and calcification of the aortic valve, ultimately hastening valvular degeneration. Larger EAT thickness on CT is linked to symptom onset in asymptomatic patients with AS.[59] In those treated with transcatheter aortic valve replacement (TAVR) for severe AS, dynamic changes in EAT volume have shown prognostic relevance. In a 2024 cohort of 258 TAVR patients, Lin et al. showed that a ≥15% rise in epicardial fat on follow-up CT (≈12 months) independently predicted more 2-year MACE, highlighting the value of tracking EAT change—not just its baseline volume.[60] Therefore, EAT is not only a contributor in AS progression but also serves as a valuable biomarker for post-TAVR risk stratification. Tracking dynamic shifts in EAT can allow clinicians to identify high-risk patients and tailor follow-up strategies. Furthermore, Akbar et al. identified an association between 2DTTE-measured EAT thickness and severe AS. They found that in both the parasternal long and short axis views, increased EAT thickness was associated with severe AS.[61]

Pulmonary Arterial Hypertension

In a 2025 retrospective cohort study using CT, higher baseline EAT volume and a larger increase over time, as measured on serial CT scans, were both linked to poorer survival outcomes in patients with pulmonary arterial hypertension (PAH).[62] In another study using MRI, EAT volume was associated with right-sided heart failure in PAH patients.[63] This relationship could suggest the role of EAT in categorizing PAH disease severity.

Autoimmune Diseases

Rheumatoid Arthritis

In rheumatoid arthritis (RA), persistent systemic inflammation significantly increases the propensity to develop subclinical atherosclerosis, regardless of the presence of traditional cardiovascular risk factors.[64]

Research demonstrates that patients with RA exhibit notably higher EAT thickness in contrast to healthy individuals using 2DTTE. Additionally, EAT thickness has been positively linked with markers of systemic inflammation such as C-reactive protein, erythrocyte sedimentation rate, and disease activity scores in RA patients. Notably, EAT thickness measured using 2DTTE was markedly decreased in individuals receiving biological RA therapy compared to those on conventional nonbiological treatments.[65] These findings reinforce the role of EAT as a reflection of systemic inflammation in RA and support its utility as a biomarker for inflammatory burden.

Systemic Lupus Erythematosus

In a cross-sectional study by Lipson et al., involving 162 systemic lupus erythematosus (SLE) patients, EAT volume measured via CT when compared to matched controls, SLE patients showed a 31% elevation ($p < 0.001$).Within the SLE group, EAT volume independently correlated with cumulative and current corticosteroid use, HDL cholesterol, and triglycerides, highlighting its potential role as a noninvasive marker of cardiometabolic risk in autoimmune populations.[66]

Human Immunodeficiency Virus Disease

In a study using CT imaging, EAT volume was found to be greater in men with human immunodeficiency virus (HIV) compared to men without. In men with HIV, duration of highly active antiretroviral therapy (HAART) was associated with increased EAT volume.[67] EAT quantification has potential to identify cardiovascular risk in individuals with HIV.

Cardiometabolic Pharmacotherapy

A systematic review and meta-analysis demonstrated that GLP-1 receptor agonists, sodium-glucose cotransporter-2 (SGLT2) inhibitors, and statins have been shown to considerably reduce EAT thickness. Studies included in this analysis used 2DTTE, CT, and MRI to measure EAT. EAT may serve as a modifiable risk factor; however, further research is needed to evaluate the long-term cardiovascular outcomes of pharmacotherapy directed toward EAT reduction.[68]

CONTROVERSIES AND LIMITATIONS

While EAT is increasingly recognized for its association with cardiometabolic risk, several challenges, and unresolved issues remain:

- *Unclear causality:* Although elevated EAT volume is strongly linked to several cardiometabolic risk factors, the precise role it plays, whether as a contributor to disease or a prognostic biomarker, remains debatable, particularly in disorders such as HFpEF and AF.

- *Imaging limitations:* The measurement of EAT differs significantly across imaging modalities. While echocardiography is widely accessible, it is limited by operator variability and provides only thickness, not volume. MRI and CT offer more accurate volumetric assessment but are costlier and less widely available.
- *Lack of standardized cutoffs:* No universally agreed-upon thresholds exist for EAT thickness or volume. Variations due to demographic determinants like age, sex, and ethnicity complicate the establishment of standardization.

CONCLUSION

Epicardial adipose tissue has established links to cardiometabolic diseases, including hypertension, diabetes, obesity, atherosclerosis, atrial fibrillation, HFpEF, and some inflammatory states. Assessment of visceral fat could be another clinically important application of EAT. Its proximity to cardiac structures enables local inflammatory and fibrotic signaling. This chapter summarizes EAT's role as both a marker and contributor to disease, reinforcing its relevance in cardiometabolic risk stratification and future therapeutic strategies in clinical practice.

REFERENCES

1. Iacobellis G, Willens HJ. Echocardiographic epicardial fat: a review of research and clinical applications. J Am Soc Echocardiogr. 2009;22(12):1311-9; quiz 417-8.
2. Iacobellis G, Corradi D, Sharma AM. Epicardial adipose tissue: anatomic, biomolecular and clinical relationships with the heart. Nat Clin Pract Cardiovasc Med. 2005;2(10):536-43.
3. Mazurek T, Zhang L, Zalewski A, Mannion JD, Diehl JT, Arafat H, et al. Human epicardial adipose tissue is a source of inflammatory mediators. Circulation. 2003;108(20):2460-6.
4. Iacobellis G, Barbaro G. The double role of epicardial adipose tissue as pro- and anti-inflammatory organ. Horm Metab Res. 2008; 40(7):442-5.
5. Rabkin SW. Epicardial fat: properties, function and relationship to obesity. Obes Rev. 2007;8(3):253-61.
6. Mahabadi AA, Berg MH, Lehmann N, Kälsch H, Bauer M, Kara K, et al. Association of epicardial fat with cardiovascular risk factors and incident myocardial infarction in the general population: the Heinz Nixdorf Recall Study. J Am Coll Cardiol. 2013;61(13):1388-95.
7. Thanassoulis G, Massaro JM, O'Donnell CJ, Hoffmann U, Levy D, Ellinor PT, et al. Pericardial fat is associated with prevalent atrial fibrillation: the Framingham Heart Study. Circ Arrhythm Electrophysiol. 2010;3(4):345-50.
8. Wong CX, Sun MT, Odutayo A, Emdin CA, Mahajan R, Lau DH, et al. Associations of Epicardial, Abdominal, and Overall Adiposity With Atrial Fibrillation. Circ Arrhythm Electrophysiol. 2016;9(12).
9. Eroğlu S. How do we measure epicardial adipose tissue thickness by transthoracic echocardiography? Anatol J Cardiol. 2015;15(5): 416 9.
10. Konwerski M, Gąsecka A, Opolski G, Grabowski M, Mazurek T. Role of Epicardial Adipose Tissue in Cardiovascular Diseases: A Review. Biology (Basel). 2022;11(3).
11. Rodrigues ÉO, Morais FF, Morais NA, Conci LS, Neto LV, Conci A. A novel approach for the automated segmentation and volume quantification of cardiac fats on computed tomography. Comput Methods Programs Biomed. 2016;123:109-28.
12. Dell'Aversana F, Tuccillo R, Monfregola A, De Angelis L, Ferrandino G, Tedeschi C, et al. Epicardial Adipose Tissue Volume Assessment in the General Population and CAD-RADS 2.0 Score Correlation Using Dual Source Cardiac CT. Diagnostics (Basel). 2025;15(6).
13. Alexopoulos N, McLean DS, Janik M, Arepalli CD, Stillman AE, Raggi P. Epicardial adipose tissue and coronary artery plaque characteristics. Atherosclerosis. 2010;210(1):150-4.
14. Kunita E, Yamamoto H, Kitagawa T, Ohashi N, Oka T, Utsunomiya H, et al. Prognostic value of coronary artery calcium and epicardial adipose tissue assessed by non-contrast cardiac computed tomography. Atherosclerosis. 2014;233(2):447-53.

15. Wang Y, Wang A, Wang L, Tan W, Xu L, Wang J, et al. Automated pericardium segmentation and epicardial adipose tissue quantification from computed tomography images. Biomedical Signal Processing and Control. 2025;100:107167.
16. Lachance C, Horton J. CADTH Horizon Scans. Photon-Counting CT: High Resolution, Less Radiation: Emerging Health Technologies. Ottawa (ON): Canadian Agency for Drugs and Technologies in Health; 2024.
17. Sagris M, Antonopoulos AS, Simantiris S, Oikonomou E, Siasos G, Tsioufis K, et al. Pericoronary fat attenuation index-a new imaging biomarker and its diagnostic and prognostic utility: a systematic review and meta-analysis. Eur Heart J Cardiovasc Imaging. 2022;23(12):e526-36.
18. Mergen V, Ried E, Allmendinger T, Sartoretti T, Higashigaito K, Manka R, et al. Epicardial Adipose Tissue Attenuation and Fat Attenuation Index: Phantom Study and In Vivo Measurements With Photon-Counting Detector CT. AJR Am J Roentgenol. 2022;218(5):822-9.
19. van Timmeren JE, Cester D, Tanadini-Lang S, Alkadhi H, Baessler B. Radiomics in medical imaging-"how-to" guide and critical reflection. Insights Imaging. 2020;11(1):91.
20. Bertaso AG, Bertol D, Duncan BB, Foppa M. Epicardial fat: definition, measurements and systematic review of main outcomes. Arq Bras Cardiol. 2013;101(1):e18-28.
21. Miller RJH, Shanbhag A, Killekar A, Lemley M, Bednarski B, Van Kriekinge SD, et al. AI-derived epicardial fat measurements improve cardiovascular risk prediction from myocardial perfusion imaging. NPJ Digit Med. 2024;7(1):24.
22. Jehn S, Roggel A, Dykun I, Balcer B, Al-Rashid F, Totzeck M, et al. Epicardial adipose tissue and obstructive coronary artery disease in acute chest pain: the EPIC-ACS study. Eur Heart J Open. 2023;3(3):oead041.
23. Zhihong G, Yuqiang Z, Linyi J, Yuling Y, Xu Y, Lei X, et al. Correlation analysis between epicardial adipose tissue and acute coronary syndrome. Sci Rep. 2025;15(1):3015.
24. Con E, Yilmaz A, Suygun H, Mustu M, Karadeniz FO, Kilic O, et al. The relationship between epicardial adipose tissue thickness and coronary artery disease progress. Bratisl Lek Listy. 2023;124(7):545-8.
25. Wang Z, Zhang J, Zhang A, Sun Y, Su M, You H, et al. The role of epicardial and pericoronary adipose tissue radiomics in identifying patients with non-ST-segment elevation myocardial infarction from unstable angina. Heliyon. 2023;9(5):e15738.
26. Kocaman SA, Baysan O, Çetin M, Kayhan Altuner T, Polat Ocaklı E, Durakoğlugil ME, et al. An increase in epicardial adipose tissue is strongly associated with carotid-intima media thickness and atherosclerotic plaque, but LDL only with the plaque. Anatol J Cardiol. 2017;17(1):56-63.
27. Guglielmo M, Lin A, Dey D, Baggiano A, Fusini L, Muscogiuri G, et al. Epicardial fat and coronary artery disease: Role of cardiac imaging. Atherosclerosis. 2021;321:30-8.
28. Braescu L, Gaspar M, Buriman D, Aburel OM, Merce AP, Bratosin F, et al. The Role and Implications of Epicardial Fat in Coronary Atherosclerotic Disease. J Clin Med. 2022;11(16).
29. Britton KA, Fox CS. Perivascular adipose tissue and vascular disease. Clin Lipidol. 2011;6(1):79-91.
30. Yu W, Zhang F, Liu B, Wang J, Shao X, Yang MF, et al. Incremental value of epicardial fat volume to coronary artery calcium score and traditional risk factors for predicting myocardial ischemia in patients with suspected coronary artery disease. J Nucl Cardiol. 2022;29(4):1583-92.
31. Mahmoud I, Dykun I, Kärner L, Hendricks S, Totzeck M, Al-Rashid F, et al. Epicardial adipose tissue differentiates in patients with and without coronary microvascular dysfunction. Int J Obes (Lond). 2021;45(9):2058-63.
32. Rosa MI, Grande AJ, Lima LD, Dondossola ER, Uggioni MLR, Hernandez AV, et al. Association Between Epicardial Adipose Tissue and Stroke. Front Cardiovasc Med. 2021;8:658445.
33. Panda S, Vimala LR, Livingstone R, Pearlin B, Irodi A, Joseph E, et al. Can epicardial and pericardial adipose tissue volume predict the presence and severity of coronary artery disease? Pol J Radiol. 2022;87:e348-53.
34. Roever L, Santos Resende E, LemosDebs Diniz A, Penha-Silva N, Lucas O'Connell J, Rodrigues de Souza F, et al. Epicardial adipose tissue and peripheral artery disease: protocol for systematic review and meta-analysis. J Integrat Cardiol. 2018;4(4).

35. Zhu R, Wang W, Gao Y, Liu J, Li B, Shan R, et al. Epicardial Adipose Tissue and Left Ventricular Hypertrophy in Hypertensive Patients With Preserved Ejection Fraction: A Multicenter Retrospective Cohort Study. J Clin Hypertens (Greenwich). 2025;27(1):e70003.
36. Eroğlu S, Sade LE, Yıldırır A, Demir O, Müderrisoğlu H. Association of epicardial adipose tissue thickness by echocardiography and hypertension. Turk Kardiyol Dern Ars. 2013;41(2):115-22.
37. Singh A, Bruemmer D. Cardiometabolic Risk. JACC: Advances. 2024;3(4):100867.
38. Manubolu VS, Lakshmanan S, Kinninger A, Ahmad K, Susarla S, Seok HJ, et al. Effect of Semaglutide on Epicardial Adipose Tissue in Type 2 Diabetes: Insights From the STOP (Semaglutide Treatment effect On coronary atherosclerosis Progression) Randomized Trial. J Am Coll Cardiol. 2024;84(9):865-7.
39. Basdas R, Martínez-Cereijo JM, Fernández ÁL, Reija L, Cabaleiro A, Bravo SB, et al. Semaglutide Modulates Proinflammatory Epicardial Adipogenesis With Paracrine Effects on hiPSC-Atrial Cardiomyocytes. JACC Basic Transl Sci. 2025:101277.
40. Aitken-Buck HM, Moharram M, Babakr AA, Reijers R, Van Hout I, Fomison-Nurse IC, et al. Relationship between epicardial adipose tissue thickness and epicardial adipocyte size with increasing body mass index. Adipocyte. 2019;8(1):412-20.
41. Ibrahim MM. Subcutaneous and visceral adipose tissue: structural and functional differences. Obes Rev. 2010;11(1):11-8.
42. Tchernof A, Després JP. Pathophysiology of human visceral obesity: an update. Physiol Rev. 2013;93(1):359-404.
43. Iacobellis G, Assael F, Ribaudo MC, Zappaterreno A, Alessi G, Di Mario U, et al. Epicardial fat from echocardiography: a new method for visceral adipose tissue prediction. Obes Res. 2003;11(2):304-10.
44. Iacobellis G, Bianco AC. Epicardial adipose tissue: emerging physiological, pathophysiological and clinical features. Trends Endocrinol Metab. 2011;22(11):450-7.
45. McGavock JM, Lingvay I, Zib I, Tillery T, Salas N, Unger R, et al. Cardiac steatosis in diabetes mellitus: a 1H-magnetic resonance spectroscopy study. Circulation. 2007;116(10):1170-5.
46. Nakanishi K, Fukuda S, Tanaka A, Otsuka K, Taguchi H, Yoshikawa J, et al. Epicardial Adipose Tissue Accumulation Is Associated With Renal Dysfunction and Coronary Plaque Morphology on Multidetector Computed Tomography. Circ J. 2016;80(1):196-201.
47. Ozturk MT, Ebinç FA, Okyay GU, Kutlugün AA. Epicardial Adiposity is Associated with Microalbuminuria in Patients with Essential Hypertension. Acta Cardiol Sin. 2017;33(1):74-80.
48. Perdomo CM, Martin-Calvo N, Ezponda A, Mendoza FJ, Bastarrika G, Garcia-Fernandez N, et al. Epicardial and liver fat implications in albuminuria: a retrospective study. Cardiovasc Diabetol. 2024;23(1):308.
49. Shamsuzzaman AS, Gersh BJ, Somers VK. Obstructive sleep apnea: implications for cardiac and vascular disease. JAMA. 2003;290(14):1906-14.
50. Song G, Sun F, Wu D, Bi W. Association of epicardial adipose tissues with obstructive sleep apnea and its severity: A meta-analysis study. Nutr Metab Cardiovasc Dis. 2020;30(7):1115-20.
51. Nakanishi K, Fukuda S, Tanaka A, Otsuka K, Taguchi H, Shimada K. Relationships Between Periventricular Epicardial Adipose Tissue Accumulation, Coronary Microcirculation, and Left Ventricular Diastolic Dysfunction. Can J Cardiol. 2017;33(11):1489-97.
52. Takahari K, Utsunomiya H, Itakura K, Yamamoto H, Nakano Y. Impact of the distribution of epicardial and visceral adipose tissue on left ventricular diastolic function. Heart Vessels. 2022;37(2):250-61.
53. Menghoum N, Badii MC, Leroy M, Parra M, Roy C, Lejeune S, et al. Exploring the impact of metabolic comorbidities on epicardial adipose tissue in heart failure with preserved ejection fraction. Cardiovasc Diabetol. 2025;24(1):134.
54. Parisi V, Conte M, Petraglia L, Grieco FV, Bruzzese D, Caruso A, et al. Echocardiographic Epicardial Adipose Tissue Thickness for Risk Stratification of Patients With Heart Failure. Front Physiol. 2020;11:43.

55. Yucel O. Relationship Between Epicardial Adipose Tissue and Atrial Fibrillation in Heart Failure With Preserved Ejection Fraction. Cureus. 2025;17(3):e80827.
56. Tsao HM, Hu WC, Wu MH, Tai CT, Lin YJ, Chang SL, et al. Quantitative analysis of quantity and distribution of epicardial adipose tissue surrounding the left atrium in patients with atrial fibrillation and effect of recurrence after ablation. Am J Cardiol. 2011;107(10):1498-503.
57. Batal O, Schoenhagen P, Shao M, Ayyad AE, Van Wagoner DR, Halliburton SS, et al. Left atrial epicardial adiposity and atrial fibrillation. Circ Arrhythm Electrophysiol. 2010;3(3):230-6.
58. Dziano J, Howie J, Ariyaratnam J, Middeldorp M, Emami M, Mishimi R, et al. Epicardial Adipose Tissue and Left Atrial Function During Exercise. Heart Lung Circulation. 2024;33:S149.
59. Davin L, Nchimi A, Ilardi F, Dulgheru R, Marchetta S, Gach O, et al. Epicardial Adipose Tissue and Myocardial Fibrosis in Aortic Stenosis Relationship With Symptoms and Outcomes: A Study Using Cardiac Magnetic Resonance Imaging. JACC Cardiovasc Imaging. 2019;12(1):213-4.
60. Lin S, Zhang Y, Wang S, Ding X, Wu J, Wang X, et al. Prognostic utility of dynamic changes in epicardial adipose tissue in patients undergoing transcatheter aortic valve replacement. Int J Cardiol. 2025;419:132697.
61. Akbar S, Bhinder J, Zagelbaum N, Zaid S, Ahmad H, Goldberg J, et al. Epicardial Adipose Tissue Predicts The Presence Of Aortic Valve Stenosis. JACC. 2020;75(11_Supplement_1):2155.
62. McCarthy BE, Feng R, Torigian DA, Tong Y, Fritz JS, Minhas JK, et al. Epicardial Adipose Tissue as an Independent Risk Factor for Mortality in Pulmonary Arterial Hypertension. Chest. 2025;167(5):1481-92.
63. Chen Y, Li J, Li F, Chen Z, Chen Z, Luo J, et al. Impact of Epicardial Adipose Tissue on Right Cardiac Function and Prognosis in Pulmonary Arterial Hypertension. Chest. 2024;165(5):1211-23.
64. Keleşoğlu Dinçer AB, Şahan HF. Increased epicardial adipose tissue thickness as a sign of subclinical atherosclerosis in patients with rheumatoid arthritis and ıts relationship with disease activity ındices. Intern Emerg Med. 2024;19(4):1015-24.
65. Lima-Martínez MM, Campo E, Salazar J, Paoli M, Maldonado I, Acosta C, et al. Epicardial fat thickness as cardiovascular risk factor and therapeutic target in patients with rheumatoid arthritis treated with biological and nonbiological therapies. Arthritis. 2014;2014:782850.
66. Lipson A, Alexopoulos N, Hartlage GR, Arepalli C, Oeser A, Bian A, et al. Epicardial adipose tissue is increased in patients with systemic lupus erythematosus. Atherosclerosis. 2012;223(2):389-93.
67. Brener M, Ketlogetswe K, Budoff M, Jacobson LP, Li X, Rezaeian P, et al. Epicardial fat is associated with duration of antiretroviral therapy and coronary atherosclerosis. Aids. 2014;28(11):1635-44.
68. Myasoedova VA, Parisi V, Moschetta D, Valerio V, Conte M, Massaiu I, et al. Efficacy of cardiometabolic drugs in reduction of epicardial adipose tissue: a systematic review and meta-analysis. Cardiovasc Diabetol. 2023;22(1):23.

CHAPTER 6

Anti-obesity Medications: Flashback and Vision Ahead

PC Manoria

ABSTRACT

Obesity is a chronic disease associated with significant metabolic and cardiovascular complications. Management includes lifestyle modification and pharmacotherapy. Several earlier anti-obesity drugs were withdrawn due to safety concerns. Currently approved agents such as orlistat, phentermine–topiramate, naltrexone–bupropion, liraglutide, semaglutide, and tirzepatide provide varying degrees of weight reduction and cardiometabolic benefits. Newer incretin-based therapies have shown substantial and sustained weight loss, and emerging agents targeting multiple metabolic pathways may further improve future obesity management.

Keywords: Obesity, anti-obesity drugs, semaglutide, tirzepatide, GLP-1 receptor agonists, pharmacotherapy

INTRODUCTION

Obesity, defined by excessive or abnormal fat accumulation, is a major risk factor for diabetes, cardiovascular disease, hypertension, and dyslipidemia. It is the second leading preventable cause of death worldwide after smoking and requires lifelong, multimodal management strategies.[1] Although recognized as a chronic disease by the World Health Organization in 1948, obesity has only recently been formally classified under the ICD-11 (code 5B81).[2] In 2021, approximately 2.11 billion adults aged ≥25 years—45.1% of the global adult population—were overweight or obese, with the highest absolute numbers reported in China, India, and the United States. Projections estimate that by 2050, 3.8 billion adults will be affected, including nearly 2 billion living with obesity.[3] Prevalence is higher in high-income countries and among women,[3,4] and the global economic burden is expected to reach USD 4.32 trillion annually by 2035.[5] Pharmacologic management of obesity has evolved from short-term appetite suppression to therapies targeting hormonal and metabolic pathways involved in energy homeostasis. This review summarizes current and emerging pharmacotherapies for obesity, focusing on mechanisms of action and their potential to improve long-term clinical outcomes.

OBESITY MANAGEMENT

Non-pharmacological Management

Lifestyle modification remains the foundation of obesity management and includes dietary intervention, physical activity, and behavioral therapy, individualized to patient characteristics and preferences.[6] Nutritional therapy focuses on personalized energy-deficit diets informed by clinical status and cultural context. Current guidelines from the American Diabetes Association and the Korean Society for the Study of Obesity recommend a daily caloric reduction of 500–750 kcal, aiming for 5–10% weight loss over 6 months. Structured low-calorie diets (1200–1800 kcal/day), using various macronutrient distributions such as low-carbohydrate, low-fat, or Mediterranean patterns, are effective provided a caloric deficit is maintained.

Meal replacements and culturally adapted dietary plans are recommended to enhance adherence.[7,8]

Physical activity plays a critical role in weight loss and long-term weight maintenance. Guidelines recommend at least 150 minutes per week of moderate-intensity aerobic exercise combined with 2–3 resistance training sessions.[8] Combined exercise modalities are more effective than either alone, and moderate-intensity programs are associated with better adherence, particularly among sedentary individuals. Although exercise timing may influence metabolic outcomes, evidence remains limited.[9]

Behavioral therapy strengthens adherence to lifestyle interventions. Structured programs comprising at least 14 sessions over 6 months—incorporating goal-setting, cognitive restructuring, and self-monitoring—are endorsed by the United States Preventive Services Task Force and the ADA.[6,9] Continued follow-up beyond 1 year, delivered through in-person or digital platforms, reduces weight regain. Emerging adjunctive approaches, such as neuromodulation, are under investigation. Overall, multidisciplinary, patient-centered care with structured follow-up is essential for sustainable weight management.

Pharmacological Management: Past

Several anti-obesity medications have been withdrawn following post-marketing safety concerns, predominantly related to cardiovascular and neuropsychiatric toxicity. Most of these agents were centrally acting drugs targeting monoaminergic pathways.

Fenfluramine and dexfenfluramine, widely used appetite suppressants often prescribed with phentermine ("fen-phen"), were withdrawn in 1997 after associations with valvular heart disease (VHD) and primary pulmonary hypertension (PPH). Echocardiographic abnormalities were reported in 24% of fen-phen users compared with none in controls, with histopathology implicating 5-HT_2B receptor-mediated valvular fibrosis.[10,11] The International Primary Pulmonary Hypertension Study demonstrated a 23-fold increased risk of PPH with use exceeding three months.[12]

Sibutramine, a serotonin-norepinephrine reuptake inhibitor, was withdrawn in 2010 following the SCOUT trial (n = 10,744), which showed a 16% increase in major adverse cardiovascular events despite modest weight loss. This outcome prompted global withdrawal and established cardiovascular outcome trials as a regulatory requirement for obesity drugs.[13,14]

Rimonabant, a cannabinoid-1 receptor inverse agonist, was suspended due to psychiatric adverse effects. In the RIO and STRADIVARIUS trials, treatment was associated with higher discontinuation rates due to depression (OR 2.5, $p = 0.01$) and anxiety (OR 3.03, $p = 0.03$), with nearly half of adverse event-related withdrawals attributed to psychiatric causes despite exclusion of patients with pre-existing mental illness.[15-17] The European Medicines Agency suspended its approval in 2008, citing an unfavorable risk-benefit profile. Additional agents were withdrawn after post-marketing surveillance confirmed unacceptable adverse effects **(Table 1)**.

Pharmacological Management: Present

Orlistat is a gastrointestinal lipase inhibitor that reduces dietary fat absorption by approximately 30% without central appetite effects. It is approved for adults with BMI ≥30 kg/m^2 or ≥27 kg/m^2 with comorbidities, and for adolescents. In long-term trials, orlistat 120 mg three times daily produced greater weight loss and significantly reduced weight regain compared with placebo, with concurrent improvements in lipid and glycemic parameters.[18,19] Efficacy has been demonstrated across populations, including Indian cohorts and insulin-treated patients with type 2 diabetes, where orlistat achieved greater reductions in

TABLE 1: List of banned anti-obesity drugs.

Drug name	*FDA approval year*	*Withdrawal year*	*Reason for withdrawal*
Fenfluramine	1973	1997	Cardiac valvulopathy and pulmonary hypertension (5-HT2B receptor activation)
Dexfenfluramine	1996	1997	Valvular heart disease and pulmonary arterial hypertension
Sibutramine	1997	2010	Increased risk of nonfatal myocardial infarction and stroke (SCOUT trial)
Rimonabant	2006 (EMA)	2008	Severe psychiatric adverse events including depression and suicidal ideation
Phenylpropanolamine (PPA)	1950s (OTC use)	2000	Increased risk of hemorrhagic stroke
Aminorex	1965	1972	Pulmonary arterial hypertension epidemic in Europe
Benfluorex	1976	2009	Valvular heart disease and heart failure
Mazindol	1973	Varies by country (2000s)	Abuse potential, elevated BP, and dependency risk
Phendimetrazine	1959	Varies by country	Abuse potential and cardiovascular effects
Methamphetamine derivatives	1950	1970	Addiction, CNS toxicity, and cardiovascular risk

body weight, HbA1c, and atherogenic lipids than placebo.[20,21] Adverse effects are predominantly gastrointestinal (e.g., oily stools, fecal urgency) and typically diminish with dietary fat restriction. Orlistat is contraindicated in pregnancy, chronic malabsorption, and cholestasis, and may impair absorption of fat-soluble vitamins and certain medications. Rare cases of hepatotoxicity and oxalate nephropathy have been reported.[22] Despite modest efficacy, orlistat remains a useful oral option for patients unsuitable for centrally acting or injectable anti-obesity therapies.

Setmelanotide is a first-in-class melanocortin-4 receptor (MC4R) agonist and the only FDA-approved therapy targeting defects in the hypothalamic leptin-melanocortin pathway causing monogenic obesity. It is approved for patients ≥2 years of age with obesity due to POMC, PCSK1, LEPR deficiencies, or Bardet-Biedl syndrome (BBS), with age- and weight-adjusted dosing.[23] In the VENTURE trial involving children aged 2–5 years (n = 12), 83% achieved a ≥0.2 reduction in BMI Z-score at 52 weeks, with a mean BMI reduction of 18% (–26% in POMC/LEPR and –10% in BBS); 91% reported reduced hunger.[24] In a separate phase 3 trial in BBS (NCT03746522; n = 38), 32.3% achieved ≥10% weight loss, 62.5% showed improved hunger scores, and the mean weight change was –2.4% at 14 weeks.[25] Common adverse effects include injection-site reactions, hyperpigmentation (via MC1R activation), nausea, and headache, with rare psychiatric events such as depression or suicidal ideation. Setmelanotide is contraindicated in patients with hypersensitivity to its components and is not approved for neonates due to benzyl alcohol-associated toxicity. Dermatologic and psychiatric monitoring is recommended during therapy.[23]

Phentermine-topiramate is a fixed-dose combination that suppresses appetite and enhances satiety. It is FDA-approved for adults (BMI ≥30 or ≥27 kg/m^2 with comorbidities) and adolescents ≥12 years, with titration up to 15/92 mg daily based on response.[26] In the 56-week CONQUER trial ($n = 2,487$), mean weight loss was 7.8% (7.5/46 mg) and 9.8% (15/92 mg) versus 1.4 kg with placebo, with 48% achieving ≥10% weight loss on the highest dose.[27] Sustained weight loss (–10.5%) and reduced progression to type 2 diabetes were confirmed in the SEQUEL extension.[28] In EQUIP, severely obese adults lost 10.9% with 15/92 mg versus 1.6% with placebo, alongside cardiometabolic improvements.[29] A BP sub-study showed a 3.3 mm Hg reduction in 24-hour systolic BP versus placebo and 4.7 mm Hg versus phentermine alone.[30] In adolescents, BMI reductions reached –10.44% (15/92 mg) with favorable lipid changes,[31] and the EQUATE trial reported 9.2% weight loss at 28 weeks.[32] Common adverse effects include paresthesia, dry mouth, insomnia, and cognitive symptoms. The drug carries boxed warnings for teratogenicity and suicidality and is contraindicated in pregnancy, glaucoma, hyperthyroidism, unstable cardiovascular disease, and recent MAOI use. Heart rate, mood, and vision should be monitored during treatment.[26]

Naltrexone-bupropion is a centrally acting fixed-dose combination that reduces appetite and food cravings via hypothalamic melanocortin pathway modulation. It is FDA-approved for adults with BMI ≥30 or ≥27 kg/m^2 with comorbidities, with titration to 32/360 mg daily over 4 weeks.[33] In COR-I and COR-II, mean weight loss was ~6.1–6.4% versus ~1.2–1.3% with placebo, with ~50% achieving ≥5% and ~25% achieving ≥10% weight loss, alongside improved hunger scores.[34,35] COR-BMOD demonstrated enhanced efficacy with behavioral therapy (9.3% vs. 5.1% weight loss), confirming additive benefit.[36] In a small BED pilot study, 45.5% achieved ≥3% weight loss with reduced binge episodes.[37] A meta-analysis of 25 trials ($n = 22,165$) confirmed significant reductions in weight (–3.67 kg) and waist circumference (–2.98 cm), with greater efficacy than bupropion alone and sustained benefit beyond 26 weeks.[38] Common adverse effects include nausea, headache, insomnia, and gastrointestinal symptoms; blood pressure and heart rate may increase, requiring monitoring. It is contraindicated in seizure disorders, uncontrolled hypertension, bulimia, opioid use, and recent MAOI exposure, and carries a boxed warning for suicidality, particularly in young adults; treatment should be discontinued if serious psychiatric or hypertensive events occur.[33]

Liraglutide is a long-acting GLP-1 receptor agonist that promotes weight loss by reducing appetite and delaying gastric emptying. Approved as Saxenda for adults (BMI ≥30 or ≥27 kg/m^2 with comorbidities) and adolescents ≥12 years (≥60 kg), it is administered once daily and titrated to 3.0 mg subcutaneously.[39] In the 56-week SCALE Obesity and Prediabetes trial ($n = 3,731$), liraglutide produced 8.0% weight loss versus 2.6% with placebo, with 63.2% achieving ≥5% and 33.1% ≥10% weight loss.[40] In adolescents, liraglutide reduced BMI by 4.6% and body weight by 4.5 kg, with significantly higher ≥5% and ≥10% BMI reductions versus placebo.[41,42] A meta-analysis ($n = 8,249$) confirmed reductions in weight, BMI, HbA1c, and blood pressure without increased hypoglycemia.[43] Common adverse effects include nausea, vomiting, and gastrointestinal symptoms, with rarer risks of tachycardia, gallbladder disease, pancreatitis, and suicidal ideation. Liraglutide carries a boxed warning for thyroid C-cell tumors and is contraindicated in medullary thyroid carcinoma, MEN 2, pregnancy, prior pancreatitis, and severe GI disease.[39] Despite daily dosing, it remains a valuable option for patients requiring daily GLP-1 therapy or unable to tolerate weekly agents.

Semaglutide is a long-acting GLP-1 receptor agonist approved as Wegovy for chronic weight management and, as of March 2024, for reducing major adverse cardiovascular events (MACE) in adults with overweight or obesity and established cardiovascular disease (CVD); it is also approved for pediatric obesity (≥12 years).[44] Administered once weekly, dosing is titrated from 0.25 to 2.4 mg to improve gastrointestinal tolerability. In STEP-1, semaglutide 2.4 mg produced 14.9% weight loss at 68 weeks versus 2.4% with placebo, with 69.1% achieving ≥10% and 32% ≥20% weight loss, alongside improvements in HbA1c, waist circumference, and blood pressure[45] **(Table 2)**. STEP-2 in type 2 diabetes showed 9.6% weight loss versus 3.4% with placebo and significant glycemic and BP reductions[46] **(Table 3)**. In the STEP-HFpEF and STEP-HFpEF DM trials, semaglutide achieved a weight reduction of

TABLE 2: STEP-1 trial outcomes.

	Semaglutide	*Placebo*	*p value*
Sample: 1961	1306	655	–
Primary outcome: • Percent body-weight change from baseline to week 68	−14.9% patients	−2.4% patients	*p* <0.001
• Reduction in body weight of 5% or more from baseline to week 68	86.4%	31.5%	*p* <0.001
Secondary endpoint: 1. Reduction in body weight of 10% or more by week 68	69.1%	12%	*p* <0.001
2. Reduction in body weight of 15% or more by week 68	50.5%	4.9%	*p* <0.001
3. Waist circumference (cm) by week 68	−13.54	−4.13	*p* <0.001
Systolic blood pressure (mm Hg) by week 68	−6.16	−1.06	*p* <0.001
Participants with body-weight reduction ≥20% at week 68	32%	1.7%	*p* <0.001
Change in glycated hemoglobin level from baseline to week 68	−0.52%	−0.17%	NA
Serious adverse events	9.8% (128)	6.4% (42)	NA
Adverse effect leading to discontinuation of drug	7% (92)	3.1% (20)	NA

TABLE 3: STEP-2 trial outcomes.

	Semaglutide 2.4 mg	*Semaglutide 1 mg*	*Placebo*	*p value*
Sample: 1210	404	403	403	–
Primary outcome: • Percent body-weight change from baseline to week 68	−9.64%	−6.99%	−3.42%	*p* <0.0001
• Reduction in body weight of 5% or more from baseline to week 68	68.8% (267)	57.1% (217)	28.5% (107)	*p* <0.0001
Secondary endpoint: 1. Reduction in body weight of 10% or more by week 68	45.6% (177)	28.7% (109)	8.2% (310)	*p* <0.0001
2. Reduction in body weight of 15% or more by week 68	25.8% (100)	13.7% (52)	3.2% (12)	*p* <0.0001
3. Waist circumference (cm) by week 68	−9.4	−6.7	−4.5	*p* <0.0001
Systolic blood pressure (mm Hg) by week 68	−3.9	−2.9	−0.5	*p* <0.0016
Change in HbA1C level from baseline to week 68	−1.6%	−1.5%	−0.4%	*p* <0.0001
Serious adverse events	9.9% (40)	7.7% (31)	9.2% (37)	NA
Adverse effect leading to discontinuation of drug	6.2% (25)	5% (20)	3.5% (14)	NA

TABLE 4: STEP HFpEF trial outcomes.

	Semaglutide	*Placebo*	*p value*
Sample: 529	263	269	–
Primary outcome:			
• Percentage change in body weight from baseline to week 52	−13.3%	−2.6	$p < 0.001$
• Change in KCCQ-CSS from baseline to week 52	16.6	8.7	$p < 0.001$
Secondary endpoint:			
1. Change from baseline to week 52 in 6-minute walk distance (m)	21.5	1.2	$p < 0.001$
2. Change from baseline to week 52 in CRP level (%)	−43.5	−7.3	$p < 0.001$
3. Waist circumference (cm) by week 52	−11.7	−2.7	NA
Change from systolic blood pressure (mm Hg) by week 52	−4.9	−2.0	NA
Reduction in body weight of 10% or more by week 52 (% of participants)	65.9%	9.5%	NA
Reduction in body weight of 15% or more by week 52 (% of participants)	43.9%	2.1%	NA
Participants with body-weight reduction ≥20% at week 52 (% of participants)	23.6%	0.4%	NA
Percentage reduction from baseline to week 52 in NT-proBNP level	−20.9	−5.3	NA
Adjudicated heart failure event (hospitalization or urgent visit for heart failure), time-to-event analysis—no. of events	1	12	
Serious adverse events	13.3% (35)	26.7% (71)	$p < 0.001$
Serious adverse effect leading to discontinuation of drug	2.3% (6)	2.3% (6)	NA

13.3% and 9.8%, respectively. It also significantly improved KCCQ-CSS, 6-minute walk distance, and CRP levels, with benefits that were consistent in participants with and without diabetes[47,48] **(Tables 4 and 5)**. The SELECT trial (n = 17,604) **(Table 6)** demonstrated a 20% reduction in cardiovascular death, MI, or stroke in adults with obesity and CVD but without diabetes, along with fewer heart-failure events and lower all-cause mortality, though discontinuation due to adverse effects was higher than placebo.[49] The most common adverse effects are gastrointestinal and typically transient. Serious risks include a boxed warning for thyroid C-cell tumors, pancreatitis, gallbladder disease, acute kidney injury, diabetic retinopathy, mild heart-rate increases, and rare mood changes or suicidal ideation.[44,49] Overall, semaglutide's robust weight-loss and cardiovascular benefits make it a leading therapy for obesity, particularly in patients with cardiovascular disease or diabetes.

Tirzepatide is a dual GIP/GLP-1 receptor agonist that reduces appetite, delays gastric emptying, and improves metabolic control via central and peripheral mechanisms. Approved as Zepbound for chronic weight management in adults with obesity or overweight with comorbidities, it also received FDA approval in 2024 for obesity-related obstructive sleep apnea (OSA). Weekly dosing starts at 2.5 mg and is titrated to 5, 10, or 15 mg (10–15 mg used for OSA).[50] In SURMOUNT-1, tirzepatide achieved 15.0–20.9% weight loss at 72 weeks versus 3.1% with placebo, with >90% achieving ≥5% and >56% ≥20% weight loss, alongside significant reductions in waist circumference and blood pressure[51] **(Table 7)**. SURMOUNT-2 showed similar efficacy in type 2 diabetes (12.8–14.7% weight loss, HbA1c ↓ >2%).[52] SURMOUNT-3 demonstrated 18.4% weight loss following prior lifestyle intervention in non-diabetic adults[53] **(Table 8)**. In the SUMMIT trial **(Table 9)**, tirzepatide reduced CV death or heart-failure

TABLE 5: STEP HFpEF DM trial outcomes.

	Semaglutide	*Placebo*	*p value*
Sample: 616	310	306	
Primary outcome: • Percentage change in body weight from baseline to week 52 • Change in KCCQ-CSS from baseline to week 52	–9.8 13.7	–3.4 6.4	*p* <0.001 *p* <0.001
Secondary endpoint: 1. Change from baseline to week 52 in 6-minute walk distance (m)	12.7	–1.6	*p* = 0.008
2. Change from baseline to week 52 in CRP level (%)	–42.0	–12.8	*p* <0.001
3. Waist circumference (cm) by week 52	-9.0	-2.6	NA
Change from systolic blood pressure (mm Hg) by week 52	-4.2	–1.7	NA
Reduction in body weight of 10% or more by week 52 (% of participants)	51.4%	10.4%	NA
Reduction in body weight of 15% or more by week 52 (% of participants)	22.4%	4.0%	NA
Participants with body-weight reduction ≥20% at week 52 (% of participants)	7.3%	1.8%	NA
Percentage reduction from baseline to week 52 in NT-proBNP level (%)	–23.2%	–4.6%	NA
Adjudicated heart failure event (hospitalization or urgent visit for heart failure), time-to-event analysis—no. of events (% of participants)	7 events (2.3%)	18 events (5.9%)	NA
Serious adverse events	17.7% (55)	28.8% (88)	*p* = 0.002
Serious adverse effect leading to discontinuation of drug	1.9% (6)	3.6% (11)	NA

TABLE 6: SELECT trial outcomes.

	Semaglutide	*Placebo*	*p value*
Sample: 17,604	8,803	8,801	
Primary outcome: Death from cardiovascular causes, nonfatal myocardial infarction, or nonfatal stroke	6.5% (569)	8% (701)	*p* <0.001
Secondary endpoint: 1. Death from cardiovascular causes	2.5% (223)	3% (262)	*p* = 0.07
2. Heart failure composite end point	3.4% (300)	4.1% (361)	NA
3. Death from any cause	4.3% (375)	5.2% (458)	NA
Hospitalization or urgent medical visit for heart failure	1.1% (97)	1.4% (122)	NA
Coronary revascularization	5.4% (473)	6.9% (608)	NA
Nephropathy composite end point	155 (1.8)	2.2% (198)	NA
Mean change in body weight over the 104 weeks	-9.39%	-0.08%	NA
Serious adverse events	33.4% (2,941)	36.4% (3,204)	*p* <0.001
Adverse effect leading to discontinuation of drug	16.6% (1,461)	8.2% (718)	*p* <0.001

TABLE 7: SURMOUNT-1 trial outcomes.

	Tirzepatide 5 mg	*Tirzepatide 10 mg*	*Tirzepatide 15 mg*	*Placebo*	*p value*
Sample: 2,539	630	636	630	643	
Primary outcome:					
1. Percentage change in body weight from baseline to week 72	−15.0 %	−19.5%	−20.9%	−3.1%	NA
2. Participants achieving ≥5% body weight reduction (%)	85.1%	88.9%	90.9%	34.5%	NA
3. Waist circumference (cm) by week 72	−14.0	−17.7	−18.5	−4.0	NA
Change from systolic blood pressure (mm Hg) by week 72	Pooled analysis of all tirzepatide doses = −7.2			−1.0	NA
Reduction in body weight of 10% or more by week 72 (% of participants)	68.5%	78.1%	83.5%	18.8%	NA
Reduction in body weight of 15% or more by week 72 (% of participants)	48.0%	66.6%	70.6%	8.8%	NA
Participants with body-weight reduction ≥20% at week 72 (% of participants)	30.0%	50.1%	56.7%	3.1%	NA
Participants with body-weight reduction ≥25% at week 72 (% of participants)	15.3%	32.3%	36.2%	1.5%	NA
Serious adverse events	6.3% (40)	6.9% (44)	5.1% (32)	6.8% (44)	NA
Adverse effect leading to discontinuation of drug	4.3% (27)	7.1% (45)	6.2% (39)	2.6% (17)	NA

TABLE 8: SURMOUNT-3 trial outcomes.

	Tirzepatide 15 mg	*Placebo*	*p value*
Sample: 579	287	292	
Primary outcome:			
• Percentage change in body weight from baseline to week 72	−18.4%	2.5%	$p<0.001$
• Participants achieving ≥5% body weight reduction (%)	87.5%	16.5%	$p<0.001$
Secondary endpoint:			
1. Change from baseline to week 72 in BMI (kg/m^2)	−7.7	1.2	$p = 0.008$
2. Change from baseline to week 72 in body weight (kg)	−21.5 kg	3.5 kg	$p<0.001$
3. Waist circumference (cm) by week 72	−14.6	0.2	$p<0.001$
Change from systolic blood pressure (mm Hg) by week 72	−5.1	4.1	NA
Reduction in body weight of 10% or more by week 72 (% of participants)	76.7%	8.9%	$p<0.001$
Reduction in body weight of 15% or more by week 72 (% of participants)	65.4%	4.2%	$p<0.001$
Participants with body-weight reduction ≥20% at week 72 (% of participants)	44.7%	2.2%	$p<0.001$
Participants with body-weight reduction ≥25% at week 72 (% of participants)	28.7%	1.2%	NA
Change in HbA1c, %	−0.5		NA
Serious adverse events	5.9% (17)	4.8% (14)	NA
Adverse effect leading to discontinuation of drug	10.5% (30)	2.1% (6)	NA

TABLE 9: SUMMIT trial outcomes.

	Tirzepatide 15 mg	*Placebo*	*p value*
Sample: 731	364	367	
Primary outcome:			
• Adjudicated death from cardiovascular causes or a worsening heart-failure event resulting in hospitalization, intravenous drugs in an urgent care setting, or intensification of oral diuretic therapy—no. (%)	9.9% (36)	15.3% (56)	$p = 0.026$
• Adjudicated death from cardiovascular causes—no. (%)	2.2% (8)	1.4% (5)	NA
• Adjudicated death from undetermined cause—no. (%)	0.5% (2)	0	NA
• Adjudicated worsening heart-failure event resulting in hospitalization, intravenous drugs in an urgent care setting, or intensification of oral diuretic therapy—no. (%)	8.0% (29)	14.2% (52)	NA
• Adjudicated worsening heart-failure event resulting in hospitalization—no. (%)	3.3% (12)	7.1% (26)	NA
• Adjudicated worsening heart-failure event resulting in intravenous diuretic therapy in an urgent care setting—no. (%)	1.4% (5)	3.3% (12)	NA
• Adjudicated worsening heart-failure event resulting in intensification of oral diuretic therapy in an outpatient setting—no. (%)	4.7% (17)	5.7% (21)	NA
• Death from any cause—no. (%)	5.2% (19)	4.1% (15)	NA
Change at 52 weeks in KCCQ-CSS	19.5 ± 1.2	12.7 ± 1.3	$p < 0.001$
Secondary endpoint:			
1. Change at 52 weeks in 6-minute walk distance (m)	26.0 ± 3.8	10.1 ± 3.9	$p < 0.001$
2. Percent change at 52 weeks in body weight (%)	−13.9 ± 0.4	−2.2 ± 0.5	$p < 0.001$
3. Percent change at 52 weeks in high-sensitivity C-reactive protein level (%)	−38.8 ± 4.5	−5.9 ± 5.3	$p < 0.001$
Change from systolic blood pressure (mm Hg) by week 72	−4.6 ± 0.8	0.1 ± 0.8	NA
Reduction NT-proBNP—ratio of geometric means (pg/mL)	0.93 ± 0.04	1.04 ± 0.04	NA

events (9.9% vs. 15.3%), improved KCCQ-CSS (+19.5) and 6-minute walk distance (+26 m), and lowered CRP and NT-proBNP, indicating robust cardiometabolic benefit in HFpEF.[54] Common adverse effects are gastrointestinal, mainly during dose escalation. Other effects include dizziness, fatigue, injection-site reactions, and alopecia. Hypoglycemia risk increases with insulin or sulfonylureas. Rare but serious risks include pancreatitis, gallbladder disease, acute kidney injury, and hypersensitivity. Tirzepatide carries a boxed warning for thyroid C-cell tumors and is contraindicated in medullary thyroid carcinoma, MEN 2, or prior severe hypersensitivity.[50]

COMPARISON OF ANTI-OBESITY DRUGS: META-ANALYSIS SUMMARY

Meta-analysis-based comparisons underscore efficacy as the primary differentiator among anti-obesity pharmacotherapies **(Table 10)**. Orlistat demonstrates the lowest mean weight loss (~10.2%) with limited metabolic benefits beyond lipid reduction, while naltrexone-bupropion (~6.1%) and liraglutide (~8%) provide modest efficacy. Phentermine-topiramate achieves intermediate weight loss (~10.9%), whereas semaglutide shows substantially greater efficacy (14.9%) and tirzepatide produces the highest

TABLE 10: Comparison of anti-obesity drug trial outcomes.

	Orlistat	*Phentermine/ topiramate*	*Naltrexone/ bupropion*	*Liraglutide*	*Semaglutide*	*Tirzepatide*
FDA approval	Adults – 1999	Adults – 2012	Adults – 2014	Adults – 2014	Adults – 2021	Adults – 2023
	Adolescents – 2003	Adolescents – 2022		Adolescents – 2020	Adolescents – 2022	
Mean weight reduction (%) vs. placebo	10.2%	10.9%	6.1%	8%	14.9%	20.9%
≥5% weight reduction in patients (%)	>70%	>60%	≈50%	>60%	>85%	>90%
Waist circumference	9.6 cm	10.9 cm	6.2 cm	8.2 cm	13.5 cm	18.5 cm
SBP	6 mm Hg	2.9 mm Hg	0.1 mm Hg	4.2 mm Hg	6.2 mm Hg	7.6 mm Hg
LDL-C	9.4%	8.4%	2%	3%	–	8.6%
DM risk prevention in population (%)	37.3%	NA	NA	NA	NA	NA
HbA1C reduction	0.5%	0%	–	1.09%	1.6%	1.69%
Patient adherence to the therapy	At 12 months – 0%	At 3 months – 36%	At 3 months – 34%	At 3 months – 52%	At 3 months – 63%	NA
		At 12 months – 13%	At 12 months – 10%	At 12 months – 17%	At 12 months – 40%	

weight reduction (20.9%), though the latter currently lacks FDA approval for cardiovascular (CV) risk reduction or adolescent use.[55] Semaglutide demonstrates consistent benefits across populations, with >85% achieving ≥5% weight loss, alongside significant improvements in HbA1c (–1.6%), systolic blood pressure (–6.2 mm Hg), and waist circumference (–13.5 cm). Tirzepatide shows comparable glycemic improvement (HbA1c –1.69%) but without an established CV indication, while liraglutide confers moderate cardiometabolic effects (HbA1c –1.09%, SBP –2.4 mm Hg).

Treatment adherence is lowest with orlistat (0%) and naltrexone-bupropion (10%), moderate with phentermine-topiramate (13%) and liraglutide (17%), and highest with semaglutide (40%), likely reflecting weekly dosing, better tolerability, and availability of an oral formulation. Semaglutide remains the only agent approved for both CV risk reduction and adolescent obesity, offering the most comprehensive clinical and regulatory profile. While tirzepatide shows promising adherence and efficacy, its long-term regulatory positioning is still evolving.

Pharmacological Management: Future

The anti-obesity drug pipeline **(Table 11)** is rapidly expanding, with next-generation therapies targeting multiple metabolic pathways beyond traditional mono-hormonal approaches. Among the most advanced candidates are oral GLP-1 receptor agonists, notably orforglipron, now in late-phase development. In ACHIEVE-1, a 40-week phase 3 trial in adults with type 2 diabetes, orforglipron (3–36 mg) reduced HbA1c by 1.3–1.6% versus 0.1% with placebo, with >65% of patients at the highest dose achieving HbA1c ≤6.5%.

TABLE 11: Anti-obesity drugs under pipeline development.

S. no.	*Drug/molecule*	*Dose*	*Company*	*Mech. of action*	*Indications other than obesity*	*Obesity trial*
1.	Orforglipron	3–36 mg	Eli Lilly	GLP-1 RA	T2D, CV outcomes in T2D (Phase-3)	Phase-3
2.	CagriSema (cagrilintide + semaglutide)	2.4 mg/2.4 mg	Novo Nordisk	GLP-1 RA + Amylin RA	T2D, CV outcomes in T2D (Phase-3)	Phase-3
3.	Survodutide	3.6–6 mg	Boehringer Ingelheim	GLP-1 RA + GCG RA	T2D, MASH (Phase-2)	Phase-3
4.	Mazdutide	4–6, 9 mg	Innovent Biologics	GLP-1 RA + GCG RA	T2D (Phase-3), CKD (Phase-1)	Phase-3
5.	Retatrutide	4–12 mg	Eli Lilly	GLP-1 RA + GIP RA + GCG RA	T2D, OA (Phase-3), CKD (Phase-1)	Phase-3
6.	Danuglipron	40–200 mg	Pfizer	GLP-1 RA	NA	Phase-2
7.	Cagrilintide	0.3–4.5 mg	Novo Nordisk	Amylin RA	MASH (Phase-1)	Phase-2
8.	PYY 1875	0.03–2.4 mg	Novo Nordisk	PYY RA	NA	Phase-2
9.	Efinopegdutide	5–10 mg	Hanmi Pharma	GLP-1 RA + GCG RA	T2D, MASH, MASLD (Phase-2)	Phase-2
10.	Pemvidutide	1.2–2.4 mg	Altimmune	GLP-1 RA + GCG RA	MASH, MASLD (Phase-2), T2D (Phase-1)	Phase-2
11.	Maridebart cafraglutide (AMG 133)	NA	Amgen	GLP-1 RA + GIPR Antagonist	NA	Phase-2
12.	NNC0165-1875 + Semaglutide	1–2 mg + 2.4 mg	Novo Nordisk	GLP-1 RA + PYY RA	NA	Phase-2
13.	Dapiglutide	4–6 mg	Zealand Pharma	GLP-1 RA + GLP 2 RA	NA	Phase-2
14.	Bimagrumab + Semaglutide	30 mg/kg + 1–2.4 mg	Versanis Bio	Activin receptor-2 inhibitor + GLP-1 RA	NA	Phase-2
15.	S-309309	NA	Shionogi	MGAT2	NA	Phase-2
16.	CT-996	NA	Carmot Therapeutics	GLP-1 RA	NA	Phase-1
17.	AZD6234	NA	AstraZeneca	Amylin RA	NA	Phase-1
18.	ZP8396	NA	Zealand Pharma	Amylin RA	NA	Phase-1
19.	HM15136	NA	Hanmi Pharma	Glucagon RA	NA	Phase-1
20.	NNC0165-1562	NA	Novo Nordisk	PYY RA	NA	Phase-1
21.	Y-14	9–36 mg	Zihip	PYY RA	NA	Phase-1

Contd...

Contd...

S. no.	Drug/Molecule	Dose	Company	Mech. of action	Indications other than obesity	Obesity trial
22.	VK2735	NA	Viking Therapeutics	GLP-1 Ra + GIP RA	MASH (Phase-1)	Phase-1
23.	SCO-094	NA	Scohia Pharma	GLP-1 RA + GIP RA	T2D, MASH	Phase-1
24.	CT-388	5–12 mg	Carnot Therapeutics	GLP-1 RA + GIP RA	T2D (Phase-1)	Phase-1
25.	Amycretin	1–100 mg	Novo Nordisk	GLP-1 RA + Amylin RA	NA	Phase-1
26.	Dacra QW II	NA	Eli Lilly	Amylin RA + Calcitonin RA	NA	Phase-1
27.	NNC0165–1562 + Semaglutide	NA	Novo Nordisk	PYY RA + GLP-1 RA	NA	Phase-1
28.	HM15211	NA	Hanmi Pharma	GLP-1 RA + GIP RA + GCG RA	MASH (Phase-2)	Phase-1
29.	NNC0247-0829	NA	Novo Nordisk	GDF15 analogue	NA	Phase-1
30.	JNJ-9090/CIN-109	NA	CinRx Pharma	GDF15 analogue	NA	Phase-1
31.	SCO-267	NA	Scohia Pharma	GPCR 40	MASH (Phase-1)	Phase-1
32.	Petrelintide	NA	Zealand Pharma	Amylin Analogue	NA	Phase-1
33.	Eloralintide	NA	Eli Lilly	Amylin Analogue	NA	Phase-2
34.	ZP6590	NA	Zealand Pharma	GIP RA	NA	Preclinical

Mean weight loss reached 7.3 kg (7.9%) without plateauing by week 40. Gastrointestinal events were the most common adverse effects, while treatment discontinuation remained low (4–8%), supporting its potential as an effective oral, non-peptide GLP-1 therapy with injectable-level efficacy.[56]

Additional high-potential agents include retatrutide (GLP-1/GIP/glucagon triple agonist), CagriSema (semaglutide plus an amylin analogue), and bimagrumab combined with semaglutide, which uniquely preserves lean mass through ActRII inhibition. Dual GLP-1–glucagon agents such as mazdutide, survodutide, and pemvidutide target both obesity and metabolic dysfunction-associated steatohepatitis (MASH). Emerging therapies—including amycretin (oral GLP-1/amylin), GDF15 analogues, PYY agonists, and mitochondrial-targeted agents—further broaden the therapeutic landscape. Driven largely by Novo Nordisk, Eli Lilly, and Amgen, >30 agents are currently in development.[57] Collectively, these innovations have the potential to approach bariatric-level outcomes and reshape obesity management through scalable, multi-pathway pharmacotherapy.

CONCLUSION

Obesity is a chronic, relapsing disease with profound metabolic and cardiovascular consequences. Recent advances in pharmacotherapy particularly incretin-based agents such as semaglutide and tirzepatide have transformed obesity management by delivering unprecedented, durable weight loss alongside meaningful cardiometabolic benefits. The dual GIP/GLP-1 receptor agonist tirzepatide, together with GLP-1 receptor agonists, has set a new benchmark for pharmacologic treatment of obesity and type 2 diabetes. As the global burden of obesity continues to rise, equitable access to these highly effective therapies will be essential. Future progress will depend on continued therapeutic innovation, integration of pharmacotherapy within multidisciplinary, patient-centered care models, and long-term strategies aimed at sustaining clinically meaningful outcomes.

REFERENCES

1. Panuganti KK, Nguyen M, Kshirsagar RK. Obesity. In: StatPearls [Internet]. Treasure Island (FL): StatPearls Publishing; 2025.
2. Rubino F, Cummings DE, Eckel RH, Cohen RV, Wilding JP, Brown WA, et al. Definition and diagnostic criteria of clinical obesity. Lancet Diabetes Endocrinol. 2025;13(3):221-62.
3. Ng M, Gakidou E, Lo J, Abate YH, Abbafati C, Abbas N, et al. Global, regional, and national prevalence of adult overweight and obesity, 1990–2021, with forecasts to 2050: a forecasting study for the Global Burden of Disease Study 2021. Lancet. 2025;405(10481):813-38.
4. Islam AS, Sultana H, Refat MN, Farhana Z, Kamil AA, Rahman MM. The global burden of overweight-obesity and its association with economic status, benefiting from STEPs survey of WHO member states: a meta-analysis. Prevent Med Rep. 2024:102882.
5. Okunogbe A, Nugent R, Spencer G, Powis J, Ralston J, Wilding J. Economic impacts of overweight and obesity: current and future estimates for 161 countries. BMJ Global health. 2022;7(9):e009773.
6. Higuera-Hernández MF, Reyes-Cuapio E, Gutiérrez-Mendoza M, Rocha NB, Veras AB, Budde H, et al. Fighting obesity: non-pharmacological interventions. Clinical nutrition ESPEN. 2018;25:50-5.
7. ElSayed NA, Aleppo G, Bannuru RR, Bruemmer D, Collins BS, Ekhlaspour L, et al. Obesity and weight management for the prevention and treatment of type 2 diabetes: standards of care in diabetes–2024. Diabetes Care. 2024;47.
8. Kim KK, Haam JH, Kim BT, Kim EM, Park JH, Rhee SY, et al. Evaluation and treatment of obesity and its comorbidities: 2022 update of clinical practice guidelines for obesity by the Korean Society for the Study of Obesity. J Obes Metab Syndr. 2023;32(1):1.
9. Wadden TA, Tronieri JS, Butryn ML. Lifestyle modification approaches for the treatment of obesity in adults. Am Psychol. 2020;75(2):235.
10. Connolly HM, Crary JL, McGoon MD, Hensrud DD, Edwards BS, Edwards WD, et al. Valvular heart disease associated with fenfluramine–phentermine. N Engl J Med. 1997;337(9):581-8.
11. Rothman RB, Baumann MH. Serotonergic drugs and valvular heart disease. Circulation. 2009;102(23):2949-57.
12. Abenhaim L, Moride Y, Brenot F, Rich S, Benichou J, Kurz X, et al. Appetite-suppressant drugs and the risk of primary pulmonary hypertension. N Engl J Med. 1996;335(9):609-16.
13. James WP, Caterson ID, Coutinho W, Finer N, Van Gaal LF, Maggioni AP, et al. Effect of sibutramine on cardiovascular outcomes in overweight and obese subjects. N Engl J Med. 2010;363(10):905-17.
14. James WP. The SCOUT study: risk-benefit profile of sibutramine in overweight high-risk cardiovascular patients. European heart journal supplements. 2005;7(suppl_L):L44-8.
15. Van Gaal LF, Scheen AJ, Rissanen AM, Rössner S, Hanotin C, Ziegler O. Long-term effect of CB1 blockade with rimonabant on cardiometabolic risk factors: two-year results from the RIO-Europe Study. Eur Heart J. 2008;29(14):1761-71.
16. Nissen SE, Nicholls SJ, Wolski K, Rodés-Cabau J, Cannon CP, Deanfield JE, et al. Effect of rimonabant on progression of atherosclerosis in patients with abdominal obesity and coronary artery disease: the STRADIVARIUS randomized controlled trial. Jama. 2008;299(13):1547-60.
17. Christensen R, Kristensen PK, Bartels EM, Bliddal H, Astrup A. Efficacy and safety of the weight-loss drug rimonabant: a meta-analysis of randomised trials. Lancet. 2007;370(9600):1706-13.
18. Sjöström L, Rissanen A, Andersen T, Boldrin M, Golay A, Koppeschaar HP, et al. Randomised placebo-controlled trial of orlistat for weight loss and prevention of weight regain in obese patients. Lancet. 1998;352(9123):167-72.

19. Hill JO, Hauptman J, Anderson JW, Fujioka K, O'Neil PM, Smith DK, et al. Orlistat, a lipase inhibitor, for weight maintenance after conventional dieting: a 1-y study. Am J Clin Nutr. 1999;69(6):1108-16.
20. Jain SS, Ramanand SJ, Ramanand JB, Akat PB, Patwardhan MH, Joshi SR. Evaluation of efficacy and safety of orlistat in obese patients. Indian J Endocrinol Metabol. 2011;15(2):99-104.
21. Kelley DE, Bray GA, Pi-Sunyer FX, Klein S, Hill J, Miles J, et al. Clinical efficacy of orlistat therapy in overweight and obese patients with insulin-treated type 2 diabetes: a 1-year randomized controlled trial. Diabetes Care. 2002;25(6):1033-41.
22. Orlistat FDA drug label. https://www.accessdata.fda.gov/drugsatfda_docs/label/2022/020766s038lbl.pdf Accessed on 13/03/2026
23. Setmelanotide FDA drug label. https://www.accessdata.fda.gov/drugsatfda_docs/label/2025/213793Orig1s008lbl.pdf Accessed on 13/03/2026
24. Argente J, Verge CF, Okorie U, Fennoy I, Kelsey MM, Cokkinias C, et al. Setmelanotide in patients aged 2–5 years with rare MC4R pathway-associated obesity (VENTURE): a 1 year, open-label, multicenter, phase 3 trial. Lancet Diabetes Endocrinol. 2025;13(1):29-37.
25. Haqq AM, Chung WK, Dollfus H, Haws RM, Martos-Moreno GÁ, Poitou C, et al. Efficacy and safety of setmelanotide, a melanocortin-4 receptor agonist, in patients with Bardet-Biedl syndrome and Alström syndrome: a multicentre, randomised, double-blind, placebo-controlled, phase 3 trial with an open-label period. Lancet Diabetes Endocrinol. 2022;10(12):859-68.
26. Phentermine and Topiramate extended release capsules FDA drug label. https://www.accessdata.fda.gov/drugsatfda_docs/label/2026/022580s031lbl.pdf Accessed on 13/03/2026
27. Gadde KM, Allison DB, Ryan DH, Peterson CA, Troupin B, Schwiers ML, et al. Effects of low-dose, controlled-release, phentermine plus topiramate combination on weight and associated comorbidities in overweight and obese adults (CONQUER): a randomised, placebo-controlled, phase 3 trial. Lancet. 2011;377(9774):1341-52.
28. Garvey WT, Ryan DH, Look M, Gadde KM, Allison DB, Peterson CA, et al. Two-year sustained weight loss and metabolic benefits with controlled-release phentermine/topiramate in obese and overweight adults (SEQUEL): a randomized, placebo-controlled, phase 3 extension study. Am J Clin Nutr. 2012;95(2):297-308.
29. Allison DB, Gadde KM, Garvey WT, Peterson CA, Schwiers ML, Najarian T, et al. Controlled-release phentermine/topiramate in severely obese adults: a randomized controlled trial (EQUIP). Obesity. 2012;20(2):330-42.
30. Bays HE, Hsia DS, Nguyen LT, Peterson CA, Varghese ST. Effects of phentermine/topiramate extended-release, phentermine, and placebo on ambulatory blood pressure monitoring in adults with overweight or obesity: a randomized, multicenter, double-blind study. Obesity Pillars. 2024;9:100099.
31. Kelly AS, Bensignor MO, Hsia DS, Shoemaker AH, Shih W, Peterson C, et al. Phentermine/topiramate for the treatment of adolescent obesity. NEJM evidence. 2022;1(6):EVIDoa2200014.
32. Aronne LJ, Wadden TA, Peterson C, Winslow D, Odeh S, Gadde KM. Evaluation of phentermine and topiramate versus phentermine/topiramate extended-release in obese adults. Obesity. 2013;21(11):2163-71.
33. Naltrexone and Bupropion extended release tablets FDA drug label. https://www.accessdata.fda.gov/drugsatfda_docs/label/2025/200063s024s026lbl.pdf Accessed on 13/03/2026.
34. Greenway FL, Fujioka K, Plodkowski RA, Mudaliar S, Guttadauria M, Erickson J, et al. Effect of naltrexone plus bupropion on weight loss in overweight and obese adults (COR-I): a multicentre, randomised, double-blind, placebo-controlled, phase 3 trial. Lancet. 2010; 376(9741):595-605.
35. Apovian CM, Aronne L, Rubino D, Still C, Wyatt H, Burns C, et al. A randomized, phase 3 trial of naltrexone SR/bupropion SR on weight and obesity-related risk factors (COR-II). Obesity. 2013;21(5):935-43.
36. Wadden TA, Foreyt JP, Foster GD, Hill JO, Klein S, O'neil PM, et al. Weight loss with naltrexone SR/bupropion SR combination therapy as an adjunct to behavior modification: the COR-BMOD trial. Obesity. 2011;19(1):110-20.

37. Grilo CM, Lydecker JA, Morgan PT, Gueorguieva R. Naltrexone+ bupropion combination for the treatment of binge-eating disorder with obesity: a randomized, controlled pilot study. Clinical therapeutics. 2021;43(1):112-22.
38. Liu Y, Han F, Xia Z, Sun P, Rohani P, Amirthalingam P, et al. The effects of bupropion alone and combined with naltrexone on weight loss: a systematic review and meta-regression analysis of randomized controlled trials. Diabetol Metabol Syndrome. 2024;16(1):93.
39. Liraglutide (SAXENDA) FDA drug label. https://www.accessdata.fda.gov/drugsatfda_docs/label/2026/206321s025lbl.pdf Accessed on 13/03/2026
40. Pi-Sunyer X, Astrup A, Fujioka K, Greenway F, Halpern A, Krempf M, et al. A randomized, controlled trial of 3.0 mg of liraglutide in weight management. N Engl J Med. 2015;373(1):11-22.
41. Kelly AS, Auerbach P, Barrientos-Perez M, Gies I, Hale PM, Marcus C, et al. A randomized, controlled trial of liraglutide for adolescents with obesity. N Engl J Med. 2020;382(22):2117-28.
42. Maselli D, Atieh J, Clark MM, Eckert D, Taylor A, Carlson P, et al. Effects of liraglutide on gastrointestinal functions and weight in obesity: a randomized clinical and pharmacogenomic trial. Obesity. 2022;30(8):1608-20.
43. Barboza JJ, Huaman MR, Melgar B, Diaz-Arocutipa C, Valenzuela-Rodriguez G, Hernandez AV. Efficacy of liraglutide in non-diabetic obese adults: a systematic review and meta-analysis of randomized controlled trials. J Clin Med. 2022;11(11):2998.
44. Semaglutide FDA drug label. https://www.accessdata.fda.gov/drugsatfda_docs/label/2026/215256s033lbl.pdf Accessed on 13/03/2026
45. Wilding JP, Batterham RL, Calanna S, Davies M, Van Gaal LF, Lingvay I, et al. Once-weekly semaglutide in adults with overweight or obesity. N Engl J Med. 2021;384(11):989-1002.
46. Davies M, Færch L, Jeppesen OK, Pakseresht A, Pedersen SD, Perreault L, et al. Semaglutide 2·4 mg once a week in adults with overweight or obesity, and type 2 diabetes (STEP 2): a randomised, double-blind, double-dummy, placebo-controlled, phase 3 trial. Lancet. 2021;397(10278):971-84.
47. Kosiborod MN, Abildstrøm SZ, Borlaug BA, Butler J, Rasmussen S, Davies M, et al. Semaglutide in patients with heart failure with preserved ejection fraction and obesity. N Engl J Med. 2023;389(12):1069-84.
48. Kosiborod MN, Petrie MC, Borlaug BA, Butler J, Davies MJ, Hovingh GK, et al. Semaglutide in patients with obesity-related heart failure and type 2 diabetes. N Engl J Med. 2024;390(15):1394-407.
49. Lincoff AM, Brown-Frandsen K, Colhoun HM, Deanfield J, Emerson SS, Esbjerg S, et al. Semaglutide and cardiovascular outcomes in obesity without diabetes. N Engl J Med. 2023;389(24):2221-32.
50. Tirzepatide (ZEPBOUND) FDA drug label. https://www.accessdata.fda.gov/drugsatfda_docs/label/2026/217806s042lbl.pdf Accessed on 13/03/2026
51. Jastreboff AM, Aronne LJ, Ahmad NN, Wharton S, Connery L, Alves B, et al. Tirzepatide once weekly for the treatment of obesity. N Engl J Med. 2022;387(3):205-16.
52. Garvey WT, Frias JP, Jastreboff AM, le Roux CW, Sattar N, Aizenberg D, et al. Tirzepatide once weekly for the treatment of obesity in people with type 2 diabetes (SURMOUNT-2): a double-blind, randomised, multicentre, placebo-controlled, phase 3 trial. Lancet. 2023;402(10402):613-26.
53. Wadden TA, Chao AM, Machineni S, Kushner R, Ard J, Srivastava G, et al. Tirzepatide after intensive lifestyle intervention in adults with overweight or obesity: the SURMOUNT-3 phase 3 trial. Nat Med. 2023;29(11):2909-18.
54. Packer M, Zile MR, Kramer CM, Baum SJ, Litwin SE, Menon V, et al. Tirzepatide for heart failure with preserved ejection fraction and obesity. N Engl J Med. 2025;392(5):427-37.
55. Gudzune KA, Kushner RF. Medications for obesity: a review. Jama. 2024;332(7):571-84.
56. Studna A (Ed). Lilly's oral GLP-1, orforglipron, demonstrated statistically significant efficacy results and a safety profile consistent with injectable GLP-1 medicines in successful Phase 3 trial (ACHIEVE-1). Eli Lilly and Company; 2025.
57. Melson E, Ashraf U, Papamargaritis D, Davies MJ. What is the pipeline for future medications for obesity? Intern J Obesity. 2024:1-9.

CHAPTER 7

Bariatric Surgery: Latest Advances and Prospects

Shashank S Shah, Elmutaz Abdalla Mekki Kanani

ABSTRACT

With its increasing popularity, bariatric surgery has evolved continuously in both its techniques and the adoption of technology. As our understanding of the complex physiological mechanisms that drive obesity and weight loss advances, it has led to the emergence of innovative therapeutic strategies based on this knowledge, thereby enhancing the tools at the disposal of the bariatric surgeons.

The progress encompasses the developments in established surgical procedures, the introduction of novel techniques, endoscopic treatments, innovations specifically targeting metabolic disorders and diabetes, as well as revisional and salvage operations, alongside improvements in safety and perioperative care that are motivated by and have profited from technological developments.

While surgery continues to be the fundamental approach for managing obesity, various endoscopic and interventional techniques present significant alternatives in specific circumstances.

With precision medicine at the forefront, the outlook seems optimistic and knowledge driven.

Keywords: Bariatric surgery advances, technological developments, therapeutic strategies, endoscopic techniques, and novel procedures

INTRODUCTION

Bariatric surgery is currently recognized as the most effective long-term intervention for severe obesity and its related metabolic comorbidities, including type 2 diabetes mellitus (T2DM), hypertension, and obstructive sleep apnea (OSA). Recent advancements in surgical techniques, minimally invasive strategies, and metabolic insights have significantly enhanced patient outcomes, safety, and accessibility. This chapter focuses on the major innovations in bariatric surgery that have taken place in the past decade, as well as those anticipated to emerge in the near future. The rapid progression of technology has become nearly impossible to keep up with, transforming every facet of life, and bariatric surgery is certainly not an exception. This chapter will cover:

- Evolution of existing surgical techniques.
- Emerging techniques.
- Endoscopic therapies.
- Metabolic and diabetes-specific advances.
- Revisional and salvage procedures.
- Safety and perioperative care advances.
- Advances in technology.
- Future prospects.

Disclaimer

This chapter does not aim to provide an exhaustive review, and an in-depth discussion on every subject exceeds its intended scope.

EVOLUTION OF EXISTING SURGICAL TECHNIQUES

Laparoscopy

The transition from open surgery to laparoscopic techniques has transformed the field of bariatric surgery. This advancement has led to a decrease in complications, a reduction in recovery times, and improved precision. Laparoscopy has motivated individuals to grapple with obesity and its health-detrimental effects to opt for bariatric surgery as the fastest and most durable solution, all while minimizing stress and cosmetic repercussions.

Single incision laparoscopic surgery (SILS) represented a significant leap forward, albeit constrained by technical difficulties such as a limited surgical field and prolonged operative time; nonetheless, it remains a viable option for selected patients.[1]

Laparoscopic Sleeve Gastrectomy Dominance

Laparoscopic sleeve gastrectomy (LSG) has emerged as the most frequently performed bariatric procedure, surpassing Roux-en-Y Gastric Bypass (RYGB), owing to its technical simplicity and comparable metabolic outcomes. Nevertheless, there are ongoing concerns regarding long-term durability, such as weight regain and exacerbation of gastroesophageal reflux disease (GERD).

Since 2013, LSG has been the most common bariatric surgery,[2] making up 65.7% of surgeries in 2022. RYGB follows in second place, accounting for 26.5% in the USA.[3] This same pattern continues in 2023.[4]

Robotic Surgery

Since its initial use in bariatric surgery just before the turn of the last century, robotic surgery has achieved remarkable milestones, evolving from robot-assisted to entirely robot-executed procedures. This transition has been rapid and substantiated by evidence. Despite the longer operative durations and relatively higher costs associated with robotic surgery, its benefits are numerous. It has demonstrated lower conversion rates and postoperative complications, attributed to improved visualization and precision in executing meticulous dissections, which is crucial in scenarios where anatomical challenges arise.

The robotic approach may be particularly beneficial for patients with high body mass index (BMI), complex bypass surgeries, previous gastrointestinal operations, and for revisional bariatric surgery. The emergence of a variety of robotic systems and advanced modern technologies is on the rise and gaining momentum.[5,6]

EMERGING TECHNIQUES

Recent advancements in bariatric surgery have been consistently introduced. The primary motivations for the development of new techniques are to enhance outcomes and minimize adverse effects while ensuring technical simplicity. Achieving effective and sustained weight loss is the foremost outcome that appeals to innovators. The novel idea behind sleeve plus operations involves adding a robust physiology-modulating element to the traditional sleeve gastrectomy to further promote weight loss and improve the metabolic response to curb T2DM. Sleeve Plus procedures allow for partial diversion of food to the distal ileum, preserve pyloric function, reduce dumping syndrome, enhance hormonal responses from the distal gut [e.g., glucagon-like peptide-1 (GLP-1) secretion], and improve glycemic control.[7] Examples of these procedures include:

- *Duodenojejunal bypass with sleeve gastrectomy (DJB-SG):* Roux-en-Y type and loop type; however, both are technically demanding.
- LSG with proximal jejunal bypass (LSG-JB).
- Single anastomosis duodenoileal bypass with sleeve (SADI-S).
- Sleeve gastrectomy with gastrojejunal bypass (SG-GJ).
- Sleeve gastrectomy with transit bipartition.

An additional focus of enhancement was addressing the shortcomings of the conventional food-rerouting methods [biliopancreatic diversion (BPD) and RYGB], which primarily fulfill the fundamental objectives of effective and sustainable weight loss, albeit at the expense of significant adverse effects. Improving these side effects and resolving the associated technical challenges could transform any procedure into optimal surgical intervention. Motivated by these considerations, Rutledge proposed the "minigastric bypass" in 1997.[8] The procedure, later referred to as the "single anastomosis gastric bypass," has evolved over time into the operation now endorsed by the International Federation for the Surgery of Obesity and Metabolic Disorders (IFSO) and the American Society for Metabolic and Bariatric Surgery (ASMBS). It is gaining popularity as an alternative to RYGB, offering similar weight loss and diabetes remission with fewer anastomoses and shorter operative times. Debate continues regarding bile reflux and long-term nutritional risks.

Vagal Nerve Blocking

vBloc® therapy represents a Food and Drug Administration (FDA)-approved implantable device designed to intermittently block vagal signaling, thereby reducing hunger. The procedure is minimally invasive, and the resultant weight loss is moderate, with a total body weight loss (TBWL) ranging from 8 to 10%.[9]

ENDOSCOPIC THERAPIES

In light of the ongoing positive trend towards reducing operative trauma, non-surgical incisionless approaches to obesity treatment have been developed. Although their effectiveness does not reach that of bariatric surgery, they can, as alternatives or adjuncts to bariatric surgery, facilitate considerable weight loss in carefully selected populations who are either not ideal candidates for surgery or are unwilling to pursue it.

The treatments encompass:

- *Intragastric balloons (IGBs)*: These include swallowable balloons and endoscopically placed IGBs.
- Endoscopic sleeve gastroplasties (ESG).
- Revisional endoscopy after bariatric surgery.

Intragastric balloons serve as temporary devices that can facilitate moderate weight loss, typically ranging from 10 to 15% TBWL. Numerous brands exist in the market, each with unique specifications and timeframes.[10]

Endoscopic sleeve gastroplasty involves the reshaping of the stomach into a sleeve through endoscopic suturing, potentially resulting in a TBWL of approximately 15–20%. A variety of endoscopic systems are currently available for this procedure, reflecting the growing interest among endoscopists.[11]

Transpyloric Shuttle, EndoBarrier, SatiSphere, and magnetic anastomosis system are some of the multiple endoscopic techniques available, although most are still experimental.

METABOLIC AND DIABETES-SPECIFIC ADVANCES

Significant glycemic improvement following surgical operations for peptic ulcer disease or upper gastrointestinal neoplasia was observed previously; however, it was not until the advent of bariatric surgery that this phenomenon was thoroughly investigated and clinically correlated with changes in the entero-endocrine hormonal system. The precise physiological mechanisms remain inadequately understood and seem to encompass intricate hormonal interactions.

The revelation of the enteroendocrine system's modulation potential in addressing obesity and diabetes has set the stage for the formulation of therapies that specifically target T2DM. Modulation can be achieved through surgical modifications of the gastrointestinal system, endoscopic interventions, or other strategies.

Ileal Interposition with Sleeve Gastrectomy

This surgical approach is essentially intended to incorporate both foregut and hindgut mechanisms, in conjunction with Ghrelin withdrawal, to ameliorate T2DM while also promoting weight loss and metabolic advantages. However, the procedure has lost popularity owing to its complexity and the scarcity of research that includes a large cohort of patients and long-term data.[12]

Duodenal Mucosal Resurfacing

Duodenal mucosal resurfacing (DMR) is an endoscopic technique that employs hydrothermal energy to ablate the duodenal mucosa, aiming to enhance insulin sensitivity and combat insulin resistance. Although the preliminary results are promising, the procedure is yet to be fully validated and remains experimental.[13]

REVISIONAL AND SALVAGE PROCEDURES

Endoscopic revision following RYGB/OAGB represents a noninvasive technique that has demonstrated some degree of success. This method employs either energy modalities, such as argon plasma coagulation (APC) or cryoablation, to promote localized fibrosis, or it may involve direct full-thickness suturing through transoral outlet reduction endoscopically (TORe) to diminish the size of the gastrojejunal anastomosis (GJA) outlet. Additionally, a combination of these two approaches has been utilized, yielding superior outcomes.[14]

Another promising technique involves the use of over-the-scope clips applied to both sides of the GJA, which has been reported to result in notably improved outcomes.[15]

Endoscopic sleeve gastroplasty can be applied to revise standard sleeve gastrectomy with good efficacy and safety.[16]

Robotic surgery offers more precision in revisional procedures.

SAFETY AND PERIOPERATIVE CARE ADVANCES

Enhanced Recovery after Bariatric Surgery Protocols

Emerging from the original enhanced recovery after surgery (ERAS) principles developed in the late twentieth century, the first set of ERAS guidelines designed for bariatric surgery (ERABS) was introduced in 2016. The rapid progression of ERABS has fostered its widespread acceptance and has established it as a common practice today.[17]

Irrespective of the specific surgical sub-specialty, all ERAS protocols aim to achieve identical goals: Optimizing patients preoperatively, reducing perioperative stress, preserving physiological function postoperatively, and facilitating a quicker recovery following surgery. This is achieved through a multidisciplinary team that delivers multimodal perioperative care across various phases, commencing from the initial outpatient consultation.[18]

Individuals suffering from obesity essentially fall in the high-risk surgical group. The ERABS framework is a holistic, multidisciplinary, patient-oriented, evidence-supported, multimodal perioperative care pathway intended to promote swift recovery from major surgical interventions by minimizing both physiological and psychological burdens. The ERABS model has the capacity to diminish morbidity rates following bariatric surgery and may also accelerate functional recovery and reduce length of stay (LOS).[17] ERABS had made it even possible to perform selected bariatric procedures as a day case.

The improvement in clinical outcomes and other measured metrics linked to compliance with ERAS guidelines has been validated by many Cochrane Reviews, including large-scale RCTs.[19,20]

Telemedicine and Digital Health

Postbariatric surgery, patients frequently encounter challenges such as struggles with dietary compliance, restricted access to consistent follow-up care, feelings of emotional isolation and diminished motivation, as well as the potential for complications including dehydration, malnutrition, or weight regain. In-person consultations may occur infrequently, resulting in a lack of support and accountability. This is where remote monitoring via telemedicine and digital health emerges as a transformative solution.

Remote patient monitoring (RPM) employs intelligent scales, wearable technology, and mobile applications to monitor various metrics, with data being sent in real-time to healthcare professionals. This facilitates prompt interventions and tailored support. Patients experience a greater sense of connection with their healthcare teams, which alleviates anxiety and enhances their confidence throughout the recovery process. Remote monitoring transcends mere convenience; it serves as a driving force for improved health outcomes. Broadly, digital health may include interventions using the internet, social media (Facebook, Twitter, Snapchat, Instagram, and WhatsApp), internet/Wi-Fi-enabled wearable devices, telemedicine, email, short messaging services (SMS), and e-learning.[21]

■ ADVANCES IN TECHNOLOGY

Technologies powered by artificial intelligence, such as machine learning, problem-solving, and predictive analytics, have enabled personalized recommendations that are customized to the unique profiles of individual patients. The capacity of these algorithms to predict patient risks associated with specific conditions, along with their role in early diagnosis and preventive care, has been transformative.[22,23] AI-driven predictive models optimize patient selection by analyzing comorbidities, genetics, and psychosocial factors. Machine learning algorithms predict postoperative complications and weight loss trajectories, facilitating precision medicine, and tailored patient management strategies.[24] However, issues related to data privacy and the susceptibility of algorithms to bias continue to pose significant challenges for these advancing technologies.[22,23]

■ FUTURE PROSPECTS

Telesurgery

Telesurgery, also known as remote surgery, is a surgical method that employs robotic technology alongside wireless networking, enabling a physician to conduct surgery on a patient despite being in different geographical locations. This system addresses the shortage of surgeons, the geographical barriers to immediate and high-quality surgical care, and the challenges of long-distance travel.

Despite its inception two decades ago and the substantial technological advancements, telesurgery continues to be an experimental rarity.[25,26]

Interventional Techniques

By offering advantages of less invasiveness, fewer possible complications, and better affordability, interventional techniques provide innovative treatment options for metabolic disorders.

Magnetic Anastomosis

A groundbreaking minimally invasive technique for the formation of a side-to-side duodenoileal magnetic compression anastomosis is designed to achieve duodenoileostomy diversion, targeting weight loss and the resolution of T2DM in adults with severe obesity. Considering the high recurrence rates of conventional endoscopic treatments and the considerable rates of bleeding and leaks that are commonly associated with traditional sutured or stapled anastomoses, the magnetic anastomosis technique presents a promising alternative. Nonetheless, it is still in the initial phases of its development in the field of bariatric surgery.[27,28]

Bariatric Embolization

Transarterial embolization targeting particular arteries that supply the ghrelin-secreting cells in the gastric fundus aims to inhibit ghrelin production and facilitate weight reduction. Additionally, it may enhance glucose metabolism; however, it remains in the experimental phase.[29]

Endovascular Denervation

The central nervous system plays a crucial role in regulating glucose metabolism through the direct innervation of various organs by autonomic nerves. Modulating the sympathetic nervous system (SNS), which is known to contribute to metabolic disorders when overactivated, represents a potential therapeutic strategy. Catheter-based neuromodulation targeting the sympathetic nerves of the islet and liver has shown metabolic advantages, thereby making denervation along the celiac and hepatic arteries an attractive option.[30]

While generally considered safe, bariatric embolization and endovascular denervation necessitate further research to address outstanding concerns and to establish high-quality evidence.

Artificial Intelligence and Precision Medicine

Personalized metabolic surgery and dietary therapies selection based on gut microbiome profiling and incretin response is under investigation.[31]

CONCLUSION

Bariatric surgery is continually advancing through the adoption of minimally invasive techniques, metabolic precision interventions, and the integration of artificial intelligence. Although conventional procedures such as RYGB and LSG are still considered the gold standards, new endoscopic and device-based therapies present viable alternatives for selected candidates.

Looking ahead, future developments are likely to focus on the modulation of the gut-brain axis, tailored surgical approaches, and the enhancement of weight loss sustainability.

REFERENCES

1. Bernadette C, Lim-Loo M, Huang CK, Chan V, Chua K. Sleeve-Plus Procedures in Asia: Duodenojejunal Bypass and Proximal Jejunal Bypass. In: Saiz-Sapena N, Oviedo M (Eds). Bariatric Surgery-From the Non-Surgical Approach to the Post-Surgery Individual Care. United Kingdom: IntechOpen; 2021.
2. Kermansaravi M, Parmar C, Chiappetta S, Shikhora S, Aminian A, Abbas SI, et al. Best practice approach for redo-surgeries after sleeve gastrectomy, an expert's modified Delphi consensus. Surg Endosc. 2023;37(3): 1617-28.
3. Clapp B, Ponce J, Corbett J, Ghanem OM, Kurian M, Rogers AM, et al. American Society for Metabolic and Bariatric Surgery 2022 estimate of metabolic and bariatric procedures performed in the United States. Surg Obes Relat Dis. 2024;20(5):425-31.
4. American Society for Metabolic and Bariatric Surgery. EASMBS Annual Meeting 2025 Exhibitor Information. [Online] Available from http://asmbs.org on 11/6/2025 [Last accessed March, 2026].
5. Velardi AM, Anoldo P, Nigro S, Navarra G. Advancements in bariatric surgery: a comparative review of laparoscopic and robotic techniques. J Pers Med. 2024;14(2):151.
6. Evans L, Cornejo J, Elli EF. Evolution of bariatric robotic surgery: revolutionizing weight loss procedures. Curr Surg Rep. 2024;12(6): 129-37.
7. Robert M, Pasquer A, Saber T. Robotic transit bipartition with sleeve gastrectomy: technical points. Obes Surg. 2022;32(6):2100-1.

8. Salgaonkar H, Sharples A, Marimuthu K, Rao V, Balaji N. One Anastomosis Gastric Bypass (OAGB). In: Lomanto D, Chen WTL, Fuentes MB (Eds). Mastering Endo-Laparoscopic and Thoracoscopic Surgery. Singapore: Springer; 2023.
9. Apovian CM, Shah SN, Wolfe BM, Ikramuddin S, Miller CJ, Tweden KS, et al. Two-Year Outcomes of Vagal Nerve Blocking (vBloc) for the Treatment of Obesity in the ReCharge Trial. Obes Surg. 2017;27(1):169-76.
10. Stavrou G, Shrewsbury A, Kotzampassi K. Six intragastric balloons: which to choose? World J Gastrointest Endosc. 2021;13(8):238-59.
11. Mauro A, Lusetti F, Scalvini D, Bardone M, De Grazia F, Mazza S, et al. A comprehensive review on bariatric endoscopy: where we are now and where we are going. Medicina (Kaunas). 2023;59(3):636.
12. Kota SK, Ugale S, Gupta N, Naik V, Kumar KV, Modi KD. Ileal interposition with sleeve gastrectomy for treatment of type 2 diabetes mellitus. Indian J Endocrinol Metab. 2012;16(4):589-98.
13. Hoyt JA, Cozzi E, D'Alessio DA, Thompson CC, Aroda VR. A look at duodenal mucosal resurfacing: rationale for targeting the duodenum in type 2 diabetes. Diabetes Obes Metab. 2024;26(6):2017-28.
14. Jaruvongvanich V, Vantanasiri K, Laoveeravat P, Matar RH, Vargas EJ, Maselli EB, et al. Endoscopic full-thickness suturing plus argon plasma mucosal coagulation versus argon plasma mucosal coagulation alone for weight regain after gastric bypass: a systematic review and meta-analysis. Gastrointest Endosc. 2020;92(6):1164-75.e6.
15. Heylen AM, Jacobs A, Lybeer M, Prosst RL. The OTSC®-clip in revisional endoscopy against weight gain after bariatric gastric bypass surgery. Obes. Surg. 2011;21(10):1629-33.
16. Maselli DB, Alqahtani AR, Abu Dayyeh BK, Elahmedi M, Storm AC, Matar R, et al. Revisional endoscopic sleeve gastroplasty of laparoscopic sleeve gastrectomy, an international, multicenter study. Gastrointest. Endosc. 2021;93(1):122-30.
17. Shah SS, Mutha S, Kharat SK, Kanani EAM, Abdalla M, Gerard A. A unique 10-year Indian Experience in Enhanced Recovery after Bariatric Surgery. J Bariatr Surg. 2024;3(1):12-6.
18. Smith TW Jr, Wang X, Singer MA, Godellas CV, Vaince FT. Enhanced recovery after surgery: A clinical review of implementation across multiple surgical subspecialties. Am J Surg. 2020;219(3):530-4.
19. Spanjersberg WR, Reurings J, Keus F, van Laarhoven CJ. Fast track surgery versus conventional recovery strategies for colorectal surgery. Cochrane Database Syst Rev. 2011(2):CD007635.
20. Bond-Smith G, Belgaumkar AP, Davidson BR, Gurusamy KS. Enhanced recovery protocols for major upper gastrointestinal, liver and pancreatic surgery. Cochrane Database Syst Rev. 2016;2:CD011382.
21. Messiah SE, Sacher PM, Yudkin J, Ofori A, Qureshi FG, Schneider B, et al. Application and effectiveness of eHealth strategies for metabolic and bariatric surgery patients: a systematic review. Digit Health. 2020;6:2055207619898987.
22. Dixon D, Sattar H, Moros N, Kesireddy SR, Ahsan H, Lakkimsetti M, et al. Unveiling the influence of AI predictive analytics on patient outcomes: a comprehensive narrative review. Cureus. 2024;16(5):e59954.
23. Janjua JI, Ghazal TM, Abushiba W, Abbas S. Optimizing patient outcomes with AI and predictive analytics in healthcare. 2024;1-6.
24. Saux P, Bauvin P, Raverdy V, Teigny J, Verkindt H, Soumphonphakdy T, et al. Development and validation of an interpretable machine learning-based calculator for predicting 5-year weight trajectories after bariatric surgery: a multinational retrospective cohort SOPHIA study. Lancet Digit Health. 2023;5(10):e692-702.
25. Choi PJ, Oskouian RJ, Tubbs RS. Telesurgery: Past, present, and future. Cureus. 2018;10(5):e2716.
26. Reddy SK, Saikali S, Gamal A, Moschovas MC, Rogers T, Dohler M, et al. Telesurgery: a systematic literature review and future directions. Ann Surg. 2024;282(22):219-27.
27. Gagner M, Abuladze D, Koiava L, Buchwald JN, Van Sante N, Krinke T. First-in-human side-to-side magnetic compression duodeno-ileostomy with the magnet anastomosis system. Obes Surg. 2023;33(8):2282-92.

28. Zhang G, Liang Z, Zhao G, Zhang S. Endoscopic application of magnetic compression anastomosis: a review. J Gastroenterol Hepatol. 2024;39(7):1256-66.
29. Khurana R, Pandey NN, Kumar S, Jagia P. Bariatric arterial embolization in patients with body mass index ranging from 25 to 40 kg/m^2: a systematic review & meta-analysis. J Cardiovasc Thorac Res. 2023;15(4):196-203.
30. Wang Z, Zhu DQ, Zhu XY, Liu DC, Cao QY, Pan T, et al. Interventional metabology: a review of bariatric arterial embolization and endovascular denervation for treating metabolic disorders. J Diabetes. 2023;15(8):665-73.
31. Chen J, Luo J, Pouwels S, Li B, Wu B, Abdelbaki TN, et al. Dietary therapies interlinking with gut microbes toward human health: past, present, and future. Imeta. 2024;3(5):e230.

SECTION 3

Diabetes Reversal/Remission

CHAPTER

8

Diabetes Remission/Reversal: Myth or Reality?

Pramod Kumar Thyparambil Aravindakshan, Viswanathan Mohan

ABSTRACT

Type 2 diabetes mellitus (T2DM) was earlier regarded as a chronic, progressive condition that inevitably required escalating therapy, often with insulin injections as well. However, emerging evidence suggests that remission of T2DM is achievable in selected individuals through intensive lifestyle interventions, weight loss, and bariatric/metabolic surgery. The American Diabetes Association (ADA) now recognizes Remission, defined as achieving glycemic targets without glucose-lowering therapy for a sustained period. The underlying mechanisms include reduction of hepatic and pancreatic fat, restoration of insulin sensitivity, and, in some cases, recovery of β-cell function. Trials such as the Diabetes Remission Clinical Trial (DiRECT) have shown remission rates approaching 50% at 1 year. In South Asians, even modest weight loss (2–5 kg) can induce remission, highlighting ethnic variations in response. However, despite these promises, long-term durability remains uncertain, with relapses to diabetes once the weight is regained. This chapter reviews the definitions, mechanisms, evidence, limitations, and future directions of diabetes remission, particularly from a South Asian perspective.

Keywords: Diabetes remission, reversal, prediabetes, type 2 diabetes mellitus, twin cycle hypothesis, South Asia

INTRODUCTION

Type 2 diabetes mellitus (T2DM) has historically been considered a lifelong disorder characterized by relentless progression. Standard teaching emphasized that patients would require lifestyle changes, oral hypoglycemic drugs, and eventually insulin. This paradigm fostered the belief that diabetes was "treatable but not curable."[1,2] However, recent advances challenge this dogma. A growing body of evidence demonstrates that T2DM can regress to a nondiabetic state under specific conditions. The American Diabetes Association (ADA) and the World Health Organization (WHO) now acknowledge remission as a legitimate therapeutic goal.[3,4] At the same time, there is considerable public hype around the concept of "reversal," often misused by commercial programs promising a "cure."[5-8] Thus, it is vital to examine whether diabetes remission is a myth or reality **(Flowchart 1)**.

DEFINITIONS AND TERMINOLOGY

The terminology surrounding diabetes remission and reversal has evolved. The term "reversal" implies a permanent cure, which is rarely achievable. The preferred term is "remission", analogous to cancer or psoriasis going into remission. According to the ADA 2021 consensus, remission is defined as glycated hemoglobin (HbA1c) < 6.5% for at least 3 months without any glucose-lowering therapy. Subcategories include partial remission (HbA1c < 6.5% for ≥1 year), complete remission (HbA1c < 5.7% for ≥1 year), and prolonged remission (≥5 years).[9] These definitions help standardize outcomes across clinical trials and clinical practice.

MECHANISMS OF REMISSION

The pathophysiological basis of remission centers on the twin cycle hypothesis, proposed by

Flowchart 1: Natural history of diabetes and remission.

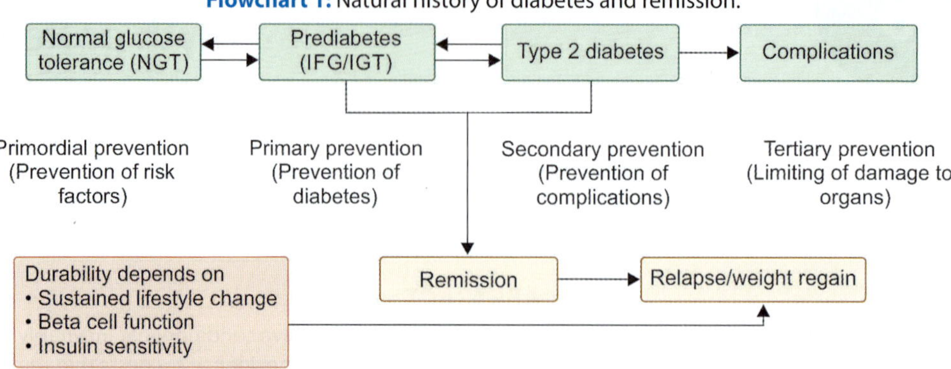

Taylor and colleagues.[10] Chronic positive energy balance leads to the accumulation of fat in the liver, resulting in hepatic insulin resistance and increased very low-density lipoprotein (VLDL) export.[11] This promotes ectopic fat deposition in the pancreas, impairing β-cell function. Profound negative energy balance, achieved by very low-calorie diets (VLCD) or bariatric surgery, reverses these cycles by reducing liver and pancreatic fat.[12] Fasting glucose levels often normalize within a week of calorie restriction, reflecting restored hepatic insulin sensitivity, while β-cell function recovers more gradually over 8–12 weeks.[13] In prediabetes, remission is driven largely by improved insulin sensitivity, whereas in T2DM, β-cell recovery is essential.[14,15]

EVIDENCE FROM CLINICAL STUDIES

Several landmark trials have established the feasibility of diabetes remission:

- The Diabetes Prevention Program (DPP, US),[16] Finnish Diabetes Prevention Study,[17] Da Qing study (China),[18] Indian Diabetes Prevention Programme (IDPP),[19] Diabetes Community Lifestyle Improvement Program (D-CLIP)[20,21] demonstrated that lifestyle intervention could prevent or delay T2DM in prediabetes.
- The DiRECT trial (UK) randomized individuals with T2DM of <6 years' duration to an intensive weight loss intervention delivered in primary care.[22] At 1 year, 46% achieved remission compared with 4% in controls. At 2 years, 36% remained in remission.[22]

The D-CLIP and Kerala DPP studies in India showed that even modest weight loss (2–5 kg) improved glycemic outcomes.[19-21] Bariatric surgery achieves remission in 60–80% of obese individuals with T2DM, though long-term relapse is common.[23] Collectively, these studies prove that remission is a clinical reality, although not universally achievable.

WHO ARE THE IDEAL INDIVIDUALS?

Not all individuals for remission with T2DM are suitable candidates for remission. The ABCDE mantra summarizes key characteristics of individuals with T2DM who can achieve remission.

- A: HbA1c not very high at baseline (e.g., <9%).
- B: Excess body weight/body mass index (BMI).
- C: Good insulin secretory reserve (as assessed by C-peptide).
- D: Short duration of diabetes (usually <8 years).
- E: Enthusiastic (highly motivated) individual

These criteria maximize the likelihood of remission. In patients with type 1 diabetes, fibrocalculous pancreatic diabetes, genetic symptoms, or advanced β-cell failure, remission of diabetes is much more difficult.

LIMITATIONS AND CHALLENGES

Despite the promise of remission, several challenges abound. Long-term durability of remission is limited: most studies report remission for 2–3 years, after which relapse (rereversal) is common if the body weight is regained.[24,25] Misleading commercial claims of a permanent cure can create unrealistic expectations.[26] Ethnic differences further complicate outcomes. South Asians achieve remission with modest weight loss but have limited β-cell reserve, increasing relapse risk.[27] Thus, while remission is possible, it requires sustained lifestyle adherence and regular medical monitoring.

PREDIABETES REMISSION: A WINDOW OF OPPORTUNITY

Prediabetes represents a stage of heightened risk but also a window of opportunity. Recent studies suggest that achieving prediabetes remission—defined as regression to normal glucose regulation—reduces the risk of incident T2DM by up to 73%.[28] In South Asians, even a 2.5–5 kg weight loss can induce remission. Mechanistically, this reflects improvements in insulin sensitivity before irreversible β-cell failure sets in.[29] Hence, targeting remission at the prediabetes stage could offer long-term protection of β-cell function and reduce diabetes incidence.

PUBLIC HEALTH AND POLICY IMPLICATIONS

If applied at scale, remission has the potential to transform diabetes care. It could reduce healthcare costs, medication burden, and complication rates. Primary care-led models, as in DiRECT, demonstrate feasibility. In India, mathematical modeling from the ICMR–INDIAB study suggests that reducing dietary carbohydrate by about 10–15% to about 50% of the calories and replacing this with protein could facilitate remission at the population level.[30] Digital health technologies,[31] mobile applications,[32] and structured coaching offer scalable tools for supporting lifestyle change.

FUTURE DIRECTIONS

Future research must clarify the long-term durability of remission and strategies to prevent relapses. Precision medicine approaches, including dietary personalization, microbiome modulation, and adjunctive use of pharmacotherapy,[33] may extend remission. Large multi-ethnic cohort studies are needed to capture variations in response. Integration of remission as a therapeutic goal in national diabetes guidelines will be crucial for widespread adoption.

CONCLUSION

Diabetes remission is no longer a myth—it is a reality for a subset of individuals with T2DM, particularly when diagnosed early and managed intensively. However, remission is not a cure. Sustainability is the key challenge, and relapses are common without continued adherence to healthy behaviors. For South Asians, where diabetes develops at younger ages and lower BMIs, remission strategies may require adaptation but hold promise even with modest weight loss. The future of diabetes care should embrace remission as a realistic, though conditional, therapeutic target.

REFERENCES

1. Mudaliar S. The evolution of diabetes treatment through the ages: from starvation diets to insulin, incretins, SGLT2 inhibitors and beyond. J Indian Inst Sci. 2023:1-11.
2. Ramachandran A, Snehalatha C, Mohan V, Viswanathan M. Remission in non-insulin dependent diabetes. J Med Assoc Thai. 1987;70(Suppl 2):185-9.
3. Shibib L, Al-Qaisi M, Ahmed A, Miras AD, Nott D, Pelling M, et al. Reversal and remission of T2DM: an update for practitioners. Vasc Health Risk Manag. 2022;18:417-43.

4. Birkenfeld AL, Mohan V. Prediabetes remission for type 2 diabetes mellitus prevention. Nat Rev Endocrinol. 2024;20(8):441-2.
5. Prasad V, Cifu A. Medical reversal: why we must raise the bar before adopting new technologies. Yale J Biol Med. 2011;84(4):471-8.
6. Lifestyle Desk. (2022). Can diabetes be reversed? Or is it remission? Indian Express. [Online] Available from https://indianexpress.com/article/lifestyle/health-specials/remission-reversal-type-2-diabetes-8323728/ [Last accessed March, 2026].
7. Salis S, Anjana RM, Unnikrishnan R, Syed S, Mohan V. Remission of type 2 diabetes: how, when, and for whom? J Assoc Physicians India. 2022;70:74-82.
8. Mohan V, Mukundan A. Remission of type 2 diabetes – what are the facts? In: Das AK, Shanmugavelu M, Saboo BD, Bantwal G, Ayyar VS (Eds). Challenging practical issues in T2DM – a dynamic approach. Bangalore: Microlabs; 2024. pp.117-22.
9. Nakhleh A, Halfin E, Shehadeh N. Remission of type 2 diabetes mellitus. World J Diabetes. 2024;15(7):1384-9.
10. Taylor R. The twin cycle hypothesis of type 2 diabetes aetiology: from concept to national NHS programme. Exp Physiol. 2025;110(7):984-91.
11. Heeren J, Scheja L. Metabolic-associated fatty liver disease and lipoprotein metabolism. Mol Metab. 2021;50:101238.
12. Juray S, Axen KV, Trasino SE. Remission of type 2 diabetes with very low-calorie diets: a narrative review. Nutrients. 2021;13(6):2086.
13. Sathananthan M, Shah M, Edens KL, Grothe KB, Piccinini F, Farrugia LP, et al. Six and 12 Weeks of Caloric Restriction Increases β Cell Function and Lowers Fasting and Postprandial Glucose Concentrations in People with Type 2 Diabetes. J Nutr. 2015;145(9):2046-51.
14. Sathish T. Precision prevention of type 2 diabetes: an approach to revitalize current lifestyle interventions. Diabetes Res Clin Pract. 2023;200:110722.
15. Thirunavukkarasu S, Taylor R, Khunti K, Tapp RJ, Raben A, Zhu R, et al. Low-calorie diets for people with isolated impaired fasting glucose. Commun Med (Lond). 2024;4(1):35.
16. Diabetes Prevention Program (DPP) Research Group. The Diabetes Prevention Program (DPP): description of lifestyle intervention. Diabetes Care. 2002;25(12):2165-71.
17. Lindström J, Louheranta A, Mannelin M, Rastas M, Salminen V, Eriksson J, et al. The Finnish Diabetes Prevention Study (DPS): lifestyle intervention and 3-year results on diet and physical activity. Diabetes Care. 2003;26(12):3230-6.
18. Gong Q, Zhang P, Wang J, Ma J, An Y, Chen Y, et al. Morbidity and mortality after lifestyle intervention for people with impaired glucose tolerance: 30-year results of the Da Qing Diabetes Prevention Outcome Study. Lancet Diabetes Endocrinol. 2019;7(6):452-61.
19. Ramachandran A, Snehalatha C, Mary S, Mukesh B, Bhaskar AD, Vijay V; et al. The Indian Diabetes Prevention Programme shows that lifestyle modification and metformin prevent type 2 diabetes in Asian Indian subjects with impaired glucose tolerance (IDPP-1). Diabetologia. 2006;49(2):289-97.
20. Weber MB, Ranjani H, Staimez LR, Anjana RM, Ali MK, Narayan KM, et al. The stepwise approach to diabetes prevention: results from the D-CLIP randomized controlled trial. Diabetes Care. 2016;39(10):1760-7.
21. Ford CN, Weber MB, Staimez LR, Anjana RM, Lakshmi K, Mohan V, et al. Dietary changes in a diabetes prevention intervention among people with prediabetes: the Diabetes Community Lifestyle Improvement Program trial. Acta Diabetol. 2019;56(2):197-209.
22. Lean ME, Leslie WS, Barnes AC, Brosnahan N, Thom G, McCombie L, et al. 5-year follow-up of the randomised Diabetes Remission Clinical Trial (DiRECT) of continued support for weight loss maintenance in the UK: an extension study. Lancet Diabetes Endocrinol. 2024;12(4):233-46.
23. Chandru S, Pramodkumar TA, Pradeepa R, Muthukumar S, Balasubramanyam M, Bhuvaneshwari R, et al. Outcomes of metabolic surgery in obese patients with type 2 diabetes with respect to impact on beta cell function, insulin sensitivity and diabetes remission - A study from south India. Diabetes Metab Syndr. 2020;14(6):1829-35.

24. Ried-Larsen M, Johansen MY, MacDonald CS, Hansen KB, Christensen R, Wedell-Neergaard AS, et al. Type 2 diabetes remission 1 year after an intensive lifestyle intervention: a secondary analysis of a randomized clinical trial. Diabetes Obes Metab. 2019;21(10):2257-66.
25. Noria SF, Shelby RD, Atkins KD, Nguyen NT, Gadde KM. Weight regain after bariatric surgery: scope of the problem, causes, prevention, and treatment. Curr Diab Rep. 2023;23(3):31-42.
26. Darke PR, Ashworth L, Main KJ. Great expectations and broken promises: misleading claims, product failure, expectancy disconfirmation and consumer distrust. J Acad Mark Sci. 2010;38(3):347-62.
27. Pramodkumar TA, Mohan V. Epidemic of cardio-metabolic disorders in South Asia: need for urgent solutions. Eur Heart J. 2025;46(29):2838-40.
28. Sandforth L, Kullmann S, Sandforth A, Fritsche A, Jumpertz-von Schwartzenberg R, Stefan N, et al. Prediabetes remission to reduce the global burden of type 2 diabetes. Trends Endocrinol Metab. 2025;36(10):899-916.
29. Sattar N, Welsh P, Leslie WS, Thom G, McCombie L, Brosnahan N, et al. Dietary weight-management for type 2 diabetes remissions in South Asians: the South Asian diabetes remission randomised trial for proof-of-concept and feasibility (STANDby). Lancet Reg Health Southeast Asia. 2023;9:100111.
30. Anjana RM, Srinivasan S, Sudha V, Joshi SR, Saboo B, Tandon N, et al. Macronutrient recommendations for remission and prevention of diabetes in Asian Indians based on a data-driven optimization model: the ICMR-INDIAB National Study. Diabetes Care. 2022;dc220627.
31. Kesavadev J, Krishnan G, Mohan V. Digital health and diabetes: experience from India. Ther Adv Endocrinol Metab. 2021;12:20420188211054676.
32. Ranjani H, Avari P, Nitika S, Jagannathan N, Oliver N, Valabhji J, et al. Effectiveness of mobile health applications for cardiometabolic risk reduction in urban and rural India: a pilot, randomized controlled study. J Diabetes Sci Technol. 2025;19322968241310861.
33. Pramodkumar TA, Pradeepa R, Jebarani S, Ganesan S, Pednekar A, Philips R, et al. Effectiveness of Glipizide and Glipizide Plus Metformin Formulation among Asian Indians with Type 2 Diabetes: a Real-World, Retrospective Electronic Medical Record Analysis. Drugs Real World Outcomes. 2025;12(3):457-66.

SECTION

4 Continuous Glucose Monitoring

CHAPTER 9

Continuous Glucose Monitoring: The Major Breakthrough in Glycemic Control

Banshi Saboo, Subhajyoti Ghosh

ABSTRACT

The monitoring and the euglycemia have never been debated since advancement of medical science. The advancement is also seen in the fields of monitoring for seeking euglycemia. It all started with Benedict's test in urine sample which was a spot test to continuous glucose monitoring. Continuous glucose monitoring (CGM) has become affordable along with better specificity to aid in daily living for people living with diabetes. Hence, this chapter will highlight the significance of CGM as a major breakthrough in life of people living with diabetes.

Keywords: Monitoring, euglycemia, CGM, living healthy with diabetes.

INTRODUCTION

The paradigm change has been witnessed in monitoring of diabetes from measuring urinary glucose to self-monitoring of blood glucose (SMBG) which eventually progressed to fulfill the unmet need, the continuous glucose monitoring. It provides estimated semi-continuous information about glucose levels via algorithms obtained from the level of interstitial fluid glucose, hence can track the pattern and trend during the period of its use. The merits and demerits of different monitoring technique are highlighted below in **Table 1**.

TABLE 1: Advantage and disadvantage of glucose monitoring technique.[1]

	Advantage	*Disadvantage*
SMBG	• Accurate measure of capillary glucose concentrations • Relatively inexpensive • Widely used and familiar	• Subject to user error and misrecorded data • Provides limited data at a single point in time • Multiple daily testing needed to effectively alter management and achieve good glycemic control (limited by patient tolerance)
CGM	• Provides a comprehensive picture of variations in glucose levels, including at times when they would normally not be measured (e.g., while sleeping, during exercise) • No "missed" readings • Provides a wide range of metrics to help guide and individualize diabetes management • Simple to use; sensor remains in place for several days • Pre-calibrated systems remove the need for daily finger-sticks	• More expensive than SMBG • Relatively complex to understand; requires training and time for familiarization • Needs high levels of compliance and interaction • Many models require multiple daily finger-sticks for calibration with SMBG • Sensor is always on the body; requires regular replacement (every 3–14 days, depending on model)

CONTINUOUS GLUCOSE MONITORING

Continuous glucose monitoring can assess the both inter and intraday fluctuations of glycemic trends. Continuous glucose monitoring (CGM) devices are minimally invasive by using a subcutaneous sensor coated with enzyme to measure interstitial glucose level, which are converted to blood glucose levels that are recorded and displayed. The readings are taken intermittently. The recorder is worn for 6–14 days based on CGM type used.

Continuous glucose monitoring has revolutionized diabetes management by providing real-time glucose monitoring. First introduced by Medtronic in 1999, CGM measures interstitial glucose every 1–5 minutes with a 4–10 minutes lag. It consists of a sensor, transmitter, and receiver. A sensor wire is inserted under the skin, transmitting glucose data via radio signals. Accuracy is maintained through periodic calibration using fingerstick blood glucose every 3, 5, or 7 days, depending on the system.

Continuous glucose monitoring is classified into blinded retrospective CGM (r-CGM) and real-time CGM (rt-CGM). R-CGM collects glucose data for therapy adjustments, while rt-CGM provides real-time readings with alerts for hypo/hyperglycemia. CGM is approved for individuals on multiple daily insulin doses, insulin pumps, or those with severe or unrecognized hypoglycemia. Three CGM types are available, viz., r-CGM, rt-CGM, and intermittent scanning CGM (isCGM). Rt-CGM continuously displays glucose data, while is CGM shows values when scanned. For the individuals with the risk of hypoglycemia, devices with alerts are recommended **(Table 2)**.

Continuous glucose monitoring can be used alone or integrated with an insulin pump as sensor-augmented pump (SAP) therapy. SAP with low glucose suspend (LGS) stops insulin for up to 2 hours during hypoglycemia and resumes upon recovery. In 2016, the FDA approved the first closed-loop system, MiniMed 670G, for patients of 14 years or older.

A hybrid closed-loop (HCL) system functions like an artificial pancreas, automatically adjusting insulin delivery based on CGM readings using a proprietary controller. Studies show HCL systems reduce hypoglycemia, especially at night, in both adults and children.

Flash glucose monitoring (FGM) system, newer innovation; provide real-time (RT) glucose reading and glucose trends with alarm to warn against hypoglycemia or hyperglycemia.

Currently available CGM are shown in **Table 3**.

TABLE 2: Difference between "retrospective" and "real time" flash glucose monitoring system.[2]

	Retrospective flash glucose monitoring	*Real time flash glucose monitoring*
Type of device	Personal use	Professional use
Sensor wear duration	Up to 14 days	Up to 14 days
Real time reading	No (retrospective)	Yes, with the scan of the sensor
How to get glucose reading?	The sensor needs to be brought to the clinic for reading	Patients can scan the sensor by themselves and get real time reading
Finger stick calibration	Not needed	Not needed
On-the-body equipment	Sensor applied by HCP, to be worn on back of patient's arm	Sensor applied by patients themselves, to be worn on back of patient's arm
Reader	HCP owned and stay in the clinic/office One reader can be used for multiple patients sensor	Patient owned one reader is paired with one sensor at a time

TABLE 3: Features of selected Food and Drug Administration (FDA)-approved and commercially available personal continuous glucose monitoring (CGM) systems.

	Dexcom G4 platinum	*Dexcom G5*	*Medtronic guardian sensor 3*	*FreeStyle libre*	*Dexcom G6*
MARD	13%	9%	9.1–10.6%	9.7%	9%
Warm up time	2 hours	2 hours	2 hours	1 hours	2 hours
Sensor wear duration	Up to 7 days	Up to 7 days	Up to 7 days	Up to 14 days	Up to 10 days
Calibration	Every 12 hours	Every 12 hours	Every 12 hours	None	None
Audible alarms, alert	Yes	Yes	Yes predictive alert	No	Yes hypoglycemia predictive alert
Labeling	Requires finger-stick confirmation	Nonadjunctive	Requires finger-stick confirmation	Nonadjunctive	Nonadjunctive
Pump integration	Animas vibe Tandem t:slim G4	Tandem t:slim X2	Medtronic MiniMed 670G hybrid closed-loop	None	Tandem t:slim Basal-IQ (PLGS)
Population	>2 years old	>2 years old	>7 years old	>18 years old	>2 years old
Acetaminophen interference	Yes	Yes	Yes	No	No

PATIENT SELECTION FOR CONTINUOUS GLUCOSE MONITORING

The 2024-25 AACE CGM Consensus recommends CGM use for individuals with type 1 diabetes (T1D) and specific characteristics, including hypoglycemia unawareness, frequent hypoglycemia, elevated HbA1c, or those requiring HbA1c lowering without increased hypoglycemia. It also supports CGM use for children and adolescents with T1D, regardless of HbA1c levels, if they are motivated and able to use the device. Additionally, CGM is recommended for individuals with type 2 diabetes (T2D) using insulin, particularly those with hypoglycemia or impaired hypoglycemia unawareness, and can be considered for those on sulfonylureas with hypoglycemia according to some experts.

For Type 1 Diabetes

- *Patients with hypoglycemia:* CGM is strongly recommended for individuals with T1D who experience hypoglycemic unawareness, frequent hypoglycemia (including severe episodes), or those whose HbA1c is above target.
- *HbA1c management:* CGM is also indicated for individuals with T1D who need to lower their HbA1c without increasing the risk of hypoglycemia.
- *Preconception and pregnancy:* CGM is recommended during the preconception period and throughout pregnancy for women with T1D.
- *Children and adolescents:* CGM is recommended for children and adolescents with T1D, especially those with HbA1c below 7.0% and those with HbA1c of 7.0% or higher who are able to use the device regularly.

For Type 2 Diabetes

- *Insulin users:* The AACE recommends considering CGM for individuals with T2D who are on insulin therapy, particularly those with hypoglycemia or impaired awareness of hypoglycemia.

- *Other medications:* Some experts suggest considering CGM for those with T2D taking sulfonylureas, especially if they experience hypoglycemia.
- *Audit of glycemic patterns:* CGM can be used as an episodic tool for auditing glycemic patterns in any person with T2D, regardless of medication, or for those wanting to understand the impact of diet and physical activity.

GENERAL CONSIDERATIONS

- *Individualized approach:* The AACE emphasizes that the choice of CGM device should be tailored to each patient's unique needs and circumstances.
- *Hospitalized patients:* In hospitalized patients with diabetes, the continuation of CGM and/or insulin pump therapy should be considered, especially if the patient is cognitively intact and has support from a knowledgeable family member or a specialized diabetes team.
- *Older adults:* For individuals 65 years of age and older with insulin-requiring diabetes, real-time continuous glucose monitoring (rtCGM) is recommended to improve glycemic control, reduce severe hypoglycemia, and improve quality of life, while still acknowledging the need for individualized goals due to potential comorbidities and reduced counter-regulatory responses.

ACCURACY OF CONTINUOUS GLUCOSE MONITORING SYSTEMS

Continuous glucose monitoring estimates blood glucose from interstitial fluid using algorithms, requiring periodic calibration with capillary glucose measurements. The time lag of approximately 7–8 minutes for adults with type 1 diabetes in fasting state[3] and 5–6 minutes in healthy individuals without diabetes.[4] Post-rigorous studies it has been stated in 2013 that minimum 95% of individual results should be within 15 mg/dL for blood glucose concentrations both ≤100 ± mg/dL and ≥100 mg/dL.

Continuous glucose monitoring accuracy is measured by mean absolute relative difference (MARD). A 4–10 minute lag exists between interstitial and blood glucose, which increases during rapid glucose changes, sometimes causing falsely high readings near hypoglycemia. Early CGMs had around 20% MARD, but advances have reduced it to a 9–14%. FGM has an 11.4% MARD, while the Dexcom G5 is under 10% **(Table 4)**.

Clinical applicability of CGM can be in the following situations:[6]

- T1DM
- T2DM on intensive insulin therapy those on MDIs or CSII therapy.
- T2DM patients experiencing repeated hypoglycemia, nocturnal hypoglycemia and or severe hypoglycemia
- Refractory hyperglycemia.
- GDM or diabetes in pregnancy

TABLE 4: Key metrics for continuous glucose monitoring (CGM) data analysis and reporting.[5]

Measures	*ATTD consensus*
Time in range • Default • Secondary	 70–180 mg/dL 70–140 mg/dL
Percentage of time in hyperglycemic range • Alert/elevated/monitor • Clinically significant/very elevated/immediate action required	 >180 (level 1) >250 (level 2)
Percentage of time in hypoglycemic range • Alert/low/monitor • Clinically significant/very low/immediate action required	 <70–54 (level 1) <54 (level 2)
Episodes of hypoglycemia/hyperglycemia (minimum no. of minutes) (with beginning and end of episode defined)	15 minutes

POSSIBLE BENEFITS OF CONTINUOUS GLUCOSE MONITORING[2]

- The monitoring helps in overall improvement of glycemic status.
- It helps to improve overnight glycemic control and prevent severe nocturnal hypoglycemia via alarms.
- The CGM reports used as educational tool for enhanced understanding of lifestyle management.
- Help in identifying alcohol-induced hypoglycemia patterns.
- Rt-CGM data can guide mealtime insulin dose, challenges with insulin timing and meal bolus.
- Continuous glucose monitoring data can help in identifying effects of complex meal on glucose levels.
- Help to manage exercise-induced hypoglycemia patterns.
- Continuous glucose monitoring data can identify the causes and effects of insulin stacking.

BARRIERS TO CLINICAL IMPLEMENTATION[7]

- The physician and clinical inertia
- Accuracy and precision
- Cost
- Sensor lifetime
- Calibration
- Commitment to intensive insulin therapy
- User experience
- Inconvenience
- Controversy regarding clinical benefits
- Lag time of interstitial fluid glucose relative to blood glucose.
- Inconsistent reporting of accuracy and precision of CGM sensors.
- Confusion regarding interpretation of glycemic variability.

COST-BENEFIT ANALYSIS OF CONTINUOUS GLUCOSE MONITORING

This chapter examines the cost-benefit analysis of CGM systems, which transform diabetes management by providing real-time glucose readings to help maintain optimal blood glucose levels.

Economic Impact

Continuous glucose monitoring systems can be costly due to device, sensors, and maintenance expenses, but their benefits, including fewer diabetes-related complications and hospitalizations, often justify the cost.

Effectiveness Studies

- *Canadian study:* A Canadian study using a Markov model found that universal CGM could result in 7,400 more people living without complications and 11,500 fewer deaths >20 years compared to SMBG. The incremental cost-effectiveness ratio (ICER) for CGM was CAD 35,017 per quality-adjusted life-year (QALY), showing CGM is cost-effective.[8]
- *Brazilian study:* A Brazilian study found that the FreeStyle Libre CGM system is cost-effective for insulin-treated Type 1 and T2D patients, with ICERs of R$ 26,267.69 per QALY for type 1 and R$ 39,692.67 per QALY for type 2. The study concluded that CGM reduces severe hypoglycemia and diabetic ketoacidosis events, enhancing quality of life.

Health Benefits

Continuous glucose monitoring shows significant improvement in glycemic control and reduction the risk of complications.

- *Improved glycemic control:* CGM systems offer continuous glucose feedback, enabling timely insulin adjustments and improved glycemic control. Users usually have lower HbA1c levels and fewer episodes of hyperglycemia and hypoglycemia compared to SMBG users.

- *Reduction in complications:* CGM users maintain optimal glucose levels, reducing the risk of complications such as retinopathy, nephropathy, and neuropathy, while also preventing acute issues such as severe hypoglycemia and diabetic ketoacidosis.

Quality of Life

Continuous glucose monitoring systems improve quality of life by reducing finger-prick tests and offering continuous monitoring, leading to higher user satisfaction, confidence, and overall well-being.[9]

RECENT ADVANCES IN CONTINUOUS GLUCOSE MONITORING

Soaring CGM and Insulin Pump use drives better Glycemic control: A pivotal John Hopkins study, published August 11, 2025, tracked nearly 2,00,000 individuals with type 1 diabetes from 2009 to 2023.

ADVANCES IN CONTINUOUS GLUCOSE MONITORING TECHNOLOGY

- *Improved accuracy and size:* Newer CGM systems, such as the Dexcom G7, offer enhanced accuracy (lower MARD values) and reduced size compared to previous generations. The Dexcom G7 combines sensor and transmitter in a single unit, making it smaller and more convenient, with a shorter warm-up period and extended wear time.[10]
- *Real-time data streaming and alerts:* CGM devices such as the FreeStyle Libre 3 provide real-time glucose readings directly to compatible smartphones, with customizable alerts and remote monitoring capabilities.
- *Extended wear time:* Some CGM systems, such as the FreeStyle Libre 2 Plus, offer longer sensor wear times (15 days), reducing the number of sensors needed per year.
- *Noninvasive CGM:* Research is ongoing into noninvasive CGM technologies, such as radiofrequency sensing, which could offer a less intrusive monitoring option.

ADVANCES IN INSULIN PUMPS

- *Automated insulin delivery (AID) systems:* AID systems, also known as hybrid closed-loop systems, integrate CGM data with insulin pump technology to automatically adjust insulin delivery based on glucose levels.
- *Hybrid closed-loop systems:* These systems require some user input, such as carbohydrate counting for mealtime boluses, but otherwise automate insulin delivery, simplifying management.[11]
- *Tubeless insulin pumps:* The Omnipod 5 is a tubeless, wearable insulin pump that connects wirelessly to a CGM sensor, offering a more discreet and convenient option.
- *Future innovations:* There is ongoing development of fully closed-loop systems that aim to be fully automated, mimicking the body's natural insulin response, and research into adjuvant medications that can further optimize glucose control when combined with AID systems.

IMPACT ON DIABETES MANAGEMENT

- *Improved glycemic control:* CGM and AID systems have consistently shown improvements in glycosylated hemoglobin (HbA1c) levels and time in range, while reducing hypoglycemic events.
- *Reduced burden of diabetes:* These technologies aim to reduce the burden of diabetes management by automating insulin delivery, minimizing the need for finger-prick

blood glucose testing, and providing more convenient monitoring options.[12]

- *Potential for remote monitoring:* Features such as remote monitoring capabilities in CGM systems facilitate communication between individuals with diabetes and their healthcare providers, enabling better support and management.[13]
- *Cost considerations:* While initial costs can be a barrier, CGM and AID systems have the potential to reduce long-term healthcare costs by preventing diabetes complications and hospitalizations.

The Food and Drug Administration approves longer-lasting insulin Dexcom CGM: G7 15-Day

The US FDA recently cleared the Dexcom G7 15-day CGM for adults, extending sensor wear time to 15.5 days. It also offers improved accuracy (MARD~8.0%) and includes a 12-hour grace period for replacement, enhancing user convenience and reducing disruptions.

KEY FEATURES AND IMPROVEMENTS

- *Extended wear time:* The G7 15-day system provides 15.5 days of wear, a 15% increase over the previous 10-day version.[14]
- *Improved accuracy:* The system boasts an 8.0% MARD, making it the most accurate CGM in its class, according to Dexcom.
- *User-friendly features:* It maintains features such as Apple Watch compatibility, automated meal, and activity logging, and a 12-hour grace period for sensor changes.
- *Integration with insulin pumps:* Dexcom is working with insulin pump partners to ensure compatibility with automated insulin delivery systems.
- *Hands-free operation:* The G7 15-day continues to offer a waterproof, hands-free design with continuous glucose level readings transmitted every 5 minutes.
- *Enhanced usability:* It allows for more comprehensive health monitoring with medication logging, in addition to activity and meal logging.

CLINICAL SIGNIFICANCE

- *Improved diabetes management:* The longer wear time and improved accuracy are expected to simplify diabetes management for users and empower them with more data for better control.
- *Reduced burden:* The extended wear time can reduce the monthly burden of sensor changes and waste.
- *Potential for increased access:* Healthcare providers are highlighting the importance of CGM access and education, with some advocating for it as standard care, which could drive higher usage and improved outcomes.

PROMISING NONINVASIVE CONTINUOUS GLUCOSE MONITORING DEVELOPED IN INDIA

Researchers at MNNIT Prayagraj and RMLIMS, Lucknow unveiled a noninvasive CGM that works without finger pricks. Placed between the thumb and index finger, this cost-effective device employs electromagnetic sensing to measure glucose in real time.

RECENT DEVELOPMENTS IN NONINVASIVE CONTINUOUS GLUCOSE MONITORING IN INDIA

- *Near-infrared (NIR) spectroscopy:* Researchers are exploring the use of NIR light to measure glucose levels noninvasively through the skin. This method involves analyzing how NIR light interacts with glucose in the interstitial fluid.
- *Mini-NIR device:* A specific example is a new mini-NIR device developed by researchers at

the SRM Institute of Science and Technology, which shows promise for accurate and painless glucose measurements.

- *Other technologies:* Other noninvasive methods being investigated include Raman spectroscopy, thermal emission spectroscopy, and microwave spectroscopy, among others.
- *Biosensors and wearables:* Research is also underway on biosensors and wearable devices that can integrate with smartphones for glucose monitoring, as well as on techniques such as impedance spectroscopy and sweat-based sensors.
- *AI and machine learning:* Machine learning models are being developed to analyze physiological signals and predict hypoglycemic events using data from wearable sensors.

CHALLENGES AND FUTURE DIRECTIONS

- *Accuracy and reliability:* Ensuring the accuracy and reliability of noninvasive glucose monitoring devices, especially in varying environmental conditions and for individuals with different physiological characteristics, remains a key challenge.
- *Regulatory approvals:* Obtaining regulatory approvals for these devices is another hurdle, as there are currently very few noninvasive CGM devices approved worldwide.
- *Integration with existing systems:* Integrating noninvasive CGM devices with existing diabetes management systems, such as insulin pumps, is crucial for effective diabetes care.
- *Data processing and analysis:* Further research is needed to improve data processing and analysis methods for optical glucose sensing techniques, as highlighted in a recent review.

CONCLUSION

Diabetes technology has revolutionized management by improving glycemic control, reducing complications, and enhancing quality of life. Despite higher initial and ongoing costs, technologies such as CGM systems, telemedicine and AI are cost-effective due to their health benefits and ability to reduce complications. These innovations justify the investment by improving outcomes and reducing the daily burden of diabetes management. Future advancements hold even more promise for improving care.

REFERENCES

1. Ajjan R, Slattery D, and Wright E. Continuous Glucose Monitoring: A Brief Review for Primary Care Practitioners. Adv Ther. 2019;36:579-96.
2. O'Connor C, and Aleppo G. Status of Continuous Glucose Monitoring Technology in Clinical Practice. In Draznin B, Edelman S, Hirsch IB, Klonoff DC (Eds). Diabetes Technology Science and Practice. Delhi: Knowledge Bridge Digital Learning Publishing; 2020. pp. 43-73.
3. Göke B, Fuder H, Wieckhorst G, Theiss U, Stridde E, Littke T, et al. Voglibose (AO-128) Is an Efficient α-Glucosidase Inhibitor and Mobilizes the Endogenous GLP-1 Reserve. Digestion. 1995;56:493-501.
4. Standl E, Schernthaner G, Rybka J, Hanefeld M, Raptis SA, Naditch L. Improved glycaemic control with miglitol in inadequately-controlled type 2 diabetics. Diabetes Res Clin Pract. 2001;51(3):205-13.
5. Danne T, Nimri R, Battelino T, Bregenstal RM, Close KL, DeVries JH, et al. International Consensus on Use of Continuous Glucose Monitoring. Diabetes Care. 2017;40:1631-640.
6. Chawla M, Saboo B, Jha S, Bhandri S, Kumar P, Kesavadev J, et al. Concensus and recommendations on Continuous glucose monitoring. J Diabetol. 2019;10:4-14.
7. Rodbard D. Continuous Glucose Monitoring: A Review of Success, Challenges and Opportunities. Diabetes Technol Ther. 2016;18(s2):3-13.
8. Siegel KR, Ali MK, Zhou X, Peng Ng B, Jawanda S, Proia K, et al. Cost-effectiveness of Interventions to Manage Diabetes: Has the Evidence Changed Since 2008?. Diabetes Care. 2020;43(7):1557-92.

9. Usoh CO, Kilen K, Keyes C, Johnson CP, Aloi JA. Telehealth Technologies and Their Benefits to People with Diabetes. *Diabetes Spectr.* 2022;35(1):8-15.
10. Yoo JH, Kim JH. Advances in Continuous Glucose Monitoring and Integrated Devices for Management of Diabetes with Insulin-Based Therapy: Improvement in Glycemic Control. Diabetes Metab J. 2023;47(1):27-41.
11. Rimon MTI, Hasan MW, Hassan MF, Cesmeci S. Advancements in Insulin Pumps: A Comprehensive Exploration of Insulin Pump Systems, Technologies, and Future Directions. Pharmaceutics. 2024;16(7):944.
12. Silva JD, Lepore G, Battelino T, Arrieta A, Castañeda J, Grossman B, et al. Real-World Performance of the MiniMed™ 780G System: First Report of Outcomes from 4120 Users. Diabetes Technol Ther. 2022;24(2):113-9.
13. Galindo RJ, Aleppo G. Continuous glucose monitoring: The achievement of 100 years of innovation in diabetes technology. Diabetes Res Clin Pract. 2020;170:108502.
14. Tucker ME. (2025). FDA Clears Dexcom G7 CGM for 15-Day Wear - Medscape - April 10, 2025. [online] Available from https://www.medscape.com/viewarticle/fda-clears-dexcom-g7-cgm-15-day-wear-2025a10008mx [Last accessed March 2026].

SECTION 5

Hypertension

CHAPTER 10

Innovations in Hypertension Management 2025

Rajeev Gupta

ABSTRACT

Uncontrolled hypertension is an important public health and clinical problem, and epidemiological studies have reported it in >75% of urban and 90% of rural populations. It is present in more than half of patients on BP lowering medicines. Implementation of step-wise BP management strategy provided by various national and international guidelines is important, and this can lead to BP control in almost 70–80%. Novel approaches for uncontrolled hypertension are available. These include using mineralocorticoid receptor antagonists (steroidal-spironolactone, eplerenone; nonsteroidal-finerenone), sacubitril-valsartan combination, and SGLT2 inhibitors in specific situations. Several biological agents are in phase-3 clinical trials and include aldosterone synthase inhibitors, angiotensinogen antagonist siRNAs, and hypertension vaccines. Renal denervation technology has now matured and is recommended in the European guidelines. This can be performed safely in resistant hypertension patients. Obesity interventions are gaining ground, and randomized clinical trials with bariatric surgery and antiobesity medicines (GLP1 receptor agonists) have reported consistent BP lowering and hypertension remission. Finally, the reduction of overall cardiovascular risk in hypertension is possible with statins, which should be prescribed in every moderate to high-risk individual with hypertension. Polypill studies have reported the usefulness of combining various cardioprotective medicines in a single pill. Lifelong adherence to hypertension therapy is the most difficult target, and support of technology and self-empowerment is crucial.

Keywords: Hypertension, resistant hypertension, renal denervation, SGLT2 inhibitors, obesity, cardiovascular risk.

INTRODUCTION

Hypertension or raised blood pressure (BP) is one of the most important risk factors for death and disease burden globally, as well as in India.[1,2] The status of hypertension control remains poor globally.[3] The situation is dismal in India and most lower-middle and low-income countries.[3] Studies from India have reported that less than half of patients with raised BP are aware of their hypertension status, about 40–50% are on treatment (lower in rural locations) and although more than half of patients with hypertension who are on treatment are under control, overall about 20–25% in urban areas and 8–12% in rural areas have controlled hypertension (<140/90 mm Hg).[4] This is despite the availability of very low-cost therapies for hypertension in our country.[5,6] Multiple strategies have been evaluated to change this state of affairs, including health policy and political interventions, focusing on social determinants of health, health-system-based approaches to promote chronic care, clinic-based approaches, and individual patient-centered interventions.[7,8] Clinic-based individual-patient-focused approaches are important as the more successful interventions can find a place in clinical practice and can translate into policies.[9]

In this review, we focus on recent innovations in pharmacological and other interventions in the management of hypertension. The interventions can be classified into two categories **(Table 1)**. In the present chapter, novel pharmacological and non-pharmacological approaches to manage difficult-to-treat hypertension or resistant hypertension are discussed. The other category of innovations is

TABLE 1: Innovations in hypertension management.

Pharmacological and other interventions	*Nonpharmacological advances*
• Medicines – *Old wine in a new bottle*: MRA – ARNI/ARB – SGLT2 inhibitors – Aldosterone synthase inhibitors – Angiotensinogen inhibitions, siRNAs – Endothelin receptor antagonists – Other biologics, vaccines • Interventions – Renal denervation – Other technologies • Obesity interventions – Bariatric surgery – GLP1 receptor agonists - Statins and Polypills for CVD risk reduction	• Strategies for diagnosis and detection – *Measurement technologies*: HBPM, ABPM, non-invasive – *New definitions and management targets*: ESH 2023, ESC 2024 – White-coat and masked hypertension – Resistant hypertension – Digital technology for target organ damage – Artificial intelligence • Adherence assessment and interventions – Noninvasive measurement technology – Drug adherence assessment – AI-based technologies

(ABPM: ambulatory blood pressure monitoring; ACEi: angiotensin converting enzyme inhibitors; ARB: angiotensin receptor blockers; CVD: cardiovascular disease; ESC: European Society of Cardiology; ESH: European Society of Hypertension; HBPM: home blood pressure monitoring; siRNA: small interfering RNA)

the availability of novel approaches for detecting, diagnosing and classifying hypertension, and strategies to promote adherence to BP-lowering medications, the major bug-bear in hypertension management. These developments are well discussed in the 2023 Guidelines of the European Society of Hypertension,[10,11] and not presented in this chapter.

STANDARD THERAPY

More than a century ago, it was recognized that raised BP was a significant contributor to cardiovascular diseases (CVD).[12,13] It was also demonstrated that raised BP can be reduced, and hypertension control can be achieved with the then extant medicines (reserpine, diuretics).[14] Following the early years, there have been rapid developments in the field of pharmacotherapy of this condition in the last few decades.[15] Multiple international and national guidelines for hypertension management and treatment, using stringent criteria, have been developed to inform practicing clinicians regarding appropriate use of drugs to achieve target BP: <140/90 by the World Health Organization (WHO) and Indian guidelines,[16,17] and <130/85 in the US and European guidelines.[18,19]

The drugs have broadly been classified into two categories—the first-line choices and supplementary drugs **(Table 2)**. Current guidelines recommend any of the first-line choices (except mineralocorticoid receptor antagonists (MRA) as the initial therapy for mild-to-moderate hypertension, either singly or as a single pill low-dose combination of 2–3 molecules.[10,16-19] Although 4-pill low-dose combinations are also available,[20] they have yet to find a place in the guidelines.[19] An important guideline is regarding the use of a single drug as monotherapy. The ESH 2023 guideline recommends that monotherapy should be reserved for use in either low-risk patients with mild hypertension (BP <150/95 mm Hg), high normal BP (BP 120–130/80) with very high CVD risk, frail individuals, or in advanced aged patients.[10] The ESH 2023 guidelines,[10] and Indian Society of Hypertension (InSH) guidelines,[16] also recommend that the single-pill combination should be taken in the morning, and

TABLE 2: Available drugs for hypertension management in India.

First line choices	*Supplementary choices*
Calcium channel blockers • *Dihydropyridine:* E.g. nifedipine, amlodipine, etc. • *Non-dihydropyridine:* E.g. verapamil, diltiazem *Angiotensin-converting enzyme inhibitors* • *First line:* E.g. enalapril, lisinopril, etc. • *Second line:* E.g., perindopril, ramipril, etc. Angiotensin receptor blockers • *First line:* Losartan, irbesartan, valsartan, etc. • *Second line:* Telmisartan, olmesartan, azilsartan, etc. *Beta blockers* • *Non-specific:* Propranolol, carvedilol, etc. • *Beta-2 receptor blockers:* Metoprolol, atenolol, bisoprolol, etc. • *Vasodilating:* Nebivolol *Diuretics* • *Thiazides:* Hydrochlorothiazide, etc. • *Thiazide like:* Chlorthalidone, indapamide, etc. • *Loop diuretics:* Furosemide, torsemide, etc. *Mineralocorticoid receptor antagonists* • *Steroidal:* Spironolactone, eplerenone, etc. • *Non-steroidal:* Finerenone, etc.	*Second line choices* • Direct renin inhibitors • *Alpha blockers:* Prazosin, doxazosin, etc. • *Central sympatholytic:* Clonidine, methyldopa, reserpine, etc. • *Direct vasodilators:* Hydralazine, minoxidil, etc. *Angiotensin receptor neprilysin inhibitors* • Sacubitril-valsartan *SGLT-2 inhibitors (adjunct)* • *Heart failure:* Dapagliflozin, empagliflozin, etc. • *CKD:* Canagliflozin, empagliflozin, etc.

CKD chronic kidney disease

to add further drugs if needed, with continued preference for single-pill combination therapies.

A step-wise approach has been recommended for the treatment of hypertension. Initial guidelines suggested ABCDE approach to hypertension management:[15] A = ACE inhibitors or ARBs, B = beta blockers, C = calcium channel blockers, D = diuretics, and E (extra drugs), using drugs shown in **Table 2**. However, after the publication of hypertension outcome trials that reported that BP lowering by any class of drugs is equally efficacious, all the international guidelines focus on BP control using any of the first-line classes of drugs. Beta-blockers have been part of the drug schema up to the 2010s, before they fell out of favor. However, with new data, there has been a re-emergence of this class of drugs, and the ESH 2023 guidelines suggest that they can be used at any level of hypertension **(Fig. 1)**.[10]

The ESH 2023 schema **(Fig. 1)**[10] is the most popular management algorithm, is widely used internationally, and has been recommended for Indian circumstances.[16] Resolve to Save Lives-Government of India algorithm is also important **(Table 3)** and can be used for the treatment of uncomplicated hypertension. This algorithm has been implemented in >10 states of India with an excellent record of efficacy.[21] ESH 2023 guidelines[10] have highlighted the fact that appropriate usage of first-line medicines can lead to hypertension control in 85–90% of the patients **(Fig. 1)**. Sadly, the prescription of these drugs in adequate doses by physicians and adherence to them by the patients is very poor.[6] We believe that these adherence-gaps need to be closed if better hypertension control rates are to be achieved in our country.

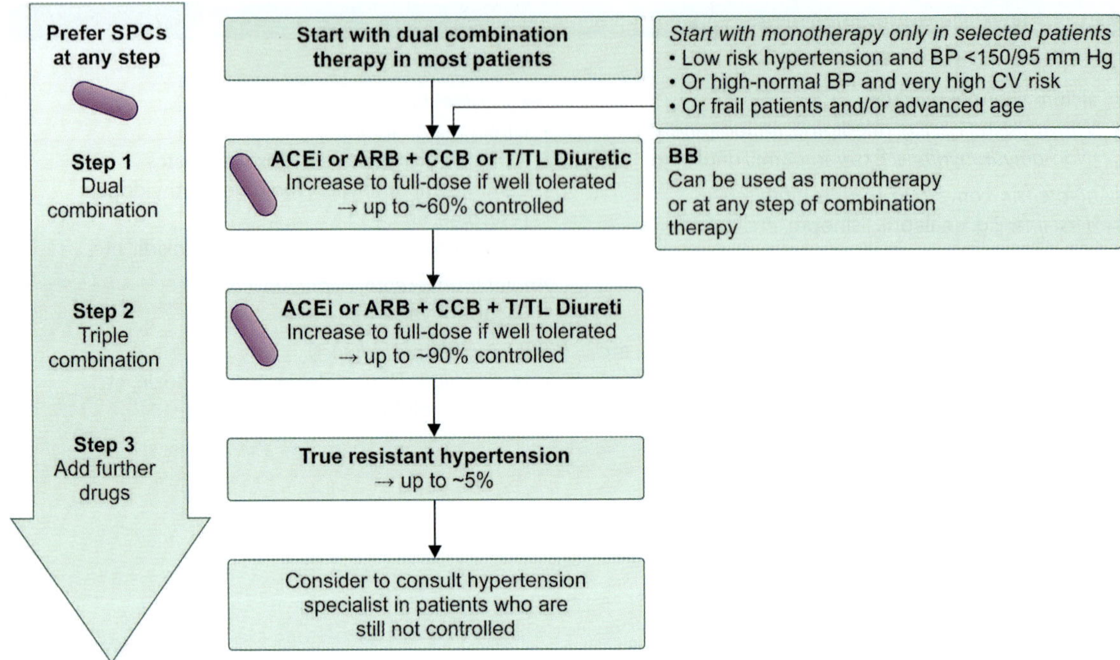

Fig. 1: European Society of Hypertension (ESH) 2023 treatment algorithm,[10] most suitable for India.

TABLE 3: India hypertension control initiative (IHCI) algorithm for blood pressure (BP) management in primary care.

	Time-frame	*Management strategy**
Stage 1	Screening	Screen all adults over a week. If BP >140/>90 mm Hg start treatment
Stage 2	Initiation	Tab Amlodipine 5 mg OD
Stage 3	Review in 1 month	If BP >140 or >90 mm Hg, increase amlodipine to 10 mg OD
Stage 4	Review in 1 month	If BP >140 or >90 mm Hg, add telmisartan 40 mg OD
Stage 5	Review in 1 month	If BP >140 or >90 mm Hg, increase telmisartan to 80 mg OD
Stage 6	Review in 1 month	If BP >140 or >90 mm Hg, add chlorthalidone 12.5 mg OD
Stage 7	Review in 1 month	If BP >140 or >90 mm Hg, increase chlorthalidone to 25 mg OD
Stage 8	Review in 1 month	If BP >140 or >90, refer to specialist

*Check compliance at every stage. OD once daily,

SECOND-LINE MEDICAL THERAPIES

Failure to control raised BP despite a proper prescription of medicines is a common occurrence. The ESH estimates that about 10% patients do not achieve the primary hypertension control target of BP <140/90.[10] More than twice these proportions fail to reach BP target of <130/80 mm Hg, the secondary target.[15-17] In real life this proportion is significantly greater and about half of patients in high income countries and less than a quarter in lower income countries achieve primary BP control target. This subgroup is the focus of intense research, as multiple issues can lead to poor BP control. They vary from a lack of focus on social determinants (poverty, illiteracy, etc.), absence of health care systems geared toward the management of long-term chronic conditions, physician-related factors (inappropriate choices) and patient-specific factors (adherence and compliance) and are beyond the scope of the present chapter.

Uncontrolled hypertension despite being on multiple medicines in appropriate dose is a common occurrence. Studies from India have reported that in tertiary-level specialist practices, poorly controlled hypertension is present in about 20% of the hypertension patient population.[22] Data from primary care in India report that less than a quarter of clinic-based hypertension patients have controlled BP. Treatment-resistant hypertension (TRH) is also an important problem. This is defined as uncontrolled BP despite the patient on at least three drugs (one of which is a diuretic) in the appropriate doses. A meta-analysis of the global data reported that one in seven patients with hypertension (about 14%) fits the definition of resistant hypertension.[23] Studies from India and most developing countries have reported TRH prevalence in 15–20%.[10] Multiple pharmacological therapies and other approaches are being evaluated in these patients and include the use of second-line and novel medicines **(Table 1)**.

Mineralocorticoid Receptor Antagonists

The MRAs have had a long history of use for diverse indications, ranging from congestive heart failure, hepatic cirrhosis, and resistant edema of multiple etiologies. In all these conditions, this class of drugs (spironolactone being the prototype) was used for potassium-sparing effects as these drugs act by binding to the mineralocorticoid receptors in kidneys, adrenals and peripheral tissues and inhibit aldosterone. These drugs prevent cardiac and vascular remodeling, decrease inflammation and improve proteinuria. They have been used in hypertension management for many years in combination with loop diuretics. However, multiple trials have reported benefits for the treatment of TRH and difficult-to-control hypertension.

Steroidal Mineralocorticoid Receptor Antagonists

Spironolactone and eplerenone are molecules approved for use in hypertension. Spironolactone is widely available in India and is an inexpensive molecule. Low-dose (25 mg/day) is effective for BP management, and higher doses (50–100 mg/day) are not required. Spironolactone has a shorter half-life (1.3–1.4 hours) than eplerenone (4–6 hours), but because the former is metabolized to three active compounds, it has a prolonged activity (14–16 hours). This is important in the presence of renal insufficiency when the dose must be reduced with a careful watch for hyperkalemia. It should not be used when eGFR is >30 mL/min/1.73 m^2.[10] Gynecomastia is an important side effect due to its antiandrogen actions and often necessitates drug discontinuation; eplerenone could be a choice in these circumstances as it has a lower incidence of gynecomastia.[10,19]

Nonsteroidal Mineralocorticoid Receptor Antagonists

The prototype of this class of drugs is finerenone. It has been intensively studied in patients with diabetic kidney disease to reduce the risk of renal function decline, cardiovascular deaths, nonfatal cardiac events, and heart failure hospitalization. This drug has lower affinity to other steroid hormone receptors than steroidal MRAs and has a lower incidence of gynecomastia, impotence and low libido. It can lead to hyperkalemia, and serum potassium levels should be monitored in cases of renal insufficiency. Although not yet recommended for use in resistant hypertension, similarities of mechanisms to steroidal MRAs prompt its inclusion as an antihypertensive drug. It has also been shown to be useful in heart failure with preserved ejection fraction (HFpEF). ESH 2023 guidelines conclude that this class of drugs may provide future alternatives to spironolactone in the treatment of resistant hypertension as they cause lower hyperkalemia and are useful in diabetic kidney disease and HFpEF.[10] ESC 2024 guidelines do not comment on nonsteroidal MRAs.[19]

Other (older) Classes

There are older drugs that can be used as supplements to standard drugs in uncontrolled hypertension **(Table 2)**. Many of them have specific indications for use in hypertension-associated comorbidities. For example, alpha-blockers are useful in renal failure-related hypertension, especially when symptoms of prostatism are present. Centrally acting drugs can be used in multiple situations, e.g., methyldopa in pregnancy, clonidine in sympathetic overactivity and renal failure, direct vasodilators in renal failure, and ganglion-blocking drugs in extreme TRH.

Sacubitril-Valsartan

The combination of angiotensin-receptor neprilysin inhibitor (ARNI) with valsartan is widely available for the treatment of heart failure across the spectrum of left ventricular ejection fraction (LVEF).[24] This combination blocks the effect of angiotensin II at the AT-1 receptor and inhibits degradation of natriuretic peptide, thus promoting peripheral vasodilatation. It was initially tried and used for hypertension, but following the exceptional success in the management of heart failure with reduced ejection fraction (HFrEF) in the PARADIGM-HF trial, the focus shifted to heart failure management.[25] A meta-analysis of 10 randomized controlled studies involving 5,931 patients reported that this combination was better than combinations of valsartan or olmesartan and amlodipine for hypertension management. It is approved for BP management in China and Japan, but not in the US or Europe.[10]

Sodium-glucose Cotransporter-2 Inhibitors

Another success story in CVD risk reduction in type-2 diabetes has been sodium-glucose cotransporter (SGLT-2) inhibitors.[10,19] These drugs are widely used in type 2 diabetes and, in addition, have found a place in the management of heart failure across the spectrum of LVEF.[26,27] Studies have shown that these drugs have mild-to-moderate antihypertensive effects. The ESC 2024 guidelines recommend this class of drugs with the level of evidence class I and strength of recommendation A (strongest possible) for two indications: (A) hypertension and chronic kidney disease, and eGFR >20 mL/min/1.73 m^2 to improve outcomes in the context of their modest BP lowering properties, and (B) hypertension with HFrEF, HFpEF, or HFmrEF in conjunction with ARBs or ACE inhibitors, beta blockers and MRAs, and symptomatic HFpEF to improve outcomes due to modest BP lowering properties.[19]

NEW APPROACH: BIOLOGICS

Aldosterone Synthase Inhibitors

This brand-new class of drugs has evolved due to multiple cardiovascular and renal benefits that have resulted from renin-angiotensin-aldosterone system (RAAS) based therapies.[28] The inhibition of aldosterone synthesis is an option to reduce the deleterious effects of aldosterone excess. Aldosterone production

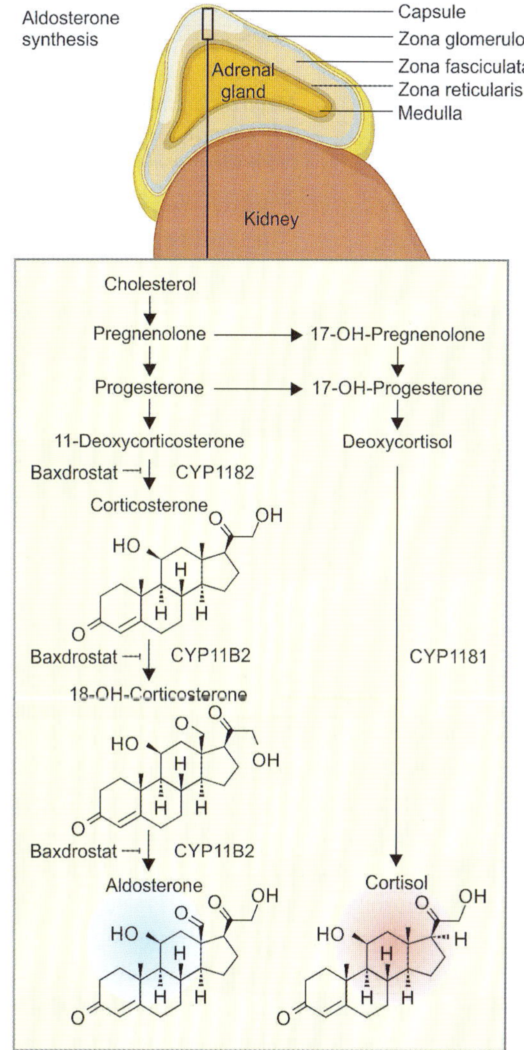

Fig. 2: Mechanisms of action of aldosterone synthase inhibitors (baxdrostat).

is controlled by the regulated transcription of *CYP11B2*, which encodes aldosterone synthase in the adrenal zona glomerulosa. This class of drugs block the conversion of cholesterol to aldosterone at multiple levels—conversion of 11-deoxycorticosterone to corticosterone, corticosterone to 18-OH-corticosterone and 18-OH corticosterone to aldosterone **(Fig. 2)**.[29] Three prototype drugs have been evaluated in phase-2 clinical trials—baxdrostat, lorundrostat, and dexfadrostat.

In preclinical and phase 1 studies, baxdrostat had 100:1 selectivity for enzyme inhibition, and baxdrostat at several dose levels reduced plasma aldosterone levels but not cortisol levels. A phase 2 trial of baxdrostat (BrigHTN), showed promising results.[30] A total of 248 patients completed the trial. Dose-dependent changes in systolic BP of –20.3 mm Hg, –17.5 mm Hg, –12.1 mm Hg, and –9.4 mm Hg were observed in the 2-mg, 1-mg, 0.5-mg, and placebo groups, respectively. It was concluded that baxdrostat in patients with TRH had dose related reduction in BP. The BP reduction was associated with decrease in plasma aldosterone level and a compensatory increase in plasma renin activity, without a reduction in the cortisol level. It had an acceptable side-effect profile, and none of the patients discontinued the trial because of hyperkalemia.

In phase-2 trial of more selective aldosterone synthase inhibitors (ASI) (lorundrostat) it was concluded that among individuals with uncontrolled hypertension, use of this drug was effective at lowering BP compared with placebo. In this study (TARGET-HTN), 200 participants were randomized. Following 8 weeks of treatment, changes in office systolic BP of –14.1, –13.2, –6.9, and –4.1 mm Hg were observed with 100 mg, 50 mg, and 12.5 mg once daily of lorundrostat and placebo, respectively. Observed reductions in systolic blood pressure in individuals receiving twice-daily doses of 25 mg and 12.5 mg of lorundrostat were –10.1 and –13.8 mm Hg, respectively.[31] Another phase 2b trial with lorundrostat has been conducted and showed that 50 mg/day reduced ambulatory BP by 6.5 mm Hg with this drug at 3 months.[32] There was greater incidence of hyperkalemia than placebo, though the proportion was lower than MRAs. Confirmatory phase-3 studies are planned. Phase 2 crossover study of another ASI, dexfadrostat, was conducted in 35 participants.

TABLE 4: Aldosterone synthase inhibitors—meta-analysis of phase-2 trials.

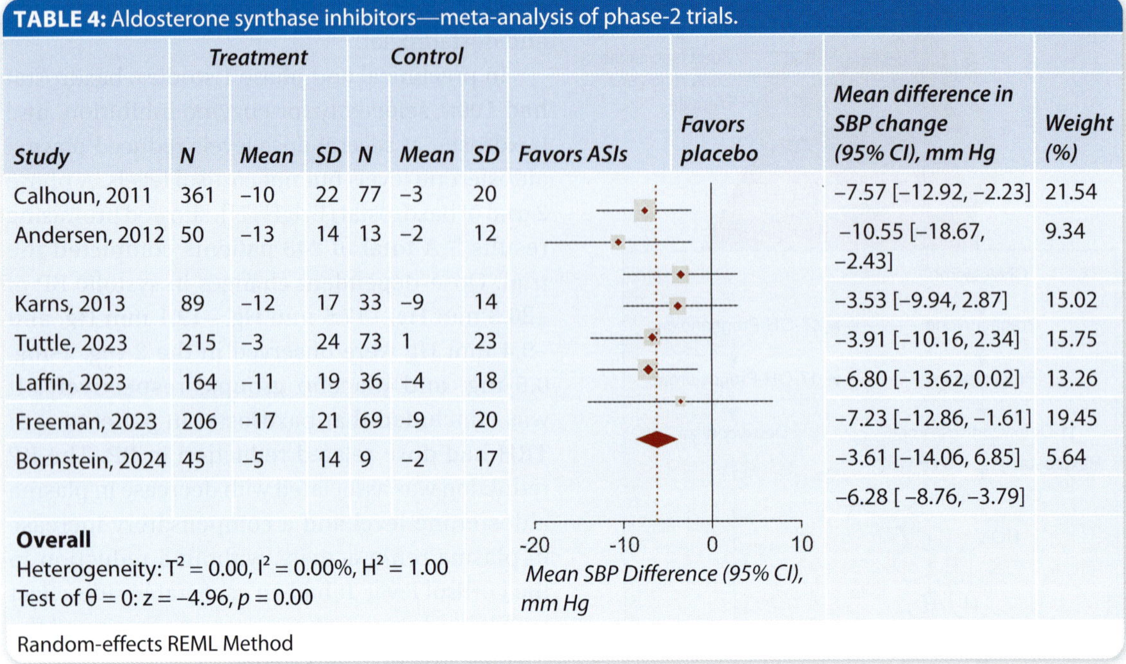

	Treatment			*Control*						
Study	*N*	*Mean*	*SD*	*N*	*Mean*	*SD*	*Favors ASIs*	*Favors placebo*	*Mean difference in SBP change (95% CI), mm Hg*	*Weight (%)*
Calhoun, 2011	361	−10	22	77	−3	20			−7.57 [−12.92, −2.23]	21.54
Andersen, 2012	50	−13	14	13	−2	12			−10.55 [−18.67, −2.43]	9.34
Karns, 2013	89	−12	17	33	−9	14			−3.53 [−9.94, 2.87]	15.02
Tuttle, 2023	215	−3	24	73	1	23			−3.91 [−10.16, 2.34]	15.75
Laffin, 2023	164	−11	19	36	−4	18			−6.80 [−13.62, 0.02]	13.26
Freeman, 2023	206	−17	21	69	−9	20			−7.23 [−12.86, −1.61]	19.45
Bornstein, 2024	45	−5	14	9	−2	17			−3.61 [−14.06, 6.85]	5.64
									−6.28 [−8.76, −3.79]	

Overall
Heterogeneity: $T^2 = 0.00$, $I^2 = 0.00\%$, $H^2 = 1.00$
Test of $\theta = 0$: $z = -4.96$, $p = 0.00$

Random-effects REML Method

It was found that this molecule corrected the aldosterone to renin ratio in patients with primary aldosteronism and corrected ambulatory BP in these patients.[33] A meta-analysis of all phase-2 studies of ASI has been conducted **(Table 4)**.[34] The study shows that ASIs reduce mean systolic BP by 6.28 mm Hg (95% CI 3.79–8.76) when used in combination of usual drugs for BP lowering.[34] Baxdrostat is in phase 3 trials. The ESH 2023 guidelines are optimistic regarding this class of drugs but strongly recommend phase-3 trials with larger cohorts and extended follow-up to determine the potential role of ASIs in clinical practice, including their role in long-term cardiovascular and renal impact.

Angiotensinogen Inhibition

Zilebesiran is a small interfering RNA (siRNA) designed to target the liver and is the newest addition to the renin-angiotensin-aldosterone system-inhibiting drugs. This subcutaneous injection posttranscriptionally silences the *AGT* gene responsible for the synthesis of angiotensinogen.[30] By preventing the progenitor protein of the renin-angiotensin-aldosterone system, zilebesiran blocks the downstream production of angiotensin II, which plays multiple roles in hypertension pathogenesis. Phase I clinical trials have demonstrated a dose-dependent efficacy of zilebesiran with BP lowering and serum angiotensinogen levels.[35] Sustained effects last for 6 months. Researchers also demonstrated a promising safety profile, as most of the adverse events were mild-to-moderate in nature. Phase II trials assessing efficacy and optimal dosing have also been performed. In a randomized controlled trial with 750+ participants with hypertension, Bakris et al.[36] reported significant BP lowering efficacy of zilebesiran at 3-months post-subcutaneous injection of 150 mg (−7.3 mm Hg), 300 mg (−10.0 mm Hg) and 600 mg (−8.9 mm Hg) as compared to placebo (+6.8 mm Hg (p <0.001). Phase 3 trials of this drug are underway and promising results of phase-2 trials pave the way

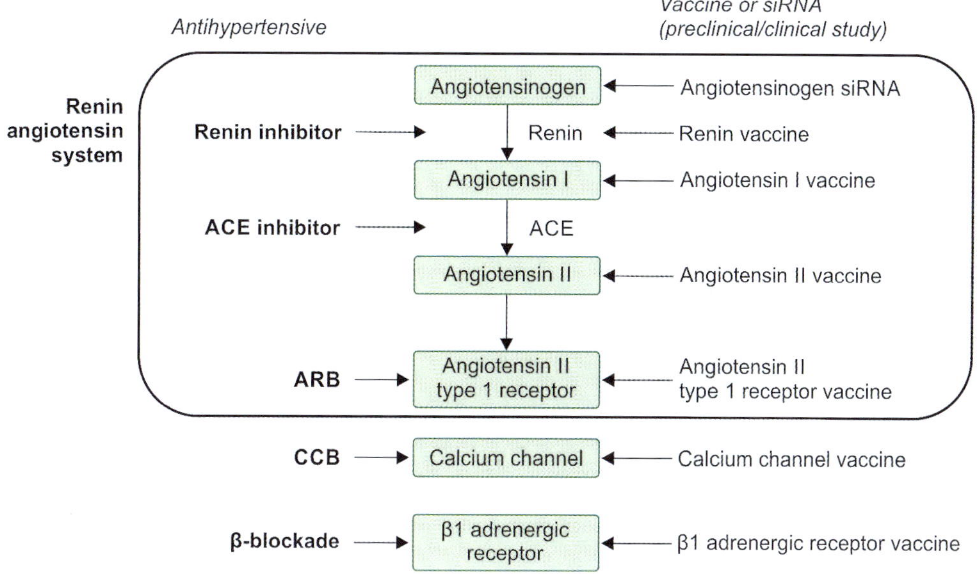

Fig. 3: Vaccines or siRNAs development for hypertension.

for periodic long-term injectable formulations in hypertension management. Cost of the therapy would be an important consideration, and formal cost-effectiveness analyses shall have to be performed before this, or similar molecules are widely used in clinical practice.

Hypertension Vaccines

This is also a biological approach for hypertension management, and as a form of immunotherapy, therapeutic vaccines have been researched in animal models for almost 50 years.[37] Most of such vaccines target the RAAS, but preclinical and phase 1 and 2 trials have produced discordant results. Vaccines for L-type calcium channel blockers have also been researched in animal models. More recently, vaccines that target beta-1 adrenergic receptors have been developed and show prevention of sympathetic stimulation-induced vascular remodeling and myocardial fibrosis **(Fig. 3)**.[38]

The target molecules for hypertension treatment are the renin-angiotensin system (angiotensinogen, angiotensin I or II, angiotensin II type 1 receptor), L-type calcium channels and β1 adrenergic receptors. The major antihypertensive drugs are renin inhibitors, ACE inhibitors, ARBs, CCBs, and β blockers. The current challenge is to develop vaccines or siRNAs for the same target molecules.[38] This is still an active area of research, and the availability of technologies for vaccine development for COVID-19 will likely catalyze hypertension vaccines.

RENAL DENERVATION THERAPY

Renovascular interventions for hypertension have had a long history. Percutaneous transluminal renal angioplasty (PTRA) has long been used for the management of secondary hypertension due to renal artery stenosis in the young. PTRA has also been used for atherosclerotic renal artery stenosis in the elderly as well as in patients with Takayasu's arteriopathy and renal arterial stenosis. A paradigm shift was the finding that radiofrequency ablation of renal arterial nerves could reduce BP. Initial preclinical

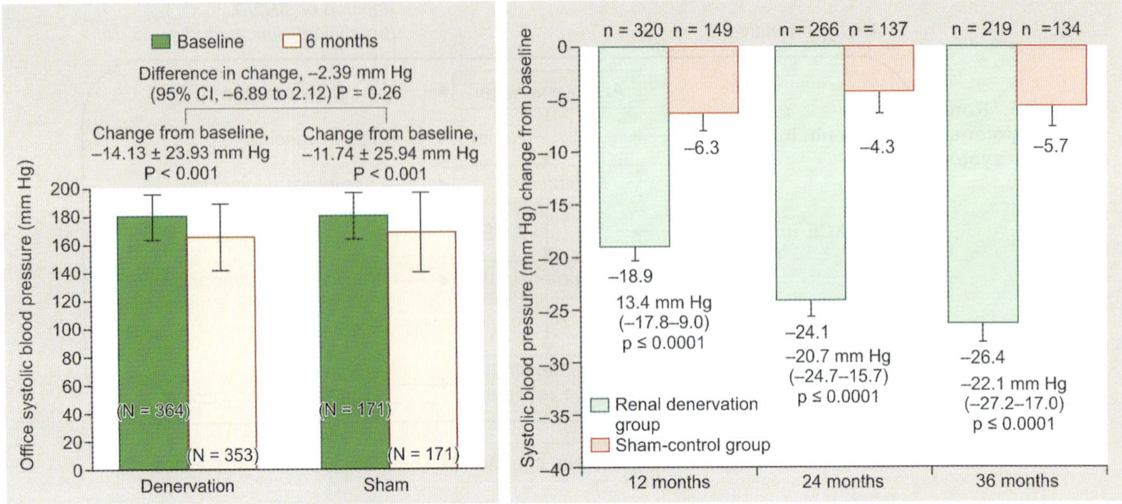

Fig. 4: Blood pressure lowering at 6 months and 36 months in the SIMPLICITY-3 trial.

trials used radiofrequency ablation of bilateral renal arterial nerves using thermal devices in a circumferential energy delivery. Multiple modifications were made to this technology, and this was successfully deployed in individuals with resistant hypertension in Europe and the USA. A significant lowering of BP, on top of medications, was observed in nonrandomized studies.[39]

In a well-conducted sham-controlled trial using this technology, SIMPLIICITY-HTN-3, did not produce significant results at 3 months follow-up **(Fig. 4)**.[40] At 6 months post-intervention, the mean reduction in office systolic BP in the intervention group was -14.1 ± 23.9 mm Hg, while it was 11.7 ± 25.9 mm Hg in the sham-controlled group **(Fig. 4)**. Prespecified follow-up of participants in this study, however, continued to show an increasingly lower systolic BP, which was in intervention versus control groups was -13.4 versus -6.3 mm Hg at 12 months, -20.7 versus -4.3 mm Hg at 24 months, and -26.4 versus -5.7 mm Hg at 36 months.[41] Meanwhile, recent randomized studies using a controlled design continue to show significantly better BP lowering in resistant hypertension **(Fig. 5)**.[39] The energy-delivery device has changed and spiral technology with ultrasound energy is being used. This technology is now well established and both the ESH 2023 and ESC 2024 guidelines have endorsed it with grade 2A recommendation.[10,19]

In India, this is an expensive technology and has a limited scope in patients with severely resistant hypertension,[42] and anecdotal evidence suggests that it is useful.[43] A recent review has summarized that renal denervation therapy has been evaluated in patients with mild, moderate or resistant hypertension; on average, it lowers BP to a similar degree as an effective antihypertensive medication **(Fig. 5)**. Both the ultrasound and radiofrequency devices can be used as an adjunctive treatment when lifestyle modifications and medications are not sufficient to control BP. It is advised that an appropriate patient selection is crucial, with a comprehensive evaluation ensuring that patients have sustained, uncontrolled hypertension and that secondary causes are appropriately investigated. Safe and appropriate implementation of RDN requires multidisciplinary teams, including hypertension specialists and well-trained interventionalists, to ensure proper evaluation, treatment and follow-up.[39,44]

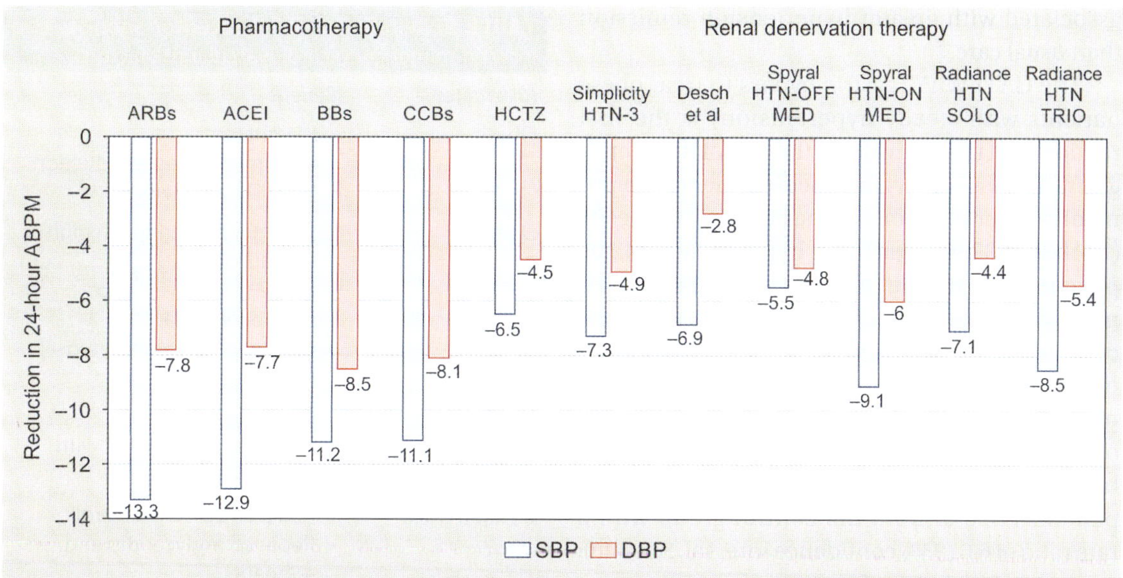

Fig. 5: Efficacy of various renal denervation techniques for lowering BP and comparison with usual BP-lowering medicines.

Source: Messerli FH, Bavushi C, Brguljan J, Burnier M, Dobner S, Elijovich F, et al. Renal denervation in the antihypertensive arsenal: knowns and known unknowns. Hypertension. 2022;40:1859-75.[39]

OBESITY MANAGEMENT: BARIATRIC SURGERY AND DRUGS

There is a direct correlation between increasing obesity and BP, both systolic and diastolic.[12,15] This has been known for decades and epidemiological studies in India have clearly demonstrated a linear relationship of BMI with systolic BP in urban and rural populations.[45] Of interest is the causal relationship of obesity with hypertension. Earlier studies failed to demonstrate this relationship due to a lack of strategies that reduced BMI significantly and persistently over a long period of time. Two interventions have been deployed for weight management and weight loss among the obese (BMI >35 kg/m^2) in recent years:[46,47] (1) bariatric surgery using sleeve gastrectomy or Roux-en-Y gastroduodenal bypass; and (2) GLP1 receptor agonists (GLP1RA) class of incretin mimetics drugs.

Bariatric Surgery

Post-hoc analysis of the STAMPEDE trial, which was a bariatric surgery trial for diabetes management in obese individuals, did not show significant BP changes despite persistent and highly significant weight loss at the end of 5 years.[47] On the other hand, in a retrospective Kaiser Permanente study there were 9,432 patients with hypertension 21–65 years old who underwent bariatric surgery during 2005–2015 and 66,651 nonsurgical matched controls. At 5 years, the unadjusted cumulative incidence of hypertension remission was 60% [95% confidence interval (CI), 58–61%] among surgery patients and 14% (95% CI, 13–14%) among controls. At 1 year, the adjusted hazard ratio for the association of bariatric surgery with hypertension remission was 10.24 (95% CI, 9.61–10.90). At 5 years, the adjusted hazard ratio was 2.10 (95% CI, 1.57–2.80). This study showed that bariatric surgery was associated with greater hypertension remission than usual care.[48]

The GATEWAY (gastric bypass to treat obese patients with steady hypertension) is the first randomized trial to evaluate the role of Roux-en-Y gastric bypass surgery and medical therapy versus medical therapy alone in patients with obesity (BMI 30.0–39.9 kg/m^2) and hypertension. 4,100 patients (70% female, mean age 43.8 ± 9.2 years, mean body mass index 36.9 ± 2.7 kg/m^2), and 96% completed a 12-month follow-up.[49] Reduction of ≥30% of the total number of antihypertensive medications while maintaining controlled BP occurred in 41 of 49 patients from the gastric bypass group (83.7%) compared with 6 of 47 patients (12.8%) from the control group with a rate ratio of 6.6 (95% confidence interval, 3.1–14.0; $p < 0.001$). Remission of hypertension was present in 25 of 49 (51%) and 22 of 48 (45.8%) patients randomized to gastric bypass, considering office and 24-hour ambulatory BP monitoring, respectively, whereas no patient submitted to medical therapy was free of antihypertensive drugs at 12 months. Final results of the GATEWAY trial have recently been published.[50] At 5-years, compared with medical therapy in the gastric-bypass surgery group there was a significantly higher rate of medication reduction (80.7% vs. 13.7%; relative risk: 5.91; 95% CI: 2.58–13.52; $p < 0.001$). The rates of hypertension remission were 2.4% versus 46.9% (relative risk: 19.66; 95% CI: 2.74–141.09; $p < 0.001$). Interestingly, the rate of apparent resistant hypertension was lower after gastric bypass surgery (0% vs. 15.2%). Larger studies are required to confirm these astounding findings. Meanwhile, it would be important to discuss the role of bariatric surgery for BP lowering in obese (BMI 30.0–39.9 kg/m^2) patients in our practice.

TABLE 5: Benefits of GLP-1 receptor agonists and incretin-mimetics on cardiovascular risk factors.

Risk factor	*Benefit*
Obesity	• Weight loss • Abdominal obesity reduction • MASLD management
Diabetes	• Diabetes prevention in high-risk individuals • Prediabetes reversal to normoglycemia • Control of glycemia in type-2 diabetes
Hypertension	• BP reduction • Hypertension reversal with weight loss
Dyslipidemia	• Reduced LDL cholesterol • Reduced triglycerides and remnants
Tobacco use	Smoking reduction
Inflammation	Decrease in hsCRP
Obstructive sleep apnea	Reduced apnea-hypopnea indices

(GIP: glucose-dependent insulinotropic peptide; GLP-1: glucagon like peptide-1; LDL: low density lipoprotein; MASLD: metabolism-associated steatotic liver disease)

Glucagon-like Peptide-1 Receptor Agonists

Recent trials with antiobesity drugs-glucagon-like peptide-1 (GLP-1) and dual GLP-1 and GIP (glucose-dependent insulinotropic polypeptide) receptor agonists have provided persuasive evidence of reduction in multiple cardiovascular risk factors, including hypertension.[51] Second-generation GLP1-RA's—liraglutide and semaglutide, have been overtaken by dual and triple incretin mimetics-tirzepatide and retatrutide. In randomized controlled trials, these molecules have reported significant weight reduction, along with control of hyperglycemia (with diabetes reversal), hypertension, hypercholesterolemia, obstructive sleep apnea (OSA) and metabolism-associated steatotic liver disease (MASLD) **(Table 5)**.[52-59] Hypertension control efficacy of these drugs has not been well discussed.[60]

We charted the systolic and diastolic BP-lowering efficacy reported in various

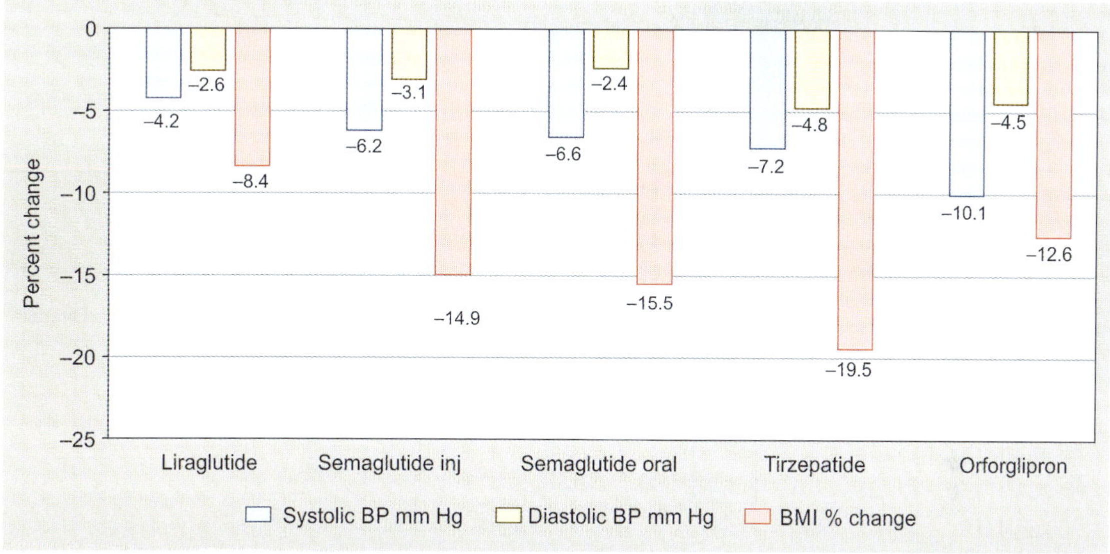

Fig. 6: Association of weight loss (% BMI) with absolute reduction in systolic and diastolic BP (mm Hg) in the intervention group in various GLP1RA trials.

GLP1RA randomized controlled trials.[52-56,59] All the trials reported significant weight loss, which was significantly more with recent GLP1RA compounds (semaglutide, tirzepatide, retatrutide, etc.). The decline of mean systolic and diastolic BP (absolute change from baseline in the intervention group) is also shown and corresponds to per cent weight loss **(Fig. 6)**. The BP-lowering efficacy of these drugs was significantly greater than placebo groups in all these trials.

Before GLPIRAs and other incretin mimetics are used for hypertension management, we need focused randomized clinical trials with cardiovascular outcomes. It is recommended that, for the present, these incretin mimetic molecules should be taken for approved indications (type 2 diabetes with obesity) only.

CARDIOVASCULAR RISK REDUCTION: STATINS AND POLYPILLS

Blood pressure control is important to prevent CVD events, however, a substantial residual risk remains. Strategies to ameliorate the residual risk include adherence to healthy lifestyles (physical activity, healthy diet, sodium restriction, potassium supplementation, weight management, and tobacco and alcohol avoidance), lipid-lowering with statins, and polypills.[61]

Lipid Management (Statins)

Low density lipoprotein cholesterol lowering is of crucial importance for CHD prevention in hypertension. Clinical trials and meta-analyses have consistently reported the benefits of LDL cholesterol lowering by drugs and the adoption of healthy lifestyles on CVD events, CVD deaths, and all-cause deaths.[62] There are only a few studies that have reported the benefits of LDL lowering with statins in uncomplicated low to moderate risk patients with hypertension. In the lipid-lowering arm of US-based ALLHAT study of >10,000 patients with hypertension who were randomized to pravastatin versus placebo, there were insignificant differences in cardiovascular events, CHD deaths or all-cause

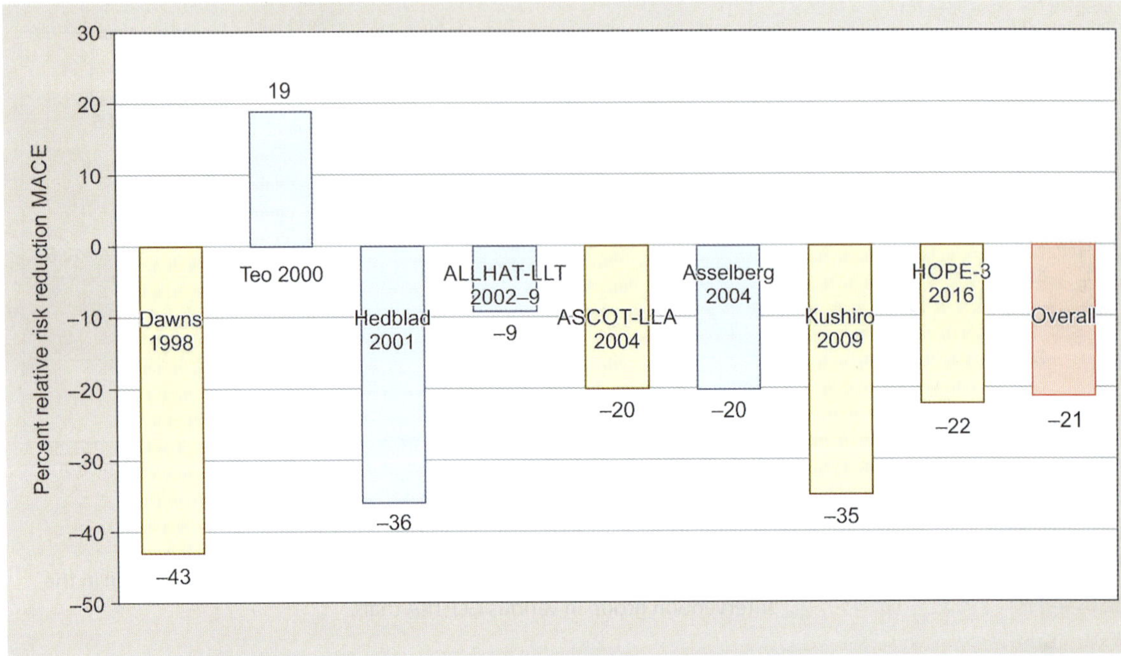

Fig. 7: Meta-analysis of randomized trials of lipid-lowering in hypertension. The overall risk reduction is 21% (95% CI 12–29%).

deaths.[63] On the other hand, in the lipid-lowering arm of the European ASCOT trial which also randomized >10,000 patients to atorvastatin versus placebo a 36% (17–50%) lower incidence of major cardiovascular endpoints was reported.[64] Subsequent large trials such as HOPE-3 and TIPS-3 also reported similar benefits.[15] A meta-analysis of trials of cholesterol lowering in uncomplicated hypertension included eight randomized studies and reported 21% (12–29%) relative risk reduction in major cardiovascular events with use of statins in uncomplicated hypertension **(Fig. 7)**.[65] This benefit was observed across all types of cardiovascular events including myocardial infarction, stroke, and cardiac deaths.

Guidelines have been slow to adopt the regular use of statins in patients with low to moderate-risk hypertension. The ESH 2023, ESC 2024, and the US guidelines recommend a risk-based approach, and LDL targets vary according to calculated risk using locally validated tools (Framingham or ACC-AHA tools in the US; SCORE and SCORE2 in Europe).[10,18,19] In the absence of locally validated risk tools in India, it is possible to use the newly developed SCORE Asia risk tool for risk classification.[66]

Polypills

Initially described as a combination of three anti-hypertensive medicines (thiazides, beta-blocker, and ACE inhibitor), aspirin, folic acid and statin, it is more pragmatically defined as a single-pill combination of antihypertensive and lipid-lowering agents. Polypills or a single-pill combination have multiple benefits, including better adherence and increased rates of BP control.[67] For primary cardiovascular disease prevention, the TIPS-3 trial used a combination of atenolol, ramipril, hydrochlorothiazide, aspirin and simvastatin as a single pill combination.

TABLE 6: Barriers and facilitators to lifestyle and medication adherence for primary prevention.

	Barriers	*Facilitators*
Healthcare system	• Low funding for noncommunicable diseases • Poor access and availability of healthcare • No insurance for outpatient management • Low-quality care • Costs	• Improvement in healthcare systems related to access, affordability, and convenience • Involvement of nonmedical professionals in healthcare • Multisystem interventions
Healthcare providers	• Lack of understanding of patient needs • Prescribing complex regimens • Failure to explain benefits and side effects • No focus on lifestyle changes • Neglecting to involve patients • Lack of continuity of care • Over-treatment	• Improving education, motivation, and cost awareness • Elimination of treatment inertia • Simplifying the medication regimen, combinations, and fixed dose combinations • Appropriate drug selection dependent on patient characteristics • Training existing community health workers, nurses, and pharmacists
Patient related	• Social isolation, especially in the elderly • Lack of motivation and commitment • Failure to realize the seriousness of the problem • Failure to sustain lifestyle changes • Multiple stakeholders and messages • Lack of quality information • Ancillary and drug costs • Universal healthcare and Insurance cover	• Patient education and counselling • Self-monitoring of adherence to lifestyles and pharmacotherapy with technology • Behavioral strategies—self-monitoring of BP and glucose, diaries, memory cues, rewards • Social support by family, health workers, physicians

In this international study (with a substantial contribution from India) at 5-year follow-up, there was a significant reduction in a composite of CVD incidence, myocardial infarction, stroke, revascularization, and cardiovascular deaths by 31% (95% CI 3–50%).[68] The polypill meta-analysis that combined three primary prevention cohorts in HOPE-3, TIPS-3, and PolyIran studies also reported a significant benefit of polypill with reduced major cardiovascular endpoints by 38% (95% CI 27–47%).[67] These findings were replicated in the hypertensive participants in the polypill trials and provide a rationale for more widespread use of this strategy.

ADHERENCE

The most important barrier in hypertension control is sustaining lifelong adherence to drugs and healthy lifestyles.[6,9] Adherence is defined as remaining attached to the medication regimen, and adequate adherence is the use of therapies >80% of the time.[69] Studies have reported that in the chronic disease setting, only about 50% of patients are adherent to therapies at 12 months, and only 20% take medication in the appropriate dose.[70]

Interview-based assessment by a health worker or physician is commonly used to assess adherence. Assessment of medication adherence is possible by other means such as electronic medication monitoring systems and biochemical measurement of drug metabolites in urine.[71] Several barriers and facilitators to adherence at various levels of healthcare exist and are outlined in **Table 6**. Outcomes of interventions to promote adherence are limited. There is some evidence that technology-based interventions, pharmacist-level interventions and health-worker-based interventions are useful in promoting adherence and influencing outcomes in hypertension.[7,8] However, robust effectiveness outcomes have not been reported in most clinical studies in India.[72]

Patient Empowerment

An important factor that promotes adherence in CHD primary prevention is self-management of risk factors.[72,73] Adherence to healthy lifestyles and pharmacological therapy in the asymptomatic state is a herculean task, and patient empowerment and personalized medicine for lifelong adherence to lifestyle changes and drug therapies may be useful. Individual empowerment and motivation is crucial and lead to healthy behavior changes in individuals.[73] Self-care is defined by the American Heart Association as a process whereby individuals and their families maintain health through health-promoting practices and managing illness.[73] Personal empowerment for self-care could be at the individual, family or community level. All these have to be strengthened to achieve adherence and compliance. Technological interventions that promote healthy lifestyle habits and dissuade unhealthy behaviors are being developed and evaluated in trials.[74-76] Technology-based strategies to promote adherence to healthy lifestyles and drug therapy are available, and given the universality of smart devices, the potential for this personalized approach is enormous.[74-77]

CONCLUSION

Uncontrolled hypertension is a major public health and clinical problem in India. Epidemiological data report that in India (and other developing countries), less than a quarter of hypertensives in urban areas and one-tenth in rural areas have their BP under control. The implementation of and adherence to the step-wise BP management strategy provided by various national and international guidelines is important **(Fig. 1)**. Universal implementation of this approach can lead to BP control in >70–80% of the patients.

Novel approaches include the use of available medicines such as mineralocorticoid receptor antagonists (steroidal—spironolactone, eplerenone; nonsteroidal—finerenone), sacubitril-valsartan combination, and SGLT2 inhibitors in specific situations. Several biological agents are in phase-3 clinical trials and include aldosterone synthase inhibitors (e.g., baxdrostat), and angiotensinogen antagonist siRNAs (e.g., zilebesiran). Renal denervation technology has now matured and is recommended in the European guidelines.[10,19] Obesity interventions are gaining ground, and randomized clinical trials with bariatric surgery and antiobesity medicines (GLP1 receptor agonists, etc.) have provided useful information regarding BP lowering. They should be reserved for hypertensives with BMI of 30.0–39.9 kg/m^2. Finally, to reduce the overall cardiovascular risk in hypertension, it is important to focus on strategies beyond BP control. Statins should be prescribed in every moderate to high-risk individual for CVD risk reduction. Polypill studies suggest the usefulness of combining various cardioprotective medicines in a single pill, both for cardiovascular benefit and promotion of adherence. Lifelong adherence to hypertension therapy is the most difficult target, and support of technology and self-empowerment is crucial in this regard.

REFERENCES

1. GBD 2021 Risk Factors Collaborators. Global burden and strength of evidence for 88 risk factors in 204 countries and 811 subnational locations, 1990–2021: a systematic analysis for the Global Burden of Disease Study 2021. Lancet. 2024; 403:2162-2203.
2. NCD Risk Factor Collaboration (NCD-RiSC). Worldwide trends in blood pressure from 1975 to 2015: a pooled analysis of 1479 population-based

measurement studies with 19.1 million participants. Lancet. 2017;389:37-55.
3. NCD Risk Factor Collaboration. Worldwide trends in hypertension prevalence and progress in treatment and control from 1990 to 2019: A pooled analysis of 1173 population-representative studies with 104 million participants. Lancet. 2021;398:957-80.
4. Gupta R, Gaur K, Ahuja S, et al. Recent studies on hypertension prevalence and control in India, 2023. Hypertens Res. 2024;47:1445-56.
5. Khatib R, McKee M, Shannon H, Chow C, Rangarajan S, Teo K, et al. Availability and affordability of cardiovascular disease medicines and their impact on use: comparison across high, middle, and low-income countries. Lancet. 2016;387:61-9.
6. Chow CK, Gupta R. Blood pressure control: a challenge to global health systems. Lancet. 2019;394:613-5.
7. Gupta R. Epidemiology of hypertension in India and public health interventions. In: Verma NS, Maheshwari A (Eds). ISH Handbook of Hypertension. New Delhi: Knowledge Bridge, 2021. pp. 1-9.
8. Gupta R, Gupta S. Social determinants' approach for hypertension control. In: Ram CVS, (Ed). Cardiological Society of India: Hypertension Reviews 2020. Noida: Incessant Nature Science Publishers, 2020. pp. 11-21.
9. Gupta R. Primary prevention of coronary heart disease: public health perspective. In: Gupta R. Heart Disease Prevention: Essays on Preventive Cardiology in India. Jaipur: Jaipur Heart Watch Foundation, 2025. pp. 1-40.
10. Mancia G, Kreutz R, Brunstrom M, Burnier M, Grassi G, Januszewicz A, et al. 2023 ESH guidelines for the management of arterial hypertension: The task force for the management of arterial hypertension of the European Society of Hypertension: Endorsed by the International Society of Hypertension (ISH) and the European Renal Association. J Hypertens. 2023; 41:1874-2071.
11. Stergiou GS, Avolio AP, Palatini P, Kyriakoulis KG, Schutte AE, Mieke S, et al. European Society of Hypertension recommendations for the validation of cuffless blood pressure measuring devices: European Society of Hypertension Working Group on Blood Pressure monitoring and cardiovascular variability. J Hypertens. 2023;41:2074-87.
12. Janeway TC. A clinical study of hypertensive cardiovascular disease. Arch Intern Med. 1913; 12:755-80.
13. Weiss S, Ellis LB. The rational treatment of hypertension. JAMA. 1930;95:846-52.
14. Hay J. The significance of raised blood pressure. BMJ. 1931;2:43-7.
15. Gupta R. Controversies in hypertension classification. In: Gupta R (Ed). Heart Disease Prevention: Essays on Preventive Cardiology in India. Jaipur: Jaipur Heart Watch Foundation. 2025;167-80.
16. Gupta R, Maheshwari A, Verma N, Narasingan SN, Tripathi K, Joshi S, et al. Indian Society of Hypertension consensus guideline for the management of hypertension 2023. Hypertens J. 2023;9:57-132.
17. World Health Organisation. Global Report on Hypertension: The Race Against a Silent Killer. 2023.
18. Whelton PK, Carey RM, Aronow WS, Casey DE Jr, Collins KJ, Dennison Himmelfarb C, et al. 2017 ACC/AHA/ AAPA/ABC/ACPM/AGS/ APhA/ASH/ ASPC/NMA/PCNA guideline for the prevention, detection, evaluation, and management of high blood pressure in adults: executive summary: a report of the American College of Cardiology/ American Heart Association Task Force on Clinical Practice Guidelines. Hypertension. 2018;71:1269-324.
19. McEvoy JW, McCarthy CP, Bruno RM, Brouwers S, Canavan MD, Ceconi C, et al. 2024 ESC guidelines for the management of elevated blood pressure and hypertension. Eur Heart J. 2024; 45:3912-4018.
20. Abuelazm M, Ali S, Saleh O, Badr A, Altobaishat O, AlBarakat MM, et al. The safety and efficacy of quadruple ultra-low-dose combination (quadpill) for hypertension treatment: a systematic review and meta-analysis of randomised controlled trials. Clin Drug Investig. 2023; 43:813-26.
21. Kaur P, Kunwar A, Sharma M, Mitra J, Das C, Swasticharan L, et al. India Hypertension Control Initiative: hypertension treatment and blood pressure control in a cohort in 24 sentinel sites. J Clin Hypertens. 2021;23:720-9.

22. Gupta R, Sharma KK, Soni S, Gupta N, Khedar RS. Resistant hypertension in clinical practice in India: Jaipur Heart Watch. J Assoc Physicians Ind. 2019;67(12):14-7.
23. Noubiap JJ, Nansseu JR, Nyaga UF, Sime PS, Francis I, Bigna JJ. Global prevalence of resistant hypertension: a meta-analysis of data from 3.2 million patients. Heart. 2019;105:98-105.
24. Rajzer P, Biegus J. Sacubitril/valsartan in a wide spectrum of heart failure patients (from mechanisms of action to outcomes in specific populations). Heart Fail Rev. 2025; 30:387-405.
25. McMurray JJV, Packer M, Desai AS, Gong J, Lefkowitz MP, Rizkala AR, et al. Angiotensin-neprilysin inhibition versus enalapril in heart failure. N Engl J Med. 2014;371:993-1004.
26. Crispino SP, Segreti A, Nafisio V, Valente D, Crisci F, Ferro A, et al. The role of SGLT2 inhibitors across all stages of heart failure and mechanisms of early clinical benefit: from prevention to advanced heart failure. Biomedicines. 2025;13:608.
27. Gupta R, Chaudhary M, Guptha S. Heart failure with preserved ejection fraction (HFpEF) in the Indian context. J Indian College Cardiol. 2025;15:42-54.
28. Leopold JA, Ingelfinger JR. Aldosterone and treatment-resistant hypertension. N Engl J Med. 2023;388:464-7.
29. Azizi M. Decreasing the effects of aldosterone in resistant hypertension: a success story. N Engl J Med. 2023; 388:461-3.
30. Freeman MW, Halvorsen YD, Marshall W, Pater M, Isaacsohn J, Pearce C, et al. Phase 2 trial of baxdrostat for treatment-resistant hypertension. N Engl J Med. 2023;388:395-405.
31. Laffin LJ, Rodman D, Luther JM, Vaidya A, Weir MR, Rajicic N, et al. Aldosterone synthase inhibition with lorundrostat for uncontrolled hypertension: the TARGET-HTN randomised clinical trial. JAMA 2023; 330:1140-50.
32. Laffin LJ, Kopjar B, Melgaard C, Wolski K, Ibbitson J, Bhikam S, et al. Lorundrostat efficacy and safety in patients with uncontrolled hypertension. N Engl J Med. 2025;392(18):1813-1823.
33. Mulatero P, Wuerzner G, Groessl M, Sconfienza E, Damianaki A, Forestiero V, et al. Safety and efficacy of once-daily dexfadrostat phosphate in patients with primary aldosteronism: a randomised, parallel group, multicentre, phase 2 trial. eClin Med. 2024;71:102576.
34. Marzano L, Merlo L, Martinelli N, Pizzolo F, Friso S. Efficacy and safety of aldosterone synthase inhibitors for hypertension: a meta-analysis of randomised controlled trials and systematic review. Hypertension. 2025; 82:e47-56.
35. Desai AS, Webb DJ, Taubel J, Casey S, Cheng Y, Robbie GJ, et al. Zilebesiran, an RNA interference therapeutic agent for hypertension. N Engl J Med. 2023; 389:228-238.
36. Bakris GL, Saxena M, Gupta A, Chalhoub F, Lee J, Stiglitz D, et al. RNA interference with zilebesiran for mild to moderate hypertension: The KARDIA-1 randomised clinical trial. JAMA 2024; 331:740-9.
37. Nakagami H, Hayashi H, Shimamura M, Rakugi H, Morishita R. Therapeutic vaccine for chronic diseases after the COVIOD-19 era. Hypertens Res. 2021; 44:1047-53.
38. Nakagami H. Challenges in the development of novel therapies, vaccines and siRNAs for the treatment of hypertension. Hypertens Res. 2023; 46:1812-1815.
39. Messerli FH, Bavushi C, Brguljan J, Burnier M, Dobner S, Elijovich F, et al. Renal denervation in the anti-hypertensive arsenal: knowns and known unknowns. Hypertension. 2022;40:1859-75.
40. Bhatt DL, Kandzari DE, O'Neill WW, D'Agostino R, Flack JM, Katzen BT, et al. A controlled trial of renal denervation for resistant hypertension. N Engl J Med. 2014;370:1393-1401.
41. Bhatt DL, Vaduganathan M, Kandzari DE, Leon MB, Rocha-Singh K, Townsend RR, et al. Long-term outcomes after catheter based renal artery denervation for resistant hypertension: final follow-up of the randomised SYMPLICITY HTN-3 trial. Lancet. 2022;400:1405-16.
42. Ram CVS. Renal denervation therapy for hypertension: all that glitters in not gold. Eur Heart J. 2022;43:2177-8.
43. Desai N, Sunilkumar S, Venkatesh CR. Resistant hypertension. In: Antani JA, Nadagouda VG, Desai N (Ed). Hypertension: known and less known facts. Hubli, Karnataka. Guru Krupa Pub. 2024;193-207.
44. Fisher NDL, Kirtane AJ. Renal denervation for hypertension. Nature Rev Cardiol. 2025 Sep;22(9):664-74.

45. Gupta R, Agrawal A, Misra A, Guptha S, Vikram NK. Metabolic cardiovascular risk factors worsen continuously across the spectrum of body mass index in Asian Indians. Indian Heart J. 2012;64:236-44.
46. Hall ME, Cohen JB, Ard JD, Egan BM, Hall JE, Lavie CJ, et al. Weight loss strategies for prevention and treatment of hypertension: A scientific statement from the American Heart Association. Hypertension. 2021;78:e38-e50.
47. Schuer PR, Bhatt DL, Kirwan JP, Wolski K, Aminian A, Brethauer SA, et al. Bariatric surgery versus intensive medical therapy for diabetes: 5-year outcomes. N Engl J Med. 2017:641-51.
48. Fisher D, Liu L, Arterburn D, Coleman KJ, Courcoulas A, Haneuse S, et al. Remission and relapse of hypertension after bariatric surgery: a retrospective study on long-term outcomes. Ann Surgery Open. 2022;3:e158.
49. Schiavon CA, Bersch-Ferrreira AC, Santucci EV, Oliveira JD, Torreglosa CR, Bueno PT, et al. Effects of bariatric surgery in obese patients with hypertension: The GATEWAY randomised trial (Gastric bypass to treat obese patients with steady hypertension). Circulation. 2018;137:1132-42.
50. Schiavon CA, Cavalcanti AB, Oliviera JD, Machado RHV, Santucci EV, Santos RN, et al. Randomised trial of the effect of bariatric surgery on blood pressure after 5 years. J Am Coll Cardiol. 2024; 83:637-48.
51. Kumar S, Blaha MJ. GLP-1 RA for cardiometabolic risk reduction in obesity- how do we best describe benefit and value? Am J Prev Cardiol. 2024; 18:100682.
52. Pi-Sunyer X, Astrup A, Fujioka K, Greenway F, Halpern A, Krempf M, et al. A randomised controlled trial of 3.0 mg of liraglutide in weight management. N Engl J Med. 2015;373:11-22.
53. Wilding JPH, Batterham RL, Calanna S, Davies M, Van Gaal LF, Lingvay I, et al. Once-weekly semaglutide in adults with overweight or obesity. N Engl J Med. 2021;384:989-1002.
54. Rosenstock J, Wysham C, Frias JP, Kaneko S, Lee CJ, Fernández Landó L, et al. Efficacy and safety of a novel dual GIP and GLP-1 receptor agonist tirzepatide in patients with type 2 diabetes: a double-blind randomised phase-3 trial. Lancet. 2021; 398:143-55.
55. Jastreboff AM, Kaplan LM, Frias JP, Wu Q, Du Y, Gurbuz S, et al. Triple-hormone receptor agonist retratrutide for obesity-a phase 2 trial. N Engl J Med. 2023;389:514-526.
56. Wharton S, Blevins T, Connery L, Rosenstock J, Raha S, Liu R, et al. Daily oral GLP-1 receptor agonist orforglipron for adults with obesity. N Engl J Med. 2023;389:877-88.
57. Malhotra A, Grunstein RR, Fietze I, Weaver TE, Redline S, Azarbarzin A, et al. Tirzepatide for the treatment of obstructive sleep apnea and obesity. N Engl J Med. 2024;391:1193-1205.
58. Loomba R, Hartman ML, Lawitz EJ, Vuppalanchi R, Boursier J, Bugianesi E, et al. Tirzepatide for metabolic dysfunction associated steatohepatitis with liver fibrosis. N Engl J Med. 2024;391:299-310.
59. Lincoff AM, Brown-Frandsen K, Colhoun HM, Deanfield J, Emerson SS, Esbjerg S, et al. Semaglutide and cardiovascular outcomes in obesity without diabetes. N Engl J Med. 2023;389:2221-32.
60. Tang H, Zhang B, Lu Y, Donahoo WT, Singh Ospina N, Kotecha P, et al. Assessing the benefit-risk profile of newer glucose lowering drugs: a systematic review and network meta-analysis of randomized outcome trials. Diabets Obes Metab. 2025;27:1444-55.
61. Gupta R. Cardiovascular protection beyond BP control in hypertension. RUHS J Health Sciences. 2023; 8:225-231.
62. Boren J, Chapman MJ, Krauss RM, Packard CJ, Bentzon JF, Binder CJ, et al. Low-density lipoproteins cause atherosclerotic cardiovascular disease: pathophysiological, genetic and therapeutic insights: a consensus statement from the European Atherosclerosis Society Consensus Panel. Eur Heart J. 2020;41:2313-30.
63. ALLHAT Officers and Coordinators for the ALLHAT Collaborative Research Group. Major outcomes in moderately hypercholesterolemic, hypertensive patients randomised to pravastatin versus usual care: The Antihypertensive and Lipid Lowering Treatment to Prevent Heart Attack Trial (ALLHAT-LLT). JAMA. 2002;288:2998-3007.
64. Sever PS, Dahlof B, Poulter NR, Wedel H, Beevers G, Caulfield M, et al. Prevention of coronary and stroke events with atorvastatin in hypertensive patients who have average or

lower than average cholesterol concentrations in the Anglo-Scandinavian Cardiac Outcomes trial- Lipid Lowering Arm (ASCOT-LLA): a multicentre randomised controlled trial. Lancet. 2003;361:1149-58.
65. Wang Y, Jiang L, Feng SJ, Tang XY, Kuang ZM. Effect of combined statin and antihypertensive therapy in patients with hypertension: a systematic review and meta-analysis. Cardiology. 2020;145: 802-12.
66. SCORE2 Asia Pacific Writing Group. Risk prediction of cardiovascular disease in the Asia-Pacific region: the SCORE2 Asia-Pacific model. Eur Heart J. 2025;46:702-15.
67. Joseph P, Roshandel G, Gao P, Pais P, Lonn E, Xavier D, et al. Fixed dose combination therapies with and without aspirin for primary prevention of cardiovascular disease: an individual participant data meta-analysis. Lancet. 2021;398: 1133-46.
68. Yusuf S, Joseph P, Dans A, Gao P, Teo K, Xavier D, et al. Polypill with or without aspirin in persons without cardiovascular disease. N Engl J Med. 2021;384:216-28.
69. Osterberg L, Blaschke T. Adherence to medication. N Engl J Med. 2005;353:487-497.
70. Ferdinand KC, Senatore FF, Clayton-Jeter H, Cryer DR, Lewin JC, Nasser SA, et al. Improving medication adherence in cardiometabolic disease: practical and regulatory implications. J Am Coll Cardiol. 2017;69:437-51.
71. Laufs U, Retting-Ewen V, Bohm M. Strategies to improve drug adherence. Eur Heart J. 2011;32: 264-8.
72. Gupta R, Wood DA. Primary prevention of ischaemic heart disease: populations, individuals and healthcare professionals. Lancet. 2019;394: 685-96.
73. Riegel B, Moser DK, Buck HG, Dickson VV, Dunbar SB, Lee CS, et al. Self-care for the prevention and management of cardiovascular disease and stroke: a scientific statement for healthcare professionals from the American Heart Association. J Am Heart Assoc. 2017;6:e006997.
74. World Health Organisation. WHO Guideline: recommendations on digital interventions for health system strengthening. Geneva. World Health Organisation. 2015.
75. Bhavnani SP, Parakh K, Atreja A, Druz R, Graham GN, Hayek SS, et al. 2017 Roadmap for innovation-ACC health policy statement on healthcare transformation in the era of digital, big data and precision health: a report of the American College of Cardiology task force on health policy statements and systems of care. J Am Coll Cardiol. 2017;70:2696-2718.
76. Topol EJ. High performance medicine: the convergence of human and artificial intelligence. Nature Med. 2019;25:44-56.
77. Mukkamala R, Shroff SG, Kyriakoulis KG, Avolio AP, Stergiou GS. Cuffless blood pressure measurement: where do we actually stand? Hypertension. 2025; 82:957-70.

SECTION 6

MASLD

CHAPTER 11

MASLD: A New Gateway to ASCVD and a Call for Integrated Care

PC Manoria, Piyush Manoria

ABSTRACT

Metabolic dysfunction-associated steatotic liver disease (MASLD) is a multisystem metabolic disorder strongly associated with atherosclerotic cardiovascular disease (ASCVD). It increases cardiovascular risk independent of traditional factors, particularly with advancing liver fibrosis. Early detection, risk stratification, lifestyle intervention, and integrated multidisciplinary care are essential to reduce both hepatic and cardiovascular morbidity and mortality.

Keywords: MASLD, ASCVD, liver fibrosis, cardiovascular risk.

INTRODUCTION

Metabolic dysfunction-associated steatotic liver disease (MASLD), formerly known as nonalcoholic fatty liver disease (NAFLD), has been traditionally looked upon as a hepatic disorder, but in reality, it is a multisystem disease with profound implications on cardiovascular health. It has emerged as a major public health problem globally as well as in India. It affects approximately 25% of the global population, with its prevalence rising from 22% in 1991 to 37% in 2019.[1] MASLD is present in up to 75% of patients with type 2 diabetes mellitus (T2D). Its prevalence is expected to increase in the future due to the ongoing epidemic of diabetes mellitus and obesity. This large metabolic burden on the young adult population will lead to a significant increase in MASLD-related disability-adjusted life years.

THE MASLD-ASCVD DUO

The hepatic consequences of MASLD revolve around steatohepatitis, fibrosis, and cirrhosis, but its systemic complications are being increasingly recognized, including atherosclerotic cardiovascular disease (ASCVD), coronary artery disease, heart failure, cardiac arrhythmias, stroke, and cardiovascular disease-related mortality. In fact, the most common cause of death in these patients is ASCVD and not liver-related complications. MASLD has become an independent risk factor for cardiovascular disease (CVD) and CVD-related mortality.[2] This risk is independent of other risk factors[3] such as age, sex, family history, dyslipidemia, obesity, hypertension, and diabetes mellitus. Fibrosis is the turning point in the natural history of MASLD, and the risk of CVD increases progressively with increasing fibrosis.[4] No doubt liver fibrosis also makes the patient progress to cirrhosis and its complications, which culminate in death.

The potential pathogenic mechanisms linking MASLD and CVD are insulin resistance, systemic inflammation, oxidative stress, intrahepatic lipid accumulation, endothelial dysfunction, decreased adiponectin, atherogenic dyslipidemia, gut microbiota, and altered bile acid metabolism. The relationship between MASLD and ASCVD is reciprocal and mutually reinforcing. MASLD amplifies cardiovascular risk through the promotion of atherogenic dyslipidemia, chronic low-grade systemic inflammation, endothelial dysfunction, and heightened oxidative stress while the metabolic components of ASCVD, such as obesity, type 2 diabetes, and hypertension, fuel the progression of MASLD. This vicious cycle highlights the importance of early detection and intervention in MASLD to reduce the cardiovascular consequences.

RECONCEPTUALIZING MASLD AS A CARDIOVASCULAR RISK FACTOR

Various studies suggest that advanced MASLD, especially in the presence of fibrosis, is an independent risk factor for cardiovascular events. Future cardiology guidelines should also emphasize the importance of hepatic steatosis in screening for CVD. This association underscores the need for a paradigm shift in how we perceive and manage MASLD, moving beyond hepatology to embrace a more holistic, integrated, multidisciplinary approach. However, a major concern is that MASLD is often asymptomatic and remains undiagnosed, as hepatic steatosis is frequently silent until late stages. This asymptomatic period results in a missed opportunity for early risk stratification and intervention. MASLD affects nearly a quarter of the global population; its implications on ASCVD prevention are substantial.

Necessity for Increased Awareness Among Physicians and Public

The need of the hour is to increase the awareness among physicians and public about the screening for MASLD in addition to the traditional cardiovascular risk factors. The screening can be done by ultrasonography of the liver, serum biomarkers, especially the Fibrosis-4 index (FIB-4), and by transient elastography. An integrated approach is needed to reduce the cardiovascular- and liver-related mortality in these patients.

Call for Early Diagnosis and Risk Stratification

The association between MASLD and ASCVD is strong; therefore, early intervention is of paramount importance. Risk stratification is crucial and is primarily performed using the FIB-4 score, categorizing patients into low risk (<1.3), intermediate risk (1.3–2.67), and high risk (>2.67) groups.

Patients at low risk can be managed with lifestyle modification, with particular emphasis on obesity management and CVD prevention. High-risk patients should be referred to a liver specialist for further evaluation and management by a multidisciplinary team to prevent progression to cirrhosis and reduce cardiovascular risk. Intermediate-risk patients should undergo further assessment with liver stiffness measurement by elastography or the enhanced liver fibrosis (ELF) blood test if available to further stratify them into low-, intermediate-, or high-risk categories, as shown in **Flowchart 1**.

A Call for Integrated Management

Effective management of MASLD requires a cohesive and integrated approach, involving hepatologists, cardiologists, endocrinologists, physicians, and primary care providers.

Lifestyle modification is the cornerstone of MASLD management, as it not only improves liver health but also significantly reduces cardiovascular risk. A very low-calorie diet (approximately 600 kcal/day) for 4 weeks has been shown to reduce liver fat from 36 to 2%. Pharmacological agents such as vitamin E, pioglitazone, and saroglitazar have been used in the treatment of MASLD for several years. In the recent past, two new molecules—resmetirom and semaglutide—have been approved by the USFDA in March 2024 and August 2025, respectively, following the MAESTRO-NASH trial[5] and the ESSENCE study.[6] Sodium-glucose

Flowchart 1: Risk stratification of MASLD.

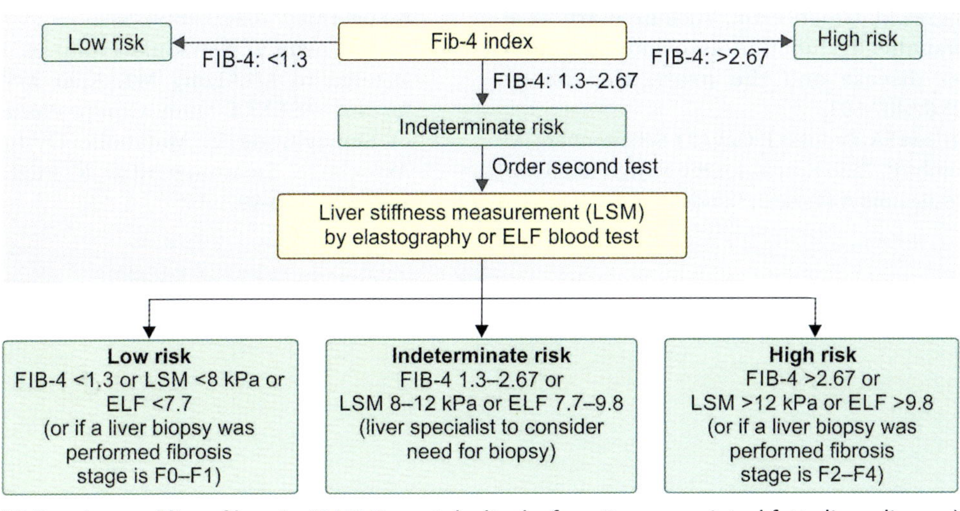

(ELF: enhanced liver fibrosis; MASLD: metabolic dysfunction-associated fatty liver disease)

cotransporter-2 inhibitors (SGLT2i) have also demonstrated beneficial effects, although they are not specifically approved for MASLD treatment.

GAPS IN MASLD AND FUTURE DIRECTIONS

Despite increasing recognition of the MASLD–ASCVD nexus, several gaps in the understanding of underlying pathophysiological mechanisms and optimal management strategies remain unresolved. Large-scale longitudinal studies are required to elucidate the causal relationship between MASLD and ASCVD and to identify reliable biomarkers capable of predicting cardiovascular outcomes in this population. In addition, public awareness of MASLD and its systemic complications must be substantially enhanced to facilitate prevention, early detection, and timely intervention for this increasingly prevalent disease.

CONCLUSION

The strong association between MASLD and ASCVD emphasizes the urgent need for early intervention, integrated care, and a renewed focus on research and public health initiatives. By addressing MASLD as a gateway to ASCVD, we can not only improve liver-related outcomes but also substantially reduce the global burden of CVD. MASLD should no longer be regarded solely as a liver-specific condition, but rather as an early clinical marker of heightened cardiovascular risk. Timely intervention is critical to prevent its downstream progression into widespread cardiovascular morbidity and mortality.

REFERENCES

1. Le MH, Yeo YH, Li X, Li J, Zou B, Wu Y, et al. 2019 Global NAFLD prevalence: a systematic review and meta-analysis. Clin Gastroenterol Hepatol. 2022;20:2809-17.e28.
2. Møller S, Kimer N, Hove JD, Barløse M, Gluud LL. Cardiovascular disease and metabolic dysfunction-associated steatotic liver disease: pathophysiology and diagnostic aspects. Eur J Prev Cardiol. 2025:zwae306.
3. Zheng H, Sechi LA, Navarese EP, Casu G, Vidili G. Metabolic dysfunction-associated steatotic liver disease and cardiovascular risk: a comprehensive review. Cardiovasc Diabetol. 2024;23(1):346.

4. Driessen S, Francque SM, Anker SD, Castro Cabezas M, Grobbee DE, Tushuizen ME, et al. Metabolic dysfunction-associated steatotic liver disease and the heart. Hepatology. 2025;82:487-503.
5. Harrison SA, Bedossa P, Guy CD, Schattenberg JM, Loomba R, Taub R, et al. for the MAESTRO-NASH Investigators A Phase 3, Randomized, Controlled Trial of Resmetirom in NASH with Liver Fibrosis. N Engl J Med. 2024;390:497-509.
6. Sanyal Arun J, Newsome Philip N, Kliers I, Østergaard LH, Long MT, Kjær MS, et al.; for the ESSENCE Study Group. Phase 3 Trial of Semaglutide in Metabolic Dysfunction–Associated Steatohepatitis. N Engl J Med. 2025;392:2089-99.

SECTION 7

Heart Failure

CHAPTER 12

Fighting the Devil of Heart Failure in Diabetes: Current Status

Siddhant Rajput, Rajesh Rajput

ABSTRACT

Heart failure (HF) is a frequent and serious cardiovascular complication in individuals with diabetes, significantly contributing to morbidity and mortality. Diabetes and HF share a bidirectional relationship driven by metabolic, inflammatory, and neurohormonal mechanisms, leading to diabetic cardiomyopathy. Early identification of at-risk individuals and stage-based evaluation are essential for prevention and timely management. Contemporary treatment strategies emphasize lifestyle modification, guideline-directed medical therapy, and glucose-lowering agents with proven cardiovascular benefit, particularly SGLT2 inhibitors. Pharmacological therapy should be individualized considering comorbidities and glycemic targets. Emerging evidence also highlights the role of metabolic surgery in improving cardiometabolic outcomes. A multidisciplinary and personalized approach is crucial for optimizing outcomes in patients with diabetes and HF.

Keywords: Diabetes mellitus, heart failure, diabetic cardiomyopathy, SGLT2 inhibitors, guideline-directed therapy, cardiometabolic risk

INTRODUCTION

Heart failure (HF) is a common comorbidity in diabetes, occurring up to 22% of the time in people with the disease.[1] Additionally, data suggest that it can occur in diabetics even when hypertension, coronary heart disease, or valvular heart disease are not present and for many diabetics; it may be the initial manifestation of cardiovascular disease. Since the prevalence of diabetes, particularly type 2 diabetes, has risen by 30% globally over the past decade and is expected to continue to rise, the burden of HF on the healthcare system will continue to increase.[2]

PREVALENCE AND INCIDENCE OF HEART FAILURE AMONG INDIVIDUALS WITH DIABETES

According to findings from several long-term observational studies of population-based cohorts with diabetes and prediabetes, such as the Framingham Heart Study and the First National Health and Nutrition Examination Survey (NHANES I) Epidemiologic Follow-up Study, men and women with diabetes or prediabetes have a two to four times higher risk of HF than people without these conditions.[3] Moreover, when evaluated in recent cohorts of millions of patients with integrated primary care, hospital admission, disease registry, and death certificate records in England, HF was the most common early sign of cardiovascular disease in adults with type 2 diabetes (T2D). During a median follow-up period of 5.5 years, type 2 diabetes was an independent risk factor for the development of HF and increased the morbidity and mortality associated with HF.[1] Recent data from the UK Prospective Diabetes Study (UKPDS) shows incidence rates of up to 11.9 per 1,000 patient-years over a 10-year follow-up period. According to data from the Scottish Diabetes Mellitus Registry, HF is also more common in people with type 1 diabetes (T1D). The Swedish National Diabetes Registry discovered that the crude incidence rate of HF hospitalization and mortality is two to five times higher for men and women with type 1 diabetes than for those without the disease, and that diastolic dysfunction is more common in these individuals. HF may be more common in people with T1D than in people with T2D, according to a recent systematic study that included 12 million participants worldwide. Even after controlling for age and other comorbidities, there is still a negative correlation between diabetes and HF.

PREVALENCE AND INCIDENCE OF DIABETES AMONG PEOPLE WITH HEART FAILURE

There is a clear reciprocal relationship between diabetes and HF. Approximately 60% of people with HF have insulin resistance,[4] and multiple large cohorts have shown that new-onset diabetes is common in this population. It is not surprising that data show a significant incidence of dysglycemia in this population, with rates ranging from 20% in community-based cohorts to 34% in pharmaceutical studies. The prevalence and incidence rates of diabetes in people with heart failure and reduced ejection fraction (HFrEF) and those with preserved ejection fraction (HFpEF) have not been directly compared in much research. Diabetes was found to be 40% common in both HFrEF and HFpEF patients in a study of hospitalized HF patients. More accurate information is needed regarding the diabetes burden distribution among people with HFrEF and HFpEF.

PATHOPHYSIOLOGY

The pathophysiology of HF in diabetics is complex and shows how different risk factors and dysregulated subcellular pathways interact, going beyond the effects of diabetes-induced hyperglycemia to cause structural and functional changes in the diabetic heart. Ventricular failure without coronary artery disease (CAD) or hypertension is known as "diabetic cardiomyopathy,"[1] and it is becoming more widely recognized. There are several possible causes of HF in diabetics, including renin-angiotensin-aldosterone system (RAAS) activation, mitochondrial dysfunction, oxidative stress, inflammation, changes in intracellular calcium homeostasis, increased production of advanced glycation end products, and changes in myocardial energy substrates, such as increased use of free fatty acids, decreased use of glucose, and increased use of oxygen, which ultimately results in decreased cardiac efficiency.[1] Triglycerides and other lipid metabolites (such as ceramides, diacylglycerol, etc.) build up in the myocardium of diabetics despite their higher rates of fatty acid utilization.

HEART FAILURE: DIAGNOSIS AND CLINICAL STAGES

Stage A: Individuals at Risk for Heart Failure

Patients who have been diagnosed with diabetes are at risk for HF and should be closely watched. At this point, the management of glycemia and other risk factors may alter (or exacerbate) the risk for clinical HF.

Stage B: Preheart Failure/Early Detection

ACC/AHA Stage B heart failure includes asymptomatic individuals who have at least one of the following: (1) Evidence of structural heart disease, (2) abnormal cardiac function, or (3) high natriuretic peptide levels or high cardiac troponin levels. Furthermore, while a single measurement of troponin or natriuretic peptide may provide useful predictive information, repeated evaluations to find increasing levels of either improve sensitivity for identifying people at increased risk for incident HF.[5] For example, two NT-proBNP measurements 6 months apart were able to identify those with T2D who were at the highest risk (both elevated), rising risk (baseline low and follow-up higher), or lower risk (6-month measurement lower) in the Examination of Cardiovascular Outcomes with Alogliptin versus Standard of Care (EXAMINE) trial.

Stages C and D: Symptomatic Heart Failure in Individuals with Diabetes

Heart failure stages C and D include People who had HF in the past or are currently exhibiting symptoms of it. In order to diagnose or rule out HF and gauge its severity, biomarker testing for BNP or NT-proBNP is recommended for individuals exhibiting dyspnea. Similar to stage B, normal BNP and NT-proBNP levels in stage C HF have a high negative predictive value, ruling out a diagnosis of decompensated HF. The positive predictive value of an elevated BNP or NT-proBNP for the diagnosis of HF is lower than the negative predictive value. Numerous noncardiac conditions, including advanced age, anemia, renal failure, obstructive sleep apnea, pulmonary hypertension, critical illness, sepsis, and severe burns, may be associated with elevated natriuretic peptide levels.

MANAGEMENT OF HEART FAILURE IN DIABETES

Lifestyle and nutritional interventions form an essential component of management in individuals with diabetes and HF **(Table 1)**.[6,7]

Pharmacologic Management of Diabetes with Heart Failure

Data from multiple extensive prospective trials involving persons with T2D, which considered HF as a secondary outcome, indicated no significant difference in HF rates between the intensive treatment group (mean HbA1c 6.4–7.0%) and the conventional therapy group [mean glycated hemoglobin (HbA1c) 7.3–8.4%].[8] Furthermore, observational studies indicate that the relationship between HbA1c levels and mortality in persons with HF is continuously U-shaped, with the lowest mortality observed in those with HbA1c levels between 7 and 8%. As a result, contemporary diabetes management guidelines differ in the specific glycemic objectives advised. For those individuals with diabetes with symptomatic HFrEF, barring contraindication, the expected components of guideline directed medical treatment (GDMT) includes: (1) Angiotensin receptor/neprilysin for HF, (2) evidenced-based β-blocker, (3) mineralocorticoid receptor antagonist (MRA), and (4) SGLT2i.[9] While the GDMT options for HFpEF are less well defined, SGLT2i is clinically proven therapy to reduce HF hospitalizations and it is reasonable to consider treatment with spironolactone or sacubitril/valsartan. Optimal glycemic targets for individuals with diabetes and HF should be tailored to account for the burden of comorbidities (including the severity of HF), the potential advantages of reducing HbA1c, the patient's life expectancy, and the possible adverse effects of intensive treatment, such as the risk of hypoglycemia, polypharmacy, treatment burden, and elevated healthcare costs and is summarized in **Table 2**.

CONSIDERATIONS ON METABOLIC SURGERY FOR DIABETES AND HEART FAILURE

Metabolic surgery is increasingly recognized as an effective intervention for severe obesity and T2D, due to its impact on metabolic regulation. Addressing cardiometabolic risk factors associated with HF involves various strategies, including weight reduction, modulation of incretins and noninsulinotropic peptides, and decreases in

TABLE 1: Lifestyle and nutrition therapies for people with diabetes and heart failure (HF).

Type of intervention	*Consensus recommendations*	*Points to remember*
Physical activity (cardiac rehabilitation)	• Regular structured exercise should be discussed • Individualize exercise training based on risk stratification, clinical assessment, and cardiopulmonary exercise testing before initiation. • Start deconditioned individuals at lower intensity with shorter sessions • Combine aerobic exercise and resistance training, ideally lifelong • Programs include exercise, education on cardiovascular risk factors, psychological support, lifestyle modification, and medical care focusing on medications with secondary cardiovascular prevention benefits • Refer eligible individuals with diabetes and HF to cardiac rehabilitation as a high priority • Home-based cardiac rehabilitation may be an alternative for clinically stable low-to-moderate risk individuals	• Improves exercise capacity, symptoms, and quality of life for people with HF • Not all individuals can participate in structured programs; identify barriers and facilitators to support patients
Serum potassium	• Clinical monitoring of potassium levels should be part of management plans • Assess serum potassium within 2–3 days and at 7 days, then at least monthly for the first 3 months and every 3 months thereafter, based on renal function and volume status stability • Educate people to avoid over-the-counter potassium supplements and potassium-based salt substitutes • Limit intake of high-potassium foods and beverages • Avoid medications that increase hyperkalemia risk [e.g., nonsteroidal anti-inflammatory drugs (NSAIDs)]	• People with diabetes are at increased risk of hyperkalemia with renin-angiotensin-aldosterone system (RAAS) blockade, including ARB and neprilysin inhibitors • Serum potassium levels independently predict mortality in HF
Smoking	• Provide smoking cessation counseling • Offer appropriate referrals for smoking support	
Dietary salt	• Lower sodium intake to <2,300 mg/day, or even <1,500 mg/day • Use DASH diet, ADA medical nutrition therapy recommendations, or AHA/ACC lifestyle management guidelines to guide sodium recommendations	Optimal salt quantity is debated and should be adapted to clinical situation, symptom severity, and baseline consumption without affecting other nutritional content

Contd...

Contd...

Type of intervention	*Consensus recommendations*	*Points to remember*
Fluid intake	• Restrict daily fluid intake to ~2 L/day for people with fluid retention or congestion not easily controlled with diuretics • Avoid severely limiting fluid to <1.5 L/day unless necessary, as it may adversely affect nutrition, renal function, and quality of life • Apply special consideration for individuals with hyponatremia	Appropriate fluid intake is debated; strict limits should be imposed only with clear fluid overload or sensitivity to fluid intake
Alcohol	• Minimize alcohol intake • Promote education on managing hypoglycemia and hypoglycemia unawareness	Alcohol intake in individuals with diabetes can increase delayed hypoglycemia risk and blunt hypoglycemia awareness
Dietary recommendations	• Tailor diets to caloric needs, personal/cultural food preferences, medications, obesity, and comorbidities • Reduce energy density to <125 kcal/100 g (compared to >160 kcal/100 g in USA/UK) • Limit saturated fat to 5–6% of total calories and eliminate transfat • Increase dietary fiber intake • Recommend a mediterranean-style diet high in MUFA as an alternative to high-carb, low-fat diets • Focus on vegetables, moderate fruits, whole grains, poultry, fish, low-fat dairy, legumes, nontropical vegetable oils, and nuts • Avoid sweets, sugar-sweetened beverages, and red meats • Follow DASH diet principles (vegetables, fruits, whole grains, low-fat milk products, nuts, fish, and lean poultry)	

(ADA: American Diabetes Association; ARB: angiotensin receptor blocker; DASH: dietary approaches to stop hypertension; MUFA: monounsaturated fatty acids)

TABLE 2: Pharmacological treatment for managing hyperglycemia in individuals with diabetes and heart failure (HF).

Drugs	*Consensus recommendations*	*Points to remember*
SGLT2i (e.g., empagliflozin, canagliflozin, and dapagliflozin)	• Reduce risk of HF hospitalizations and major cardiovascular outcomes in individuals with T2D and established ASCVD or high ASCVD risk.[10] • Dapagliflozin and empagliflozin reduce CV death and worsening HF in HFrEF (with or without diabetes) • Canagliflozin and dapagliflozin recommended in T2D with CKD and albuminuria (UACR ≥200 mg/g) • Benefit seen in both HFrEF and HFpEF, and in CKD even without significant albuminuria	• Recommended for T2D with high ASCVD risk, HF, or CKD, *regardless* of glucose-lowering needs • *Mechanisms:* Natriuresis, reduced plasma volume, lowered BP, decreased aortic stiffness, weight loss, reduced oxidative stress, and inflammation • *Risk:* Urinary/genital infections and dehydration • Avoid initiating in those on a *very-low-carb* diet • Initiate early in *stage B* HF; expected component of care in *stage C/D*
GLP-1RA	• Less established benefit in HF vs. SGLT2i • Consider if SGLT2i is contraindicated or not tolerated, including in advanced CKD • May be added to SGLT2i for improved glycemic control, with indirect benefits (weight, BP, and CKD) and low hypoglycemia risk	• May improve LVEF, LVESV, and LV filling pressure • *Potential CV effects:* RAAS inhibition, lowered oxidative stress and BP, improved endothelial function, reduced triglycerides/LDL[11] • *Risk: GI-related side effects*
Metformin	• Safe and effective in absence of contraindications • Favored over sulfonylureas when additional glycemic control is needed • Low risk of hypoglycemia and weight gain	• Associated with reduced all-cause hospitalization in HF • Lower HF hospitalization risk vs. sulfonylureas, including in reduced EF • May cause *GI side effects*
Sulfonylureas	Should be used cautiously and *only if* therapies with proven HF benefit are unavailable	Increased risk of *severe/recurrent hypoglycemia* and *weight gain*
Insulin	Use only when necessary, with caution	May increase risk of *hypoglycemia* and *weight gain*
DPP-4 inhibitors	*Not recommended* in T2D with stage B, C, or D HF	
TZDs	• *Not recommended* in stage B HF • *Contraindicated* in stage C or D HF	Increase risk of *fluid retention and weight gain*

(ASCVD: atherosclerotic cardiovascular disease; CKD: chronic kidney disease; SGLT2i: sodium-glucose cotransporter 2 inhibitors; UACR: urine albumin-to-creatinine ratio)

lipotoxicity, inflammation, and insulin resistance. In addition to reduction in risk factors pertinent to HF, the substantial reduction in body weight linked to metabolic surgery is directly correlated with a decrease in major cardiovascular events among individuals with HF, particularly those with (HFpEF). Additionally, metabolic surgery has been associated with the reversal of cardiac remodeling, leading to enhancements in both systolic and diastolic function.

CONCLUSION

Heart failure remains a major and often underrecognized complication in diabetes, reflecting a complex bidirectional relationship between the two conditions. Current evidence highlights the importance of early detection, lifestyle optimization, and guideline-directed therapies, especially agents with proven cardiovascular benefit such as SGLT2 inhibitors. A stage-based and individualized management approach is essential to effectively combat the growing burden of HF in people with diabetes and improve long-term clinical outcomes.

REFERENCES

1. Park JJ. Epidemiology, pathophysiology, diagnosis and treatment of heart failure in diabetes. Diabet Metab J. 2021;45:146-57.
2. American Diabetes Association. Introduction: Standards of Medical Care in Diabetes—2022. Diabetes Care. 2022;45(Suppl.1):S1-2.
3. Ohkuma T, Komorita Y, Peters SAE, Woodward M. Diabetes as a risk factor for heart failure in women and men: a systematic review and meta-analysis of 47 cohorts including 12 million individuals. Diabetologia. 2019;62:1550-60.
4. Shen J, Greenberg BH. Diabetes management in patients with heart failure. Diabetes Metab J. 2021;45:158-72.
5. Pandey A, Vaduganathan M, Patel KV, Ayers C, Ballantyne CM, Kosiborod MN, et al. Biomarker-based risk prediction of incident heart failure in pre-diabetes and diabetes. JACC Heart Fail. 2021;9:215-23.
6. Khan MS, Khan F, Fonarow GC, Sreenivasan J, Greene SJ, Khan SU, et al. Dietary interventions and nutritional supplements for heart failure: a systematic appraisal and evidence map. Eur J Heart Fail. 2021;23:1468-76.
7. American Diabetes Association. Cardiovascular disease and risk management: Standards of Medical Care in Diabetes—2021. Diabetes Care. 2021;44(Suppl. 1):S125-50.
8. Skyler JS, Bergenstal R, Bonow RO, Buse J, Deedwania P, Gale EA, et al.; American Diabetes Association; American College of Cardiology Foundation; American Heart Association. Intensive glycemic control and the prevention of cardiovascular events: implications of the ACCORD, ADVANCE, and VA diabetes trials: a Position Statement of the American Diabetes Association and a Scientific Statement of the American College of Cardiology Foundation and the American Heart Association. Diabetes Care. 2009;32:187-92.
9. Diabetes Canada Clinical Practice Guidelines Expert Committee; Connelly KA, Gilbert RE, Liu P. Treatment of diabetes in people with heart failure. Can J Diabetes. 2018;42(Suppl. 1):S196-200.
10. Zelniker TA, Wiviott SD, Raz I, Im K, Goodrich EL, Bonaca MP, et al. SGLT2 inhibitors for primary and secondary prevention of cardiovascular and renal outcomes in type 2 diabetes: a systematic review and meta-analysis of cardiovascular outcome trials. Lancet. 2019;393:31-9.
11. Heuvelman VD, Van Raalte DH, Smits MM. Cardiovascular effects of glucagon-like peptide 1 receptor agonists: from mechanistic studies in humans to clinical outcomes. Cardiovasc Res. 2020;116:916-30.

CHAPTER 13

Heart Failure with Preserved Ejection Fraction: A Cardiologist's Perspective

Pankaj Manoria, Somyata Somendra, Vineet Sankhla

ABSTRACT

Recognition and management of heart failure with preserved ejection fraction (HFpEF) remain challenging due to its multifactorial origin and strong association with systemic comorbidities. Patients commonly present with exertional limitation and congestion despite normal systolic function, requiring careful clinical evaluation supported by imaging and diagnostic scoring systems. Contemporary management prioritizes volume control, optimization of blood pressure and metabolic risk factors, and treatment tailored to underlying phenotypes. Recent therapeutic advances, particularly sodium-glucose cotransporter 2 (SGLT2) inhibitors and obesity-directed therapies, have improved symptom burden and reduced hospitalization risk, marking a transition toward individualized management strategies in HFpEF.

Keywords: HFpEF, heart failure management, diastolic dysfunction, comorbidity-driven disease, SGLT2 inhibitors, personalized therapy.

INTRODUCTION

Heart failure with preserved ejection fraction (HFpEF) represents a complex clinical syndrome characterized by the presence of heart failure (HF) symptoms and signs despite a left ventricular ejection fraction (LVEF) ≥50%. Unlike classical systolic heart failure, the central abnormality in HFpEF is diastolic dysfunction—the inability of the ventricle to fill adequately without a rise in filling pressures.[1-3]

Over the past two decades, HFpEF has transitioned from a "diagnosis of exclusion" to a distinct pathophysiological entity, with specific hemodynamic, structural, and molecular mechanisms. HFpEF now accounts for > 50% of all heart failure cases worldwide, with an increasing burden owing to aging populations, hypertension, obesity, and diabetes.[4-6]

EPIDEMIOLOGY

The HFpEF is highly prevalent in elderly populations, especially among women and patients with metabolic comorbidities. In community studies, its prevalence increases exponentially after 60 years of age, paralleling hypertension and atrial fibrillation (AF). The lifetime risk of developing HFpEF is estimated to exceed 20% after age 65, and women constitute nearly two-thirds of this population.[4,7]

Important epidemiologic observations include:

- Hypertension is the single strongest antecedent, present in > 80% of cases.
- Obesity and diabetes mellitus contribute to systemic inflammation and microvascular dysfunction.
- Atrial fibrillation is both a risk factor and a consequence of elevated filling pressures.
- Chronic kidney disease (CKD) and coronary artery disease (CAD) are frequent comorbidities.

The incidence and mortality of HFpEF continue to rise, whereas outcomes in heart failure with reduced ejection fraction (HFrEF) have improved due to disease-modifying therapies.

Thus, HFpEF has emerged as the dominant phenotype of HF in developed countries.

PATHOPHYSIOLOGY

Overview

The HFpEF is not a single disease but a syndrome with multiple phenotypes. The central hemodynamic feature is elevated left ventricular (LV) filling pressures at rest or during exertion, secondary to impaired relaxation, increased stiffness, or both.[8-11]

Normal Diastolic Physiology

Normal LV filling depends on rapid active relaxation and passive distensibility. During early diastole, LV pressure falls quickly due to elastic recoil and "untwisting" of the myocardium, allowing efficient suction of blood from the left atrium (LA). A compliant ventricle can accommodate volume at low pressures, maintaining pulmonary venous pressure below 15 mm Hg.

Diastolic Dysfunction in Heart Failure with Preserved Ejection Fraction

In HFpEF, diastolic relaxation is slowed and incomplete, and the LV becomes stiffer, leading to a leftward shift of the diastolic pressure-volume relationship.

Key abnormalities include:

- Prolonged relaxation and delayed isovolumic pressure decay.
- Reduced early diastolic suction, making filling highly dependent on atrial contraction.
- Elevated LV end-diastolic pressure, transmitted backward to the pulmonary veins.
- Increased LV wall thickness and mass, with concentric remodeling and preserved chamber volume.

These abnormalities explain exertional dyspnea; even small rises in venous return during exercise result in disproportionate pulmonary pressure increases.

Structural and Cellular Remodeling

HFpEF is characterized by:

- Concentric LV hypertrophy, increased wall thickness, and normal or reduced LV volumes.
- Left atrial enlargement, reflecting chronic elevation of LV filling pressure.
- Interstitial fibrosis, increased collagen deposition, and cardiomyocyte hypertrophy.
- Microvascular inflammation and endothelial dysfunction, leading to reduced nitric oxide bioavailability and titin hypophosphorylation, increase stiffness.
- Systemic inflammation secondary to obesity, diabetes, and aging *alters* myocardial energetics and calcium handling.

Extracardiac Contributions

Abnormalities are not limited to the LV:

- Pulmonary hypertension and right ventricular (RV) dysfunction arise from chronic elevation of LA pressure.[11]
- Arterial stiffness and impaired vasodilator reserve increase afterload.
- Skeletal muscle dysfunction and impaired oxygen utilization contribute to exercise intolerance.

CLINICAL FEATURES AND DIAGNOSIS OF HEART FAILURE WITH PRESERVED EJECTION FRACTION

Clinical Features

The HFpEF presents with symptoms and signs of heart failure (HF) in the presence of a normal or near-normal LVEF ≥ 50%. The cardinal features—*dyspnea, exercise intolerance, and fatigue*—result from elevated left ventricular (LV) filling pressures and impaired diastolic reserve.

The clinical manifestations can be insidious, often precipitated or worsened by comorbidities and acute stressors such as infection, arrhythmia, or uncontrolled hypertension.[12]

Symptoms

- *Exertional dyspnea and fatigue*—the earliest and most common complaints, related to limited cardiac output augmentation and pulmonary venous hypertension.
- *Orthopnea and paroxysmal nocturnal dyspnea (PND)*—secondary to elevated LV filling pressures and pulmonary congestion.
- *Peripheral edema and weight gain*—indicate systemic venous congestion and right ventricular (RV) involvement.
- *Exercise intolerance*—multifactorial, due to impaired chronotropic reserve, skeletal muscle abnormalities, and vascular stiffness.
- *Palpitations*—often due to atrial fibrillation (AF), which coexists in up to 40–60% of HFpEF cases.

Overall, the *clinical presentation of HFpEF mirrors that of HFrEF*, though often more subtle. Dyspnea and fatigue dominate, with symptoms often precipitated by exertion or comorbidities.[13]

Physical Signs

Clinical examination may reveal elevated jugular venous pressure, pulmonary rales, S4 gallop, hepatomegaly, or peripheral edema. A significant proportion of patients show evidence of *hypertensive heart disease*, obesity, or metabolic syndrome, reflecting underlying systemic contributors **(Table 1)**.

TABLE 1: Common clinical features and their mechanistic correlates.

Clinical features	*Underlying mechanism*
Exertional dyspnea, fatigue	Elevated left ventricular (LV) filling pressure, reduced cardiac reserve
Orthopnea, paroxysmal nocturnal dyspnea (PND)	Pulmonary venous congestion
Peripheral edema, weight gain	Systemic venous hypertension, right ventricular (RV) dysfunction
Palpitations	Atrial fibrillation, loss of atrial contribution
Exercise intolerance	Impaired chronotropic response, vascular stiffness, skeletal myopathy
Angina-like chest discomfort	Microvascular ischemia, LV hypertrophy

PRECIPITATING FACTORS AND ASSOCIATED RISK

The HFpEF typically arises in a *vulnerable substrate* with comorbidities such as hypertension, diabetes, obesity, and CKD. Acute decompensation often follows identifiable triggers.

- *Atrial fibrillation:* Loss of atrial contraction and rapid ventricular response raise LV filling pressures.[14]
- *Uncontrolled hypertension:* An abrupt afterload increase leads to pulmonary congestion.
- *Ischemia:* Even a minor supply-demand mismatch impairs relaxation and diastolic filling.
- *Volume overload or renal dysfunction:* Salt retention augments venous pressures.
- *Infection, anemia, thyroid disorders, or tachyarrhythmia:* Exacerbate hemodynamic stress and decompensation.

These triggers are particularly deleterious in elderly women with hypertension and metabolic disease, where diastolic compliance is already impaired.

DIAGNOSTIC EVALUATION

The HFpEF remains a *clinical diagnosis supported by objective evidence* of elevated filling pressures, structural heart disease, or natriuretic peptide elevation, in the absence of alternate causes such as valvular, infiltrative, or pericardial disease. Diagnosis integrates *clinical context, biomarkers, imaging, and hemodynamic testing.*[12-15]

When to Suspect HFpEF

The HFpEF should be suspected in patients with *symptoms of HF* and preserved LVEF, especially if they have:

- Age ≥ 60 years
- Hypertension or obesity
- AF, CAD, diabetes, or CKD

Stepwise Diagnostic Approach

- *Clinical suspicion*—unexplained dyspnea, preserved LVEF, presence of comorbidities.
- *Rule out mimics*—pulmonary disease, anemia, pericardial constriction, obesity-hypoventilation, or high-output HF.
- *Echocardiography*—evidence of diastolic dysfunction [E/e′ > 9, left atrial (LA) enlargement, left ventricular (LV) hypertrophy].
- *Natriuretic peptides*—B-type natriuretic peptide (BNP) ≥ 35 pg/mL or NT-proBNP ≥ 125 pg/mL in sinus rhythm; higher thresholds in AF.
- *Supportive imaging or invasive data*—elevated LV end-diastolic or pulmonary capillary wedge pressure (≥15 mmHg at rest or ≥25 mm Hg with exercise).

Diagnostic Scoring Systems

H_2FPEF Score[12]

This score combines six variables to estimate the probability of HFpEF in patients with unexplained dyspnea **(Table 2)**.

TABLE 2: H_2FPEF Score.

Variable	*Points*
Body mass index (BMI) >30 kg/m^2	2
≥2 antihypertensive medications	1
Atrial fibrillation	3
Pulmonary artery systolic pressure >35 mm Hg	1
Age >60 years	1
E/e′ >9	1

Interpretation:

- *0–1:* Low probability (≤25%)
- *2–5:* Intermediate (up to 70%)
- *≥6:* High probability (≥90%)

The score is validated for noninvasive clinical settings and can guide referral for diastolic stress testing or invasive hemodynamic assessment.

HFA–PEFF Algorithm[15]

The *heart failure association (HFA)-PEFF diagnostic algorithm* proposes a stepwise approach combining clinical, echocardiographic, and biomarker domains.

Step 1: Pretest assessment—HF symptoms with preserved EF (Table 3)

Step 2: Scoring Domains

Scoring:

- ≥5 points → HFpEF confirmed
- 2–4 points → Indeterminate → perform stress echo or invasive testing
- ≤1 point → HFpEF unlikely

Step 3: Role of Exercise and Invasive Testing

When noninvasive findings are inconclusive, *exercise echocardiography, or right heart catheterization* may demonstrate an abnormal rise in LV filling pressures [pulmonary capillary wedge pressure (PCWP) ≥25 mm Hg during exercise], confirming HFpEF. These tests help differentiate HFpEF from noncardiac causes of exertional dyspnea, such as deconditioning or pulmonary disease.[16,17]

TABLE 3: Heart failure symptoms with preserved ejection fraction.

Domain	Major criteria (2 points)	Minor criteria (1 point)
Functional	E/e' ≥15; TR velocity > 2.8 m/s	E/e' 9–14; GLS <16%
Morphologic	Left atrium (LA) volume index >34 mL/m²; left ventricular (LV) mass index ↑	Relative wall thickness >0.42
Biomarker	NT-proBNP >220 pg/mL (sinus rhythm)/>660 pg/mL (AF)	NT-proBNP >125–220 pg/mL

(NT-proBNP: Natriuretic peptides—B-type natriuretic peptide)

TABLE 4: Diagnostic framework for HFpEF.

Component	Key criteria/thresholds
Symptoms and signs	Dyspnea, fatigue, orthopnea, edema
LVEF	≥50%
Structural abnormality	Left ventricular (LV) hypertrophy, left atrium (LA) enlargement
Functional abnormality	E/e' >9–15, TR >2.8 m/s
Biomarkers	BNP ≥ 35 pg/mL or NT-proBNP ≥ 125 pg/mL
Hemodynamics	PCWP ≥ 15 mm Hg at rest or ≥25 mm Hg on exercise

(BNP: B-type natriuretic peptide; HFpEF: Heart failure with preserved ejection fraction; NT-proBNP: Natriuretic peptides—B-type natriuretic peptide; LVEF: Left ventricular ejection fraction; PCWP: pulmonary capillary wedge pressure)

Key Diagnostic Insights

- *Obesity and AF lower the diagnostic sensitivity of natriuretic peptides*, necessitating reliance on imaging and hemodynamics rather than biomarkers alone.
- *Diastolic stress testing*, unmasking exercise-induced elevation in LV filling pressures, is increasingly used in specialized centers.
- *Multimodality imaging* [echo, cardiac magnetic resonance imaging (MRI)] helps identify mimics such as amyloidosis or hypertrophic cardiomyopathy.
- *HFpEF mimics*—valvular disease, constrictive pericarditis, high-output states, or infiltrative cardiomyopathies—must be systematically excluded **(Table 4)**.

The stepwise diagnostic approach to HFpEF is illustrated in **Flowchart 1**.

THERAPEUTIC PRINCIPLES IN HEART FAILURE WITH PRESERVED EJECTION FRACTION

The HFpEF is a *heterogeneous syndrome*, driven by systemic inflammation, cardiometabolic dysfunction, myocardial stiffness, microvascular disease, and extracardiac comorbidities. Unlike HFrEF, *no therapy convincingly reduces mortality* across the entire HFpEF spectrum. Management, therefore, focuses on:

- Reducing *heart failure hospitalizations*
- Improving *symptoms, functional capacity, and quality of life* **(Table 5)**

Treating *phenotype-specific drivers* (obesity, diabetes, CKD, AF, hypertension).

PHARMACOTHERAPY AND DEVICE-BASED THERAPIES

Recent trials have shifted HFpEF treatment from nihilism to *selective disease-modifying therapy*, led by SGLT2 inhibitors and obesity-targeted agents.

Pharmacotherapy

First-line disease-modifying therapy: SGLT2 inhibitors

Rationale: The SGLT2 inhibitors are the only drug class with consistent, guideline-endorsed benefit

Flowchart 1: Stepwise diagnostic approach to heart failure with preserved ejection fraction (HFpEF).

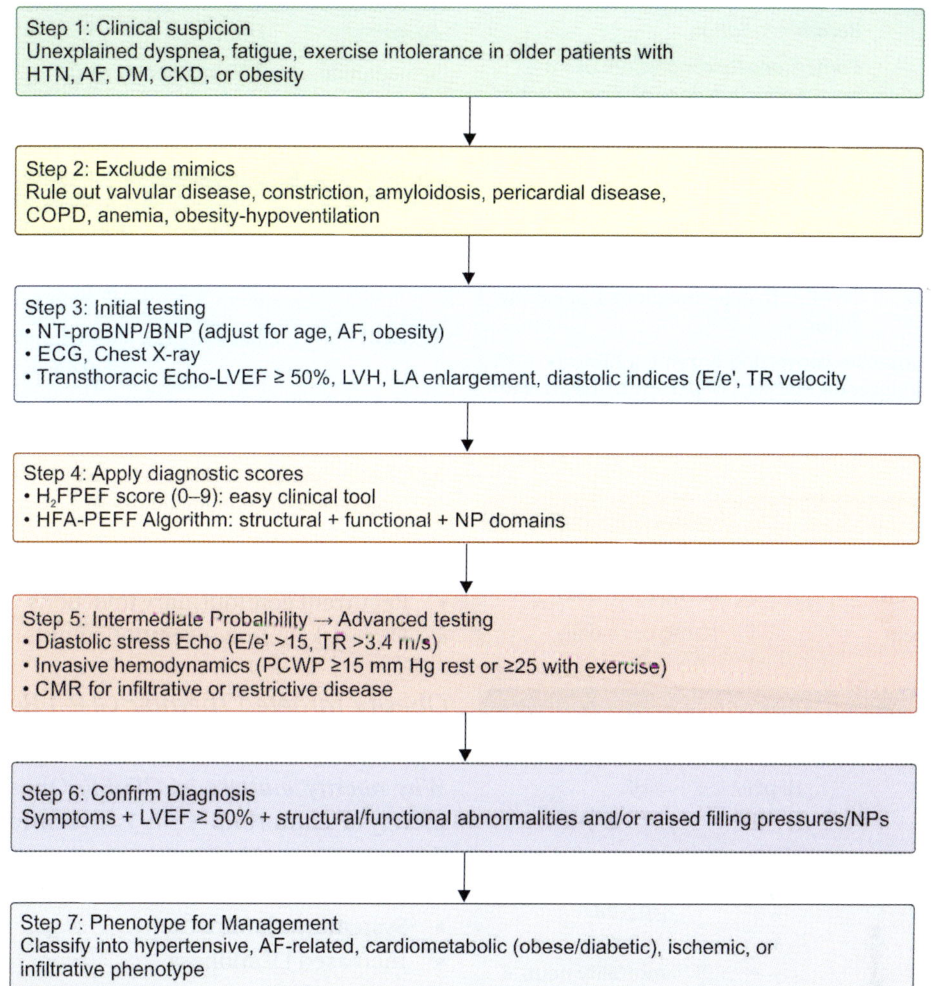

(AF: Atrial Fibrillation; CKD: Chronic Kidney Disease; CMR: Cardiac Magnetic Resonance; COPD: Chronic Obstructive Pulmonary Disease; DM: Diabetes Mellitus; ECG: Electrocardiogram; HTN: Hypertension; LVEF: Left Ventricular Ejection Fraction; PCWP: Pulmonary Capillary Wedge Pressure; PR: Pressure/Rate)

in HFpEF across a broad LVEF range.[18,19] Their benefit appears independent of diabetes status and likely reflects pleiotropic effects on:

- Cardiac loading conditions
- Renal function
- Inflammation and myocardial energetics

Indication:

- HFpEF (LVEF ≥ 50%)
- New York Heart Association (NYHA) class II–III symptoms

Agents and dosing **(Table 6)**:

A *class effect* is assumed; patients already on another SGLT2 inhibitor can continue the same agent.

Key clinical trial evidence **(Table 7)**:

Quality-of-life scores (KCCQ) consistently improved, with *no significant mortality reduction.*

TABLE 5: General measures in the treatment of HFpEF.

Strategy	*Recommendation*
Diuretics	*Cornerstone for congestion:* Use the lowest effective dose of loop diuretics
Blood pressure control	Target <130/80 mm Hg; ACEi/ARB preferred for hypertension
Lifestyle	Salt restriction, regular exercise, and weight reduction
Vaccination	Influenza, pneumococcal vaccines
Avoid drugs	NSAIDs, thiazolidinediones, or excess fluids

(ACEi: Angiotensin-converting enzyme inhibitors; ARB: Angiotensin receptor blockers; HFpEF: Heart failure with preserved ejection fraction; NSAIDs: Nonsteroidal anti-inflammatory drugs)

TABLE 6: Agents and dosing.

Drug	*Dose*
Empagliflozin	10 mg once daily
Dapagliflozin	10 mg once daily

TABLE 7: Key clinical trial evidence.

Trial/meta-analysis	*Population*	*Key outcome*
EMPEROR-Preserved, DELIVER	HFpEF/ HFmrEF	↓ HF hospitalization
Meta-analysis (HFpEF + HFmrEF)	12,000 pts	HF hospitalization: HR *0.74* All-cause mortality neutral

(HF: Heart failure; HFpEF: Heart failure with preserved ejection fraction)

Safety considerations:

Avoid:

- Type 1 diabetes
- Prior or high risk of diabetic ketoacidosis (DKA)
- Pregnancy

Use with caution:

- Volume depletion or hypotension
- eGFR <20 mL/min/1.73 m² or rapidly declining renal function

TABLE 8: Agents and dosing.

Agent	*Titration*
Semaglutide	0.25 mg weekly → up to 2.4 mg
Tirzepatide	2.5 mg weekly → up to 15 mg

TABLE 9: Key trials evidence in HFpEF.

Trial	*Population*	*Main findings*
STEP-HFpEF	Obese HFpEF	↑ KCCQ, ↑ 6-MWD, ↓ HF events
SUMMIT	Obese HFpEF	HF hospitalization HR 0.44
Meta-analysis	HFpEF	Worsening HF HR 0.56

(HF: Heart failure; HR: Heart rate; HFpEF: Heart failure with preserved ejection fraction; 6-MWD: 6-minute walk distance)

- Recurrent genitourinary infections
- High risk for foot ulceration or amputation

Obesity-targeted Therapy: GLP-1 Receptor Agonists

Why obesity matters in HFpEF: Obesity is not merely a comorbidity—it is a central disease driver in many HFpEF phenotypes, contributing to:

- Systemic inflammation
- Increased LV stiffness
- Impaired exercise capacity

Indication:

- HFpEF with body mass index *(BMI)* ≥*30 kg/m²*
- Particularly effective when *BMI* ≥ *35 kg/m²*

Agents and dosing[20,21] **(Table 8)**

Can be safely combined with SGLT2 inhibitors as shown by Key Trial **(Table 9)**.

Weight loss ranged from *~10 to 13%*, far exceeding lifestyle intervention trials, with parallel improvements in:

- Exercise capacity
- Symptom burden
- Health-related quality of life

Limitations:

- Gastrointestinal (GI) intolerance leading to discontinuation (≈4–5%).
- Long-term HF outcomes beyond symptom improvement remain under study.

Secondary Therapy: Mineralocorticoid Receptor Antagonists

Role in HFpEF: Mineralocorticoid receptor antagonists (MRAs) offer modest reductions in HF hospitalization, particularly in carefully selected patients, but do not reduce mortality.[22,23]

Indication:

- *Persistent New York Heart Association (NYHA) II–III symptoms despite:*
    - Diuretics
    - SGLT2 inhibitor ± GLP-1 RA

Eligibility:

- Serum K^+ ≤4.7 mEq/L
- eGFR ≥ 30 mL/min/1.73 m^2

  Agents and dosing **(Table 10)**

  Key evidence **(Table 11)**

Important caveat: TOPCAT showed strong *regional heterogeneity*, raising concerns about adherence and diagnostic accuracy outside the Americas.

TABLE 10: Agents and dosing.

Agent	*Starting dose*	*Target*
Spironolactone	12.5 mg daily	25–50 mg
Eplerenone	25 mg daily	50 mg
Finerenone	eGFR-based	Up-titrate

(eGFR: estimated glomerular filtration rate)

TABLE 11: Key evidence.

Trial	*Key result*
TOPCAT	↓ Heart failure (HF) hospitalization (HR *0.83*)
FINEARTS	↓ HF events (rate ratio *0.82*)
Meta-analysis	HF hospitalization HR *0.82*

Adverse effects:

- Hyperkalemia
- Worsening renal function
- Blood pressure reduction is usually minimal.

Therapies with Limited or Selective Roles

Sacubitril–valsartan:

- *PARAGON-HF:* Borderline reduction in HF hospitalization[24]
- No mortality benefit
- Higher hypotension and angioedema risk
- May benefit *selected subgroups* (lower EF range, recent HF admission)

ACE inhibitors/ARBs:

- *Not disease-modifying in HFpEF*
- Useful for comorbidities (HTN, CKD, CAD)
- PEP-CHF, CHARM-Preserved, I-PRESERVE: neutral on major outcomes

β-blockers:

- No proven HFpEF benefit
- *Indicated for:*
    - AF rate control
    - Chronic coronary syndrome
    - Hypertension

Calcium channel blockers:

- Symptom-directed use (e.g., hypertension)
- No HF-specific benefit

Ineffective or Harmful Therapies in HFpEF (Table 12)

TABLE 12: Ineffective or harmful therapies in HFpEF.

Therapy	*Evidence*
Nitrates	↓ activity (NEAT-HFpEF)
PDE-5 inhibitors	Neutral or harmful (RELAX, tadalafil trials)
Digoxin	No benefit (DIG ancillary)
Endothelin antagonists	Neutral

(PDE-5: phosphodiesterase type 5)

TABLE 13: Management of comorbidities.

Comorbidity	*Management focus*
Atrial fibrillation	Rate/rhythm control, anticoagulation; rhythm restoration improves symptoms
Hypertension	Strict control reduces hospitalization
Diabetes	Prefer SGLT2 inhibitors or GLP-1 agonists
Obesity/OSA	Weight loss, CPAP improve hemodynamics
Coronary artery disease	Revascularize if ischemia contributes to HF
CKD/anemia	Optimize volume and correct contributing factors

(CKD: Chronic kidney disease; CPAP: continuous positive airway pressure; GLP-1: Glucagon-like peptide-1; OSA: Obstructive sleep apnea; SGLT2: sodium-glucose transporter 2 inhibitors)

Device-based Therapies

Remote Pulmonary Artery Pressure Monitoring

Role: Highly selected patients with recurrent HF admissions despite optimal therapy.[25]

Evidence:

- CHAMPION and related trials suggest ↓ HF hospitalization
- *Limitations:*
    - Mixed HF populations
    - COVID-era confounding
    - Lack of blinding

Not Recommended for Routine HFpEF Rare

Interatrial Shunt Devices

- Reduce LA pressure acutely[26]
- Long-term trials failed to show benefit and raised safety concerns
- *Not recommended*

Pacing Strategies

- No consistent benefit in HFpEF[27]
- Pacemakers should be implanted *only for standard rhythm indications*
- Experimental pacing strategies remain investigational

The management of comorbidities are given in **Table 13**.

Exercise and Cardiac Rehabilitation

Structured *aerobic exercise* improves peak VO_2 and quality of life. Programs combining *endurance and resistance training* show the greatest benefit in diastolic filling and vascular function.

PROGNOSIS (TABLE 14)

- *5-year mortality* ≈50%, similar to HFrEF.[4,7]
- *Predictors of poor outcome:* advanced age, AF, CKD, pulmonary hypertension, and recurrent hospitalizations.
- *Sudden cardiac death* is less frequent than in HFrEF; deaths are mainly from noncardiac causes (renal failure, infection, stroke).
- LVEF ≥50%. (Many pivotal trials enrolled LVEF ≥40–45%; benefit often greatest at *lower* EF within the "preserved" spectrum).

PHARMACOLOGICAL TREATMENT OF HFpEF

The Stepwise pharmacological management of HFpEF is outlined in **Flowchart 2**.

TABLE 14: Heart failure with preserved ejection fraction (HFpEF) pharmacotherapy (disease-modifying + phenotype-directed) aligned to the European Society of Cardiology (ESC)/American College of Cardiology (ACC).

Therapy class	*Who to use (typical wording)*	*Guideline position (ESC/ACC-AHA-HFSA)*	*Key trial evidence (headline)*	*Expected benefit (what to tell patients)*	*Practical dosing*	*Key safety/ monitoring*
SGLT2 inhibitor (empagliflozin/ dapagliflozin)	Symptomatic HFpEF (often NYHA II–III), regardless of diabetes status	ESC 2023: *Recommended* for HFpEF to reduce HF hospitalization/ CV death (Class I, LOE A). ACC/AHA/ HFSA 2022: *Can be beneficial* in HFpEF to reduce HF hospitalizations and CV mortality (Class 2a)	Meta-analysis (HFpEF + HFmrEF): HF hospitalization HR 0.74; all-cause mortality neutral; QoL improves	Modest reduction in HF hospitalizations; QoL improvement; mortality benefit not clearly shown in HFpEF	Empagliflozin 10 mg OD or dapagliflozin 10 mg OD	Avoid T1DM, pregnancy; avoid/ high caution with prior DKA risk, volume depletion/ hypotension, eGFR <20, rapidly falling kidney function, recurrent complicated GU infections; counsel genital mycotic infection risk
GLP-1 receptor agonist (semaglutide/ tirzepatide)—*obesity phenotype*	HFpEF with body mass index (BMI) ≥ 30 (often higher benefit at BMI ≥ 35) + lifestyle weight loss	Not yet a core "HF guideline GDMT" pillar in ESC/ACC HF guidelines; increasingly recommended in HFpEF phenotype/obesity management pathways (expert consensus rather than Class/LOE)	Tirzepatide trial (BMI ≥30, LVEF ≥50): HF hospitalization HR 0.44, QoL (KCCQ) +6.9 points vs placebo at 52w; more GI discontinuation. Semaglutide (STEP-HFpEF): ↑KCCQ, ↑6-MWD, ↓urgent HF visits; weight loss ~10–13%	Large improvements in symptoms/ QoL and exercise capacity, meaningful weight loss; HF events signal favorable; mortality neutral to date	Semaglutide: start 0.25 mg weekly, uptitrate q4w to 2.4 mg. Tirzepatide: start 2.5 mg weekly, uptitrate q4w to 15 mg	Gastrointestinal (GI) intolerance (nausea/vomiting/ diarrhea), gallbladder disease risk; monitor weight, BP, volume status; continue long-term if tolerated; can combine with SGLT2i

Contd...

Contd…

Therapy class	*Who to use (typical wording)*	*Guideline position (ESC/ACC-AHA-HFSA)*	*Key trial evidence (headline)*	*Expected benefit (what to tell patients)*	*Practical dosing*	*Key safety/ monitoring*
MRA (spironolactone/ eplerenone/ finerenone)	Persistent symptoms despite diuretic + SGLT2i (± GLP-1 RA in obesity) and eligible renal/K+ profile	ACC/AHA/HFSA 2022: MRAs *may be considered* in HFpEF (Class 2b). (ESC: MRAs used selectively; strongest HFpEF "disease-modifying" recommendation is SGLT2i.)	TOPCAT: HF hospitalization HR 0.83; mortality neutral; hyperK/ creatinine ↑. FINEARTS (finerenone): ↓ urgent/unplanned HF events (rate ratio 0.82); mortality neutral. Meta-analysis: HF hospitalization HR 0.82; mortality neutral	Small reduction in HF hospitalizations; minimal BP effect; no proven mortality benefit	Spironolactone 12.5 mg OD, titrate q2w to 25–50 mg. Eplerenone 25 → 50 mg OD. Finerenone eGFR-based dosing	Start only if K ≤4.7 and eGFR ≥30. If K >5.0, reduce/stop. Check K/Cr at ~3–7 days, 1 month, then periodically; avoid high-K diet/ NSAIDs where possible
ARNI (sacubitril/ valsartan)	Selected HFpEF patients (often lower EF within HFpEF, women, recent HF admission) where BP tolerates	ACC/AHA/HFSA 2022: ARNI *may be considered* (Class 2b). (ESC: more selective use; strongest HFpEF recommendation remains SGLT2i)	PARAGON-HF: borderline ↓ HF hospitalizations (rate ratio 0.85, CI up to 1.00); mortality neutral; hypotension/ angiedema ↑; hyperK/renal events ↓	Possible reduction in HF hospitalizations in selected subgroups; not a universal HFpEF therapy	Standard ARNI initiation/ titration per BP/renal function	Watch for hypotension, angioedema, renal function; avoid with a history of angioedema; washout after ACEi
ARB (e.g., candesartan/ irbesartan)	Mainly for hypertension/ CKD/diabetes; HFpEF role is modest/ uncertain	ACC/AHA/HFSA 2022: ARBs *may be considered* (Class 2b)	CHARM-Preserved: borderline ↓ HF hospitalizations; I-PRESERVE neutral	BP control + comorbidity management; HF outcomes inconsistent	Usual HTN/CKD dosing	Renal function/K monitoring; BP targets as per HTN guidance

Contd…

Contd...

Therapy class	***Who to use (typical wording)***	***Guideline position (ESC/ACC-AHA-HFSA)***	***Key trial evidence (headline)***	***Expected benefit (what to tell patients)***	***Practical dosing***	***Key safety/ monitoring***
ACE inhibitor	For other indications (post-MI, CKD, diabetes, HTN), not primary HFpEF therapy	Not recommended as HFpEF-specific disease-modifying therapy (use for comorbidity indications)	PEP-CHF: primary endpoint neutral; some functional improvement signals	Symptom/functional benefit inconsistent; HF outcomes not robust	Standard ACEi dosing	Renal function/K; cough/ angioedema
β-blocker	AF rate control, chronic coronary syndrome, HTN	Not HFpEF-specific outcome-modifying; used for comorbidities	Individual patient meta-analysis: no clear benefit in sinus rhythm LVEF ≥ 50%	Symptom control via HR/BP; no proven HFpEF outcome benefit	Agent-specific	Bradycardia, fatigue; adjust in chronotropic incompetence
Calcium channel blocker	Later-line HTN therapy; angina if appropriate	Symptom/HTN management only	—	BP/angina control; no HFpEF outcome benefit	Agent-specific	Edema, bradycardia (non-DHP)
Not recommended for HFpEF treatment: Organic nitrates; PDE-5 inhibitors; digoxin (unless AF rate control); endothelin antagonists	Avoid routine use for HFpEF symptom/ outcome improvement	ACC/AHA/HFSA 2022: Avoid routine nitrates/PDE-5i (Class 3: No Benefit).	NEAT-HFpEF: isosorbide mononitrate ↓ daily activity; RELAX etc.: PDE-5i neutral; DIG ancillary: no outcome benefit	No outcome benefit; some may worsen activity tolerance	—	Use only for non-HFpEF indications (angina, AF rate control, etc.)

(ARNI: angiotensin receptor–neprilysin inhibitor; COR: class of recommendation; HTN: Hypertension; LOE: level of evidence; KCCQ: Kansas City Cardiomyopathy Questionnaire; 6-MWD: 6-minute walk distance; MRA: mineralocorticoid receptor antagonist; SGLT2i: sodium–glucose cotransporter-2 inhibitor)

Flowchart 2: Stepwise pharmacological management of heart failure with preserved ejection fraction (HFpEF).

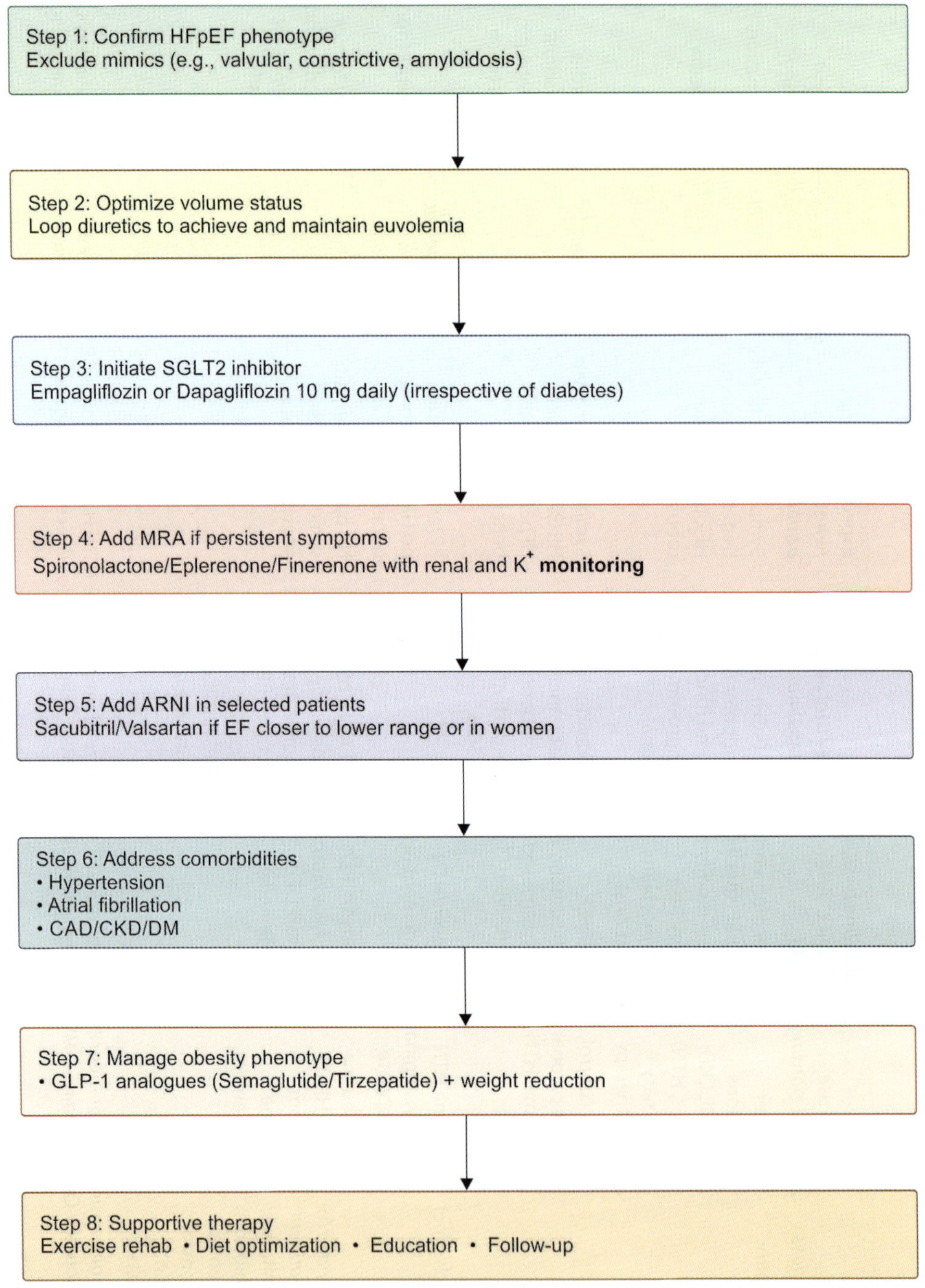

(CAD: Coronary artery disease; CKD: Chronic kidney disease; CPAP: Continuous positive airway pressure; DM: Diabetes mellitus; GLP-1: Glucagon-like peptide-1; HFpEF: Heart failure with preserved ejection fraction; SGLT2: sodium-glucose transporter 2 inhibitors)

CONCLUSION

The HFpEF represents a shift in heart failure care from single-drug therapy to comprehensive risk and comorbidity management. Accurate clinical recognition, structured diagnostic evaluation, and targeted treatment of associated metabolic and cardiovascular conditions form the basis of effective care. Emerging therapies have improved symptom control and reduced hospitalizations, but long-term outcome improvement depends on individualized, patient-centered management strategies.

REFERENCES

1. Borlaug B, Sharma K, Shah S, Ho J. Heart failure with preserved ejection fraction: JACC scientific statement. J Am Coll Cardiol. 2023;81:1810-34.
2. Redfield M. Heart failure with preserved ejection fraction. N Engl J Med. 2017;376:897-907.
3. Borlaug BA. Evaluation and management of heart failure with preserved ejection fraction. Nat Rev Cardiol. 2020;17:559-73.
4. Bhatia RS, Tu JV, Lee DS, Austin PC, Fang J, Haouzi A, et al. Outcome of heart failure with preserved ejection fraction in a population-based study. N Engl J Med. 2006;355:260-9.
5. Heidenreich P, Bozkurt B, Aguilar D, Allen LA, Byun JJ, Colvin MM. 2022 AHA/ACC/HFSA guideline for the management of heart failure. Circulation. 2022;145:e895-1032.
6. McDonagh T, Metra M, Adamo M, McDonagh T, Metra M, Adamo M. 2021 ESC Guidelines for the diagnosis and treatment of acute and chronic heart failure. Eur Heart J. 2021;42:3599-726.
7. 2021 ESC Guidelines for the diagnosis and treatment of acute and chronic heart failure. Eur Heart J. 2021;42:3599-726.
8. Owan TE, Redfield MM. Epidemiology of diastolic heart failure. Prog Cardiovasc Dis. 2005;47:320–32.
9. Kitzman DW, Little WC, Brubaker PH, others. Pathophysiological characterisation of isolated diastolic heart failure. JAMA. 2002;288:2144–50.
10. Zile MR, Bennett TD, St John Sutton M, others. Transition from chronic compensated to acute decompensated heart failure: pathophysiological insights obtained from continuous monitoring of intracardiac pressures. Circulation. 2008;118:1433.
11. Mohammed SF, Hussain I, Mirzoyev SA, others. Coronary microvascular rarefaction and myocardial fibrosis in heart failure with preserved ejection fraction. Circulation. 2015;131:550.
12. Lam CS, Roger VL, Rodeheffer RJ, others. Pulmonary hypertension in heart failure with preserved ejection fraction: a community-based study. J Am Coll Cardiol. 2009;53:1119.
13. Reddy Y, Carter R, Obokata M, others. A simple, evidence-based approach to help guide the diagnosis of heart failure with preserved ejection fraction. Circulation. 2018;138:861-70.
14. Reddy Y, Kaye D, Handoko M, others. Diagnosis of heart failure with preserved ejection fraction among patients with unexplained dyspnea. JAMA Cardiol. 2022;7:891-9.
15. Zakeri R, Chamberlain AM, Roger VL, Redfield MM. Temporal relationship and prognostic significance of atrial fibrillation in heart failure patients with preserved ejection fraction: a community-based study. Circulation. 2013;128:1085.
16. Pieske B, Tschöpe C, de Boer R, others. How to diagnose heart failure with preserved ejection fraction: the HFA-PEFF diagnostic algorithm. Eur Heart J. 2019;40:3297-317.
17. Obokata M, Kane G, Reddy Y, others. Role of diastolic stress testing in the evaluation for heart failure with preserved ejection fraction. Circulation. 2017;135:825-38.
18. Borlaug B, Nishimura R, Sorajja P, others. Exercise hemodynamics enhance the diagnosis of early heart failure with preserved ejection fraction. Circ Heart Fail. 2010;3:588–95.
19. Anker S, Butler J, Filippatos G, others. Empagliflozin in heart failure with a preserved ejection fraction. N Engl J Med. 2021;385:1451-61.
20. Solomon S, McMurray J, Claggett B, others. Dapagliflozin in heart failure with mildly reduced or preserved ejection fraction. N Engl J Med. 2022;387:1089-98.
21. Kosiborod M, Abildstrøm S, Borlaug B, others. Semaglutide in patients with obesity-related heart failure with preserved ejection fraction. N Engl J Med. 2023;389:1069-80.

22. Packer M, Zile M, Kramer C, others. Tirzepatide for heart failure with preserved ejection fraction and obesity. N Engl J Med. 2025;392:427-39.
23. Pitt B, Pfeffer M, Assmann S, others. Spironolactone for heart failure with preserved ejection fraction. N Engl J Med. 2014;370:1383-92.
24. Solomon S, McMurray J, Vaduganathan M, others. Finerenone in heart failure with mildly reduced or preserved ejection fraction. N Engl J Med. 2024;391:1475-85.
25. Solomon S, McMurray J, Anand I, others. Angiotensin-neprilysin inhibition in heart failure with preserved ejection fraction. N Engl J Med. 2019;381:1609-20.
26. Abraham W, Adamson P, Bourge R, others. Wireless pulmonary artery haemodynamic monitoring in chronic heart failure. The Lancet. 2011;377:658-66.
27. Shah S, Borlaug B, Chung E, others. Interatrial shunt device for HFpEF: REDUCE LAP-HF II. The Lancet. 2022;399:1130-40.
28. Reddy YNV, Koepp KE, Carter R, others. Rate-Adaptive Atrial Pacing for Heart Failure With Preserved Ejection Fraction. JAMA. 2023;329:801-10.

SECTION 8

Chronic Kidney Disease

Managing Hyperkalemia in Heart Failure and Chronic Kidney Disease: Overcoming Roadblocks with Best Practices

Dilip A Kirpalani, Hardik K Shah, Sana M Sahigara, Ashok L Kirpalani

ABSTRACT

Hyperkalemia is a frequent and clinically significant complication in patients with heart failure and chronic kidney disease, often limiting the optimal use of guideline-directed therapies. This chapter reviews potassium homeostasis, causes and recognition of hyperkalemia, emergency and chronic management strategies, and recent advances in potassium-binding agents that help overcome therapeutic barriers and improve long-term outcomes.

Keywords: Hyperkalemia, heart failure, chronic kidney disease, potassium balance, RAAS inhibitors, potassium binders

INTRODUCTION

The two most important cations in the body are sodium and potassium. Predominantly potassium exists in the cells and sodium outside the cells, i.e., in the extracellular fluid including interstitial fluid, plasma, and lymph. Within the cell, potassium maintains the function of the cells particularly muscle, heart, and nerve cells. It is kept within the cells by sodium-potassium pump which prevents sodium from going inside the cell and prevents potassium from leaking out. 2% of the potassium of the body, however, exists in the extracellular fluid. Its concentration normally ranges between 3.5 and 5 mEq/L. Together with sodium, the acid-base balance of the extracellular fluid, i.e., plasma and interstitial fluid is maintained within a range of pH 7.4. It is important to keep the potassium within the above range because changes outside this range can have profound effects on the heart, muscle, and nerves affecting the health of the patient. Extreme disturbances of the serum potassium level can be life threatening.

The serum potassium is maintained within range by balancing of intake, distribution, and excretion. The most important organs in maintaining the potassium balance are the kidneys, adrenal glands, and various cellular mechanisms.

POTASSIUM INTAKE AND ABSORPTION FROM GUT

Potassium is absorbed mainly in small intestine and average oral intake is 50–150 mEq/day. In the healthy state, excess potassium is rapidly excreted from the kidneys. The normal kidneys handle potassium by first filtering it in the glomerulus then reabsorbing it in the proximal convoluted tubule and the loop of Henle and finally secreting it in the distal convoluted tubule and collecting ducts under the control of aldosterone which is secreted by the adrenal gland. At this level, sodium and potassium play "jugalbandi" using the tubules and various pumps like the sodium-potassium ATPase to maintain a perfect balance when in good health. Potassium is also excreted from the colon particularly in chronic kidney disease (CKD) and it is this function that makes it possible to remove excess potassium from the gut by using cation exchange resins to which I will allude subsequently.

DEFINITIONS

Normokalaemia: 3.5–5 mEq/L

Hyperkalemia >5 mEq/L: Usually seen in acute kidney injury (AKI), CKD, aldosterone deficiency state such as Addison's disease, adrenal tumors causing hypoaldosteronism, severe acidosis, severe tumor lysis and severe sepsis due to cell breakdown.

Hypokalemia <3.5 mEq/L: Usually seen in starvation, diuretic usage, and corticosteroid excess, i.e., Cushing's disease, Conn's syndrome (aldosterone secreting tumor of adrenal glands), and various hereditary disorders.

Pseudohyperkalemia: This is a laboratory artefact producing high serum potassium level. It occurs when potassium is checked in the serum not plasma. It is due to lysis of the cellular components of the blood, i.e., red cells, white cells, and platelets after collection and after being put into the vacutainer or bulb. It is not a true hyperkalemia but can cause panic and unnecessary excess treatment and, therefore, it should be clarified immediately after reading the potassium report so that potentially no harmful treatment is initiated. Potassium gets released from red cells by hemolysis, destruction of white cells and platelets after the collection process. It is known to occur when serum is not immediately centrifuged and is kept sometimes overnight before being tested for potassium. It can also occur in patients who have severe thrombocytosis or leukocytosis due to lymphoproliferative disorders, leukemia, etc. The following can cause this problem:

- Mechanical trauma to red cells during the phlebotomy
- High platelets and WBC count
- Errors in sample transport
- Delay in centrifugation
- Some rare familial conditions such as hemolytic anemias.

It should be suspected when the clinical condition does not corroborate and the ECG is not fitting in to the diagnosis. Under those circumstances, a fresh sample should be taken in heparinized (Green top) vacutainer and repeated.

SIGNIFICANCE OF POTASSIUM DISORDERS

Both hyperkalemia and hypokalemia lead to disruption of cardiac muscle function and the conduction system of the heart. Both can produce life-threatening arrhythmia and in extremes arrest the heart. The skeletal musculature also is affected by both hypo- and hyperkalemia leading to "periodic paralysis". In the past, when digitalis was the mainstay of CHF treatment, the incidence of hypokalemia in patients receiving digitalis and diuretics resulted in major arrhythmias and caused morbidity and fatality. Prevention of hypokalemia by administration of oral potassium and/or potassium-sparing diuretics was a frequent practice. Before the era of renin angiotensin aldosterone blocking agents, the major danger to the heart was from hypokalemia particularly for those patients who were receiving digitalis and diuretics. Today, the armamentarium for heart failure treatment has changed. More frequent potassium imbalances in the form of hyperkalemia are due to drugs like RAAS inhibitors, including ACE-i, ARBs, DRIs, mineralocorticosteroid receptor antagonists (MRAs), nonsteroidal MRAs, and MRA synthetase blockers. These are the new pillars of heart failure care together with sodium-glucose cotransporter-2 inhibitor (SGLT2-i). SGT2-is are usually potassium neutral and may protect from hyperkalemia induced by RAAS inhibitors. The subject of potassium abnormalities is vast and the purpose of this small chapter is to highlight what is new in the armamentarium of medicines available to manage potassium abnormalities. New drugs for overcoming hyperkalemia now make it possible to remove the roadblocks in the drug treatment of CKD and CHD. Therefore, this chapter will now concentrate only on hyperkalemia with special emphasis on:

- Recognition of hyperkalemia
- Management of acute life-threatening hyperkalemia
- Management of chronic hyperkalemia
- Prevention of hyperkalemia.

RECOGNITION OF HYPERKALEMIA

When to Expect and Anticipate Hyperkalemia

1. *Advanced CKD and advanced heart failure:* In early CKD stage I and II [when glomerular filtration rate (GFR) is >60], hyperkalemia is not common per se but when using drugs which cause hyperkalemia, i.e., potassium-sparing diuretic such as MRAs, ACE-is, ARBs, DRIs, nonsteroidal anti-inflammatory drugs (NSAIDs), one can expect, anticipate, and take preventive measures such as dietary restrictions of high-potassium diet, frequent estimation of serum potassium level, correction of hyperglycemia in diabetics, and correction of acidosis. In diabetics with stages I–III CKD, one may expect hyperkalemia due to type IV renal tubular acidosis (RTA) which is due to sclerosis of the JG apparatus leading to low renin and low aldosterone also known as hyporeninemic hypoaldosteronism. Therefore, there is greater need for vigilance in diabetic patients even in early CKD. In other patients of CKD, hyperkalemia usually comes when the urine output becomes less and CKD IV and V develop.
2. In the management of CKD, these drugs are used both as antihypertensives and also as an antiproteinuric which dual action makes them the first-line drugs used to prevent deterioration of kidney function.
3. Patients receiving ACE-is, ARBs, and MRAs in the management of heart failure. This group of drugs is now considered as the pillar in every patient of heart failure with reduced ejection fraction (HFrEF) and also in heart failure with mildly reduced ejection fraction (HFmrEF). The combination of sacubitril with valsartan (ARNI) is one of the newer pillars of HFrEF treatment and its usage is accompanied by hyperkalemia.
4. The usage of these drugs is often hindered by the development of hyperkalemia. The older K^+ binders are useful for overcoming immediately the hyperkalemia that develops in 48–72 hours, but the older binders are limited in their utility because when used for a longer period of time they cause severe unpleasant side effects and should not be used. The development of newer potassium binders has made it possible to keep using these binders in combination with the above RAAS-blocking agents for months and years.
5. Many patients of CKD also have heart failure, i.e., HFrEF/HFmrEF due to chronic ischemic cardiomyopathy and/or myocardial fibrosis-related cardiomyopathy. Recent research has identified chronic heart failure as a disease entity on its own and this responds to aldosterone inhibition by MRAs. The earlier MRAs such as spironolactone and eplerenone have many adverse and toxic effects due to the steroidal nature of their structure. Newer MRAs have been developed which are nonsteroidal (NsMRAs), e.g., Finerenone group and aldosterone synthetase inhibitors (MRA-ASI). They are expected to have lesser incidence of hyperkalemia but are not completely free from it and so concomitant use with newer potassium binders would protect the patient from unwanted hyperkalemia.

6. *Chronic liver disease ± gastrointestinal (GI) bleed*: In such patients who have refractory edema and anasarca, the administration of adequate doses of MRA ± beta-blockers to overcome fluid retention is hindered by the development of hyperkalemia.
7. *Post-chemotherapy*: The breakdown of cells with chemotherapy in oncology, e.g., tumor lysis syndrome results in severe life-threatening hyperkalemia.
8. Patients of AKI of any origin especially those who already have underlying CKD develop severe life-threatening hyperkalemia, e.g., NSAID toxicity.
9. Diabetics with hyperosmolar state and DKA
10. Any GI bleed.

In all these ten situations, hyperkalemia can be prevented by preemptive use of newer potassium binders.

Clinical Presentation of Hyperkalemia

- *History:* Most patients are asymptomatic and are detected unexpectedly on laboratory multi-metabolic analysis such as SMA-12, total body profile, renal profile, and other such profiles.

  When hyperkalemia produces symptoms, it is always life threatening, i.e.:

  "The Kuch Kuch Hota Hai syndrome"—the patient is unable to describe clearly what he feels but he feels unwell, the sense of doom, severe muscle weakness, and various muscular symptoms which he cannot describe.
- *Examination:* Sinus bradycardia, acidotic breathing (Kussmaul), either dehydration or overhydration
- In a diabetic an urgent blood glucose and ECG must be done in the doctor's clinic.
- ECG changes in hyperkalemia **(Table 1)**
- When does hyperkalemia become emergency?
  - Serum potassium >7 mEq/L
  - Extreme muscle weakness resulting in muscle paralysis
  - Other cardiac arrhythmias
  - Ongoing GI bleed immediately after chemotherapy (emergency measures to be initiated without waiting for warning signals to develop)
  - In patients on MHD, do not wait for confirmations, start dialysis immediately.

Emergency Management of Hyperkalemia when First Detected

- Salbutamol inhalation 100 µg/dose 2 puffs—this is the easiest first measure because it does not need IV line. Repeat every half hour while waiting to reach the hospital.
- Injection calcium gluconate by IV 10 mL of 10% solution calcium gluconate in dextrose. Inject slowly over 5–7 minutes. Patient will feel hot.
- In diabetics, check blood glucose, if blood glucose high, i.e., more than 180, give 10–12 U regular insulin depending on the blood glucose level IV.
- In nondiabetics, start 100 cc 25% dextrose and add 6–8 U regular insulin short-acting IV in the drip and give over 10 minutes.
- After giving insulin in diabetic and nondiabetics, keep a watch on blood glucose over 2 hours as patient may get hypoglycemia and need another 100 cc 25% dextrose to overcome that hypoglycemia.
- If possible, give 50 cc 7.5% sodium bicarbonate IV in patients who are not in obvious cardiac failure or fluid overload.
- As soon as you reach hospital, put patient on monitor and keep in ICU with resuscitation apparatus stand by. The ECG pattern should change rapidly.
- If patient with heart failure or fluid overload, give furosemide/torsemide IV push 40 mg.

TABLE 1: ECG changes associated with varying degrees of hyperkalemia.

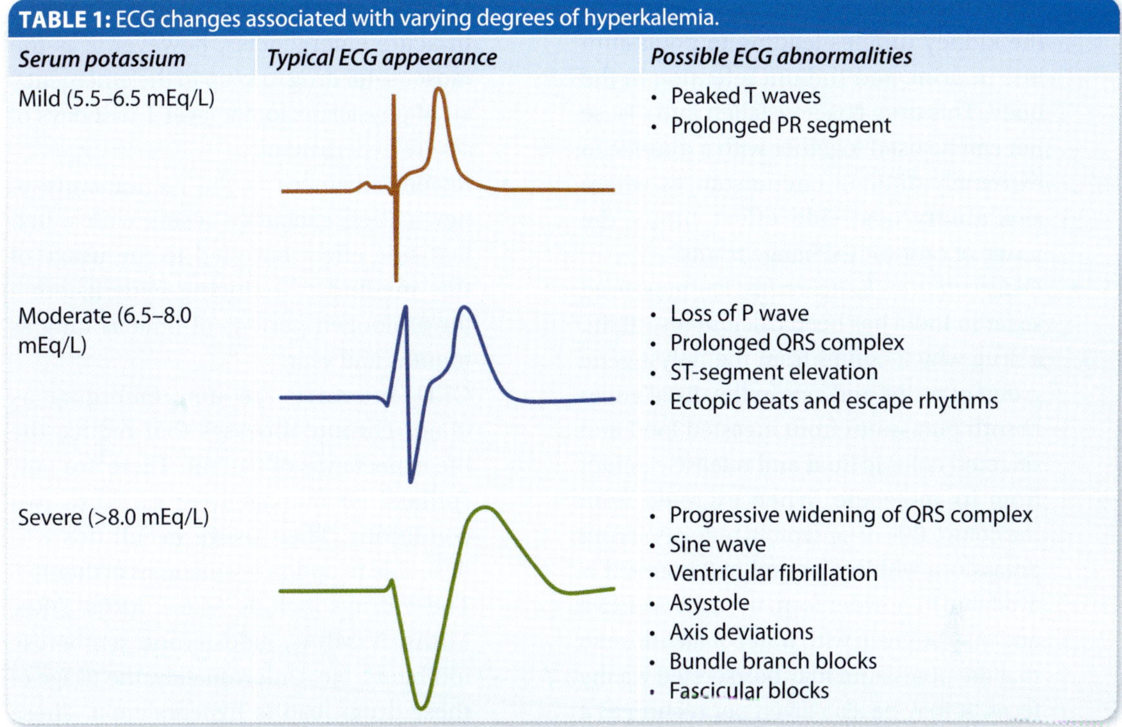

Serum potassium	*Typical ECG appearance*	*Possible ECG abnormalities*
Mild (5.5–6.5 mEq/L)		• Peaked T waves • Prolonged PR segment
Moderate (6.5–8.0 mEq/L)		• Loss of P wave • Prolonged QRS complex • ST-segment elevation • Ectopic beats and escape rhythms
Severe (>8.0 mEq/L)		• Progressive widening of QRS complex • Sine wave • Ventricular fibrillation • Asystole • Axis deviations • Bundle branch blocks • Fascicular blocks

- Immediately give, by mouth, 1 sachet 15 g calcium polystyrene sulfonate potassium binder with water or 30 g with water as retention enema if patient is unconscious or nasogastric (NG) tube not available.

Management of Hyperkalemia in Chronic States

- The first step in the management of hyperkalemia in chronic state is lifestyle modification with diet. The diet of such a patient who is chronically hyperkalemic due to whatever reasons should best be prescribed by qualified dietitian. The physician should inform the dietitian of the metabolic state of the patient. It is best to prescribe the diet by filling up a form addressed to the dietitian. This is particularly important in patients with CKD because those patients will also have other limitation in the diet such as control of salt, fluid intake, glucose control, calories, and lipid control. The dietitian should also be aware of the medications that the patient is receiving and which may interact with the potassium in the diet such as diuretic, RAAS inhibitors, NSAIDs, etc. Sample prescription is enclosed herewith as **Appendix 1**.
- The dietitian will give the list of what foods to avoid, which are rich in potassium, and how to "leach" potassium from the food **(Appendix 2 and 3)**.
- It is advisable to predict and preempt hyperkalemia by making the patient aware of what is hyperkalemia and how to avoid certain food items and leach the potassium out of others.
- Until recently, there were only two medications available for chronic hyperkalemia:
  - Fludrocortisone (synthetic mineralocorticosteroid resembling aldosterone)

which exchanges sodium for potassium in the kidney tubules leading to potassium loss in urine and sodium retention in the body. This drug has now fallen into disuse but can be used together with a diuretic in extremely difficult circumstances where availability/cost/side effect limits the usage of cationic exchange resins.

- *Older cation exchange resins:* The most used so far in India has been calcium resonium, a drug which comes from the polystyrene group of resins and acts in the distal gut to absorb potassium from ingested food and secreted colonic fluid and release calcium from its molecule. When excreted from the colon, this drug rapidly reduces serum potassium within a period of 2 hours. It is available in powder form in sachets of 15 g and may be given with water or lactulose so that the potassium may be excreted via the feces. It may be also given per rectum as a retention enema for up to 45 g dissolved in water and/or administered with lactulose if the patient is unable to swallow or take orally for any reason. This method can be very useful in unconscious patient or when very quick action is required. An earlier polystyrene resin called sodium resonium has now fallen into disuse because it exchanges sodium for potassium instead of calcium for potassium. With this earlier resin, there was a risk of sodium in the gut being absorbed and causing volume overload and worsening hypervolemia, hypertension, and heart failure.
- The major limitation for usage of calcium resonium is that it tends to give major GI side effects if used for >48–72 hours. Patient can develop severe constipation, colonic ileus, intestinal obstruction, and severe outcomes there from. Its prolonged use in chronic hyperkalemia has been known to developing colonic malignancy. In acute emergencies, however, it is the most useful drug to keep in the emergency kit of physicians to tide over 1 or 2 days of severe hyperkalemia.
- Recent advances in the manufacture of new cation exchange resins with much less side effect have led to the usage of this method of reducing hyperkalemia for prolonged periods of time as long as months and year.
- CKD and CHF are now emerging as major chronic illnesses that reduce the life expectancy of patient. There are new "pillars" of management of these two conditions. Their usage in full doses is desirable to optimize outcomes of therapy. These drugs include ACE-i, ARBs, DRIs, MRAs, NsMRAs, aldosterone synthetase inhibitors, etc. Unfortunately, the usage of these drugs lead to hyperkalemia. These drugs are prescribed for domiciliary care and the patient may revisit the doctor after many months. During the intervening period, the original underlying causative illnesses such as diabetic nephropathy, ischemic cardiomyopathy, etc. may worsen the internal milieu of the patient and predispose to hyperkalemia. Therefore, hyperkalemia acts as a roadblock to the management of CHF and CKD. With the advent of newer resins such as patiromer and *Sodium zirconium cyclosilicate* which can be used for prolonged periods of time without side effect, the management of CHF and CKD has become efficient.
- *Patiromer:* Patiromer is a polymer which is not absorbed in the gut and exchanges potassium for calcium in the distal colon allowing removal of potassium through the feces and thereby reducing serum potassium levels. Unlike calcium resonium,

it is slow acting and takes about 4–7 hours to start acting and its maximum effect lasts up to 48 hours. It should not be used in emergency situation requiring immediate lowering of potassium level. The drug is to be taken with food but 3 hours away from any medications. The efficacy as a normokalaemic agent has been proved by OPAL-HK and AMETHYST-DN trials. This drug can be used almost permanently but care should be taken for frequent re-estimation of potassium because of following side effects:

- Hypokalemia
- Hypomagnesemia
- GI symptoms and uneasiness with constipation and sometimes diarrhea and nausea.

Its major advantage over zirconium is that it is not sodium retaining and does not cause aggravation of hypertension, edema, and heart failure.

- *Sodium zirconium cyclosilicate:* This is another new nonpolymeric cationic exchanger for treatment of hyperkalemia. It selectively binds to intestinal sodium and hydrogen and exchanges potassium in the colon where potassium is highest. Potassium has priority over calcium and magnesium. The initial dose recommended is 10 g three times a day for about 2 days followed by maintenance dose of 5–15 g once a day. This medicine must be taken before or after 2 hours of any other medication. Clinical trials such as HARMONIZE and ZS-003 have demonstrated safe normokalemia within 2 hours of oral administration. The drug can be used over months and years. It is given orally and comes out in the feces having bound the potassium. Both patiromer and zirconium are very useful in concomitant administration with RAAS inhibitor, and other pillars of CHF care such as ARNI and MRAs like Finerenone. Its major advantage over patiromer is that it starts producing its action within about 2 hours as compared to 4–7 hours of patiromer. However, it is still slower than calcium resonium which would be the first choice in acute hyperkalemia as an emergency measure. Its major disadvantage over patiromer is that it exchanges sodium for potassium and the sodium gets absorbed from the gut causing fluid retention. Data from studies show that the sodium retention is not extremely high but more data is required after clinical experience in phase IV trials particularly in our country where diet is already excessive in salt. Other side effects are similar to patiromer but probably milder on the gut. Frequent estimations of serum potassium must be done to prevent hypokalemia. Fortunately, zirconium will soon be available in India whereas patiromer still has a long way to clear the formalities. Both these drugs are keenly awaited to remove the roadblocks that exist for the management of chronic hyperkalemia, CKD, and CHF.

Concluding summary for tackling hyperkalemia:

When potassium is high:

- *Assess urgency and:*
  - Rule out pseudohyperkalemia
  - *If there are ECG changes or K^+ >6.5 mmol/L:* Initiate emergency therapy (IV calcium, insulin/glucose, beta agonist, and calcium resonium) as a last resort emergency dialysis.
  - *If stable:* Admit patient to ICU 24 hours after first dose of calcium resonium
  - If the patient is already on maintenance hemodialysis, send urgently for immediate hemodialysis

- *Acute management (stable, moderate hyperkalemia):*
  - Withold potassium raising drugs if possible
  - Start calcium resonium 15–45 g oral or per-rectal for about 6–24 hours
  - Recheck potassium at 4–6 hours and 24 hours
  - Start emergency dialysis therapy if potassium not normalized
- *Chronic management:*
  - Initiate newer potassium binders if available, if not consider fludrocortisone
  - Reinstate RAAS inhibitor at guideline doses if tolerated
- Provide dietary counseling (individualized)
- *Long-term strategy:*
  - Address acidosis, constipation, uncontrollable diabetes, and reversible drug causes
  - Continue regular monitoring and adjust binder dose to maintain K^+ between 4 and 5 mmol/L
  - Continue dietary management

CONCLUSION

Hyperkalemia remains an important clinical challenge in patients with CKD and heart failure, particularly when using RAAS-inhibiting therapies that are essential for improving outcomes. Prompt recognition, assessment of urgency, and appropriate acute management are critical to prevent life-threatening complications. Long-term management requires dietary counseling, regular monitoring of potassium levels, and careful adjustment of medications. The availability of newer potassium-binding agents such as patiromer and sodium zirconium cyclosilicate provides an effective strategy for maintaining normokalemia and enables continued use of guideline-directed therapies in CKD and heart failure.

ACKNOWLEDGMENTS

Acknowledgments to Dr Umaira Ansari, and Mr Ivor D'souza

FURTHER READING

1. Bakris GL, et al. Management of hyperkalemia in patients with CKD and heart failure. J Am Coll Cardiol. 2021.
2. Kosiborod M, et al. Efficacy and safety of sodium zirconium cyclosilicate for treatment of hyperkalemia. NEJM. 2014.
3. Packham DK, Rasmussen HS, Lavin PT, El-Shahawy MA, Roger SD, Block G, et al. Sodium zirconium cyclosilicate in hyperkalemia. N Engl J Med. 2015;372(3):222-31.
4. Pitt B, et al. Hyperkalemia and the use of RAAS inhibitors in patients with cardiovascular disease, renal disease, and/or diabetes. Am J Med. 2022.
5. Weir MR, Bakris GL, Bushinsky DA, Mayo MR, Garza D, Stasiv Y, et al. Patiromer in patients with kidney disease and hyperkalemia receiving RAAS inhibitors. N Engl J Med. 2015 Jan 15;372(3): 211-21.

Appendix 1: Sample Diet Prescription of Instructions to Dietitian

PATIENT NAME: Mr. XXX 08.10.2025

AGE: 72 Yrs. SEX: Male

Physical Examination:

Weight: 85 kg **Height:** 5ft 7inch **BMI:** 29.4 kg/m^2

Diagnosis: CKD- DNeph, eGFR: 37 ml/min **Duration:** Until next visit.

Serum creatinine: 1.9 mg% **Serum potassium:** 5.9 mEq/L

Diabetic/Non-Diabetic: Diabetic

Diet Advised:

Salt intake: 4 g/day Protein: 0.8 g/kg of ideal weight Potassium: Zero

Fat: Low Caloric Intake: 1200 Fluid Volume: 1200 ml

Others: 1. Patient is vegetarian.
2. Reduce weight.

For diet related queries, please contact dietician

Appendix 2: Content of Potassium in Various Food Items

Food groups	*Low (<150)*	*Medium (<250)*	*High (>250)*
Cereals	• Maida (wheat refined) • Varagu (rada/Kodu millet) • Samai (vari/little millet) • Rice flakes • Rice puffs • Rice parboiled • Rice milled	• Wheat vermicelli • Brown rice	• Wheat whole • Ragi (finger millet) • Quinoa • Amaranth (Rajgira) • Bajra (pearl millet) • Barley • Jowar (foxtail millet) • Maize
Pulses	Nil	Nil	All
Milk and products	Milk: Cows, buffalo, paneer	Nil	Khoa
Nonveg	Eggs	• Chicken wings • Chicken breast • Chicken drumstick • Bombay duck (Bombil) • Rohu	• All other meats (goat, beef, and pork) • All types of shell fishes • Organ meats
Nuts	Nil	Nil	All
Oil seeds	Nil	Nil	All
Fruits	• Apple • Jambu (white, purple) • Pear • Pineapple • Papaya • Guava • Strawberry	• Blackberry • Cherry • Fig • Amla • Grapes • Sweet lime • Litchi • Mango • Muskmelon • Orange • Plum • Pomegranate • Star fruit	• Apricot • Avocado • Bael fruit • Black currant • Raisins • Tamarind • Dates • Banana • Custard apple • Jackfruit • Peach • Chiku
Vegetables (cooked)	• Green capsicum • Bottle gourd (Dudhi) • Lettuce • Parvar • Ridge gourd (Turai) • Snake gourd (Padwal) • Tinda • Ivy gourd (Tindli) • Ash gourd (kohla) • Bitter gourd (karela) • Pumpkin	• Cabbage • Fenugreek • Brinjal • Cucumber • Pea • Tomato • Zucchini • Onion • Cauliflower • Capsicum (red/yellow)	• Coriander • Mint • Spinach • Chawli beans • Corn • Drum sticks • Lady finger • Jackfruit (raw) • Broad beans • Cluster beans • Field beans • French beans • Raw banana • Beetroot • Carrot • Potato • Radish • Sweet potato • Tapioca • Water chestnut

Source: Indian Food Composition Table (IFCT, 2017)

Appendix 3: How to Leach Vegetables and Remove Potassium

Leaching:

- All vegetables, especially green leafy vegetables and roots like potato, sweet potato, etc., should be LEACHED, that is, peel, chop into small pieces, soak it in ample of water for 3–4 hours at room temperature
- Discard this water and then boil in fresh water
- Once boiled, discard the water once again, place the vegetable on a strainer or wrap it in a muslin cloth
- Squeeze out every drop of water. This step is crucial because potassium is water soluble and removing the water eliminates excess potassium
- Dals can also be leached in a similar manner
- But, remember leaching only removes some potassium, not all. High potassium foods still need to be restricted

Appendix 3: How to Leach Vegetables and Remove Potassium

SECTION 9

Pharmacotherapy

CHAPTER

15

Sodium-glucose Cotransporter Inhibitors: Multifaceted Blockbuster Drug in Diabetes and Heart Failure

Akshat Banga, Prakash Deedwania

ABSTRACT

Sodium-glucose cotransporter-2 (SGLT2) inhibitors have redefined cardiometabolic therapeutics by delivering reproducible benefits that extend well beyond glucose lowering. Initially developed as antihyperglycemic agents, SGLT2 inhibitors consistently reduce heart failure (HF) hospitalization across the spectrum of left ventricular ejection fraction (LVEF), slow chronic kidney disease (CKD) progression, and improve patient-reported health status, effects that are largely independent of baseline diabetes status. Their clinical impact is anchored in integrated physiology: proximal tubular blockade of sodium-glucose reabsorption induces glucosuria with natriuresis and osmotic diuresis, lowers interstitial congestion with modest blood pressure reduction, and triggers favorable neurohormonal and renal hemodynamic changes that mitigate glomerular hyperfiltration. Concurrently, pleiotropic mechanisms, including improved myocardial energetics and metabolic flexibility, attenuation of inflammation and oxidative stress, and favorable vascular and endothelial effects, likely contribute to rapid and durable reductions in HF events. Landmark cardiovascular outcome trials first revealed early separation of HF hospitalization curves, establishing a class effect. Subsequent HF-specific randomized trials confirmed meaningful reductions in composite HF endpoints in HF with reduced, mildly reduced, and preserved ejection fraction, alongside consistent renal protection. In contemporary practice, SGLT2 inhibitors are foundational therapy in heart failure with reduced ejection fraction (HFrEF) and heart failure with preserved ejection fraction (HFpEF), increasingly prioritized early in HF hospitalization once hemodynamic stability is achieved, and recommended across guideline documents in HF, diabetes, and CKD. Despite robust efficacy and favorable safety profiles, implementation gaps persist in clinical practice. This chapter reviews the biology and pharmacology of SGLT inhibition, mechanistic pathways underlying cardiovascular and renal protection, clinical trial evidence in HF and diabetes, safety considerations, contemporary guideline recommendations, and future directions.

Keywords: SGLT2 inhibitors; heart failure; diabetes mellitus; chronic kidney disease; cardiorenal syndrome; guideline-directed medical therapy.

INTRODUCTION

Heart failure (HF) and type 2 diabetes mellitus (T2DM) represent intersecting global epidemics and a major public health challenge, with each condition amplifying the morbidity and mortality of the other. Diabetes increases the lifetime risk of developing HF by nearly twofold, while HF independently predicts excess mortality and morbidity among patients with diabetes.[1] This bidirectional relationship is driven by shared pathophysiologic mechanisms including insulin resistance, neurohormonal activation, inflammation, and microvascular dysfunction, culminating in diabetic cardiomyopathy characterized by myocardial fibrosis, energetic inefficiency, and both reduced and preserved ejection fraction phenotypes.[2,3]

For decades, glucose-lowering strategies focused solely on glycemic control, with conventional agents like sulfonylureas and thiazolidinediones failing to improve, and occasionally worsening, HF outcomes (e.g., fluid retention with thiazolidinediones), underscoring that glycemic control alone does not ensure cardiovascular (CV) protection.[2] The advent of sodium-glucose cotransporter-2 (SGLT2) inhibitors marked a transformative shift from glycemia-centric to cardioprotective therapy.[4,5] Initially developed to reduce renal glucose reabsorption, large-scale cardiovascular outcome trials (CVOTs) designed to demonstrate CV safety unexpectedly revealed profound reductions in heart failure hospitalization (HFH) and CV death.[6-8]

The paradigm shifted with SGLT2 inhibitors. Following landmark dedicated HF trials demonstrating benefit across the EF spectrum regardless of diabetes status, SGLT2 inhibitors dapagliflozin and empagliflozin have been incorporated into contemporary HF guidelines as one of four foundational pillars of therapy, alongside renin-angiotensin system inhibition, β-blockers, and mineralocorticoid receptor antagonists.[9,10] While canagliflozin and ertugliflozin show consistent HF benefits in CVOT populations, dual SGLT1/2 inhibition (e.g., sotagliflozin) may add mechanistic breadth but requires continued clarification of benefit-risk across indications.

This chapter synthesizes current evidence supporting SGLT2 inhibitors as multifaceted cardiometabolic agents, emphasizing their biological rationale, mechanistic underpinnings, clinical efficacy across HF phenotypes, safety profile, and future therapeutic directions.

SODIUM-GLUCOSE COTRANSPORTER BIOLOGY AND PHARMACOLOGY

Transporter Isoforms and Tissue Distribution

The sodium-glucose cotransporter family comprises two principal isoforms with distinct physiologic roles **(Table 1)**. SGLT2, a low-affinity, high-capacity transporter, is predominantly expressed in the S1 segment of the proximal renal tubule where it mediates approximately 90% of filtered glucose reabsorption.[11] SGLT1, conversely, is a high-affinity, low-capacity transporter found primarily in intestinal brush borders, with additional expression in myocardium, platelets,

TABLE 1: Sodium-glucose cotransporter (SGLT) isoforms and tissue distribution.

Characteristic	*SGLT1*	*SGLT2*	*Clinical implications*
Primary location	Small intestine (brush border)	Kidney (proximal tubule)	SGLT1: Postprandial glucose control; SGLT2: Renal glucosuria
Glucose affinity	High (Km ~0.4 mM)	Low (Km ~2 mM)	SGLT1: Efficient at low glucose; SGLT2: Proportional to glucose load
Capacity	Low (V_{max} ~0.3 mmol/min)	High (V_{max} ~4.4 mmol/min)	SGLT2: Handles majority of renal glucose reabsorption
Na + Glucose stoichiometry	2:1	1:1	SGLT1: Greater sodium coupling per glucose molecule
Cardiovascular expression	Myocardium, platelets, endothelium	Minimal direct cardiac expression	SGLT1: Potential direct cardiac/vascular effects
Inhibition effects	↓ Intestinal glucose absorption	↓ Renal glucose reabsorption	Complementary mechanisms for glucose lowering
Selectivity of sotagliflozin	IC50 ~36 nM	IC50 ~1.8 nM	~20-fold selectivity for SGLT2 over SGLT1

and vascular endothelium.[12] These transporters differ in their sodium-glucose stoichiometry (SGLT2 1:1 and SGLT1 2:1), conferring differential effects on local sodium flux and cellular ion homeostasis.[13] Inhibition of SGLT2 induces glycosuria and natriuresis, while partial SGLT1 inhibition affects intestinal glucose absorption and postprandial glycemic excursions.

Available Agents and Selectivity Profiles

Currently approved SGLT2 inhibitors include empagliflozin, dapagliflozin, canagliflozin, and ertugliflozin, each exhibiting varying degrees of SGLT2 selectivity ranging from approximately 250-fold (canagliflozin) to over 2,000-fold (empagliflozin and ertugliflozin).[14] Sotagliflozin represents dual SGLT1/2 inhibition, additionally targeting intestinal SGLT1, offering modest incremental glycemic and potentially cerebrovascular benefits, albeit with increased gastrointestinal adverse effects.[15,16] **Figure 1** illustrates the mechanism of action and physiologic effects of SGLT inhibition.

All agents enable once-daily oral dosing with steady-state achievement within 3-5 days.[14] Empagliflozin and dapagliflozin carry the most extensive HF evidence and guideline support, with regulatory approvals spanning heart failure with reduced ejection fraction (HFrEF), heart failure with preserved ejection fraction (HFpEF), and chronic kidney disease (CKD) indications.[17,18]

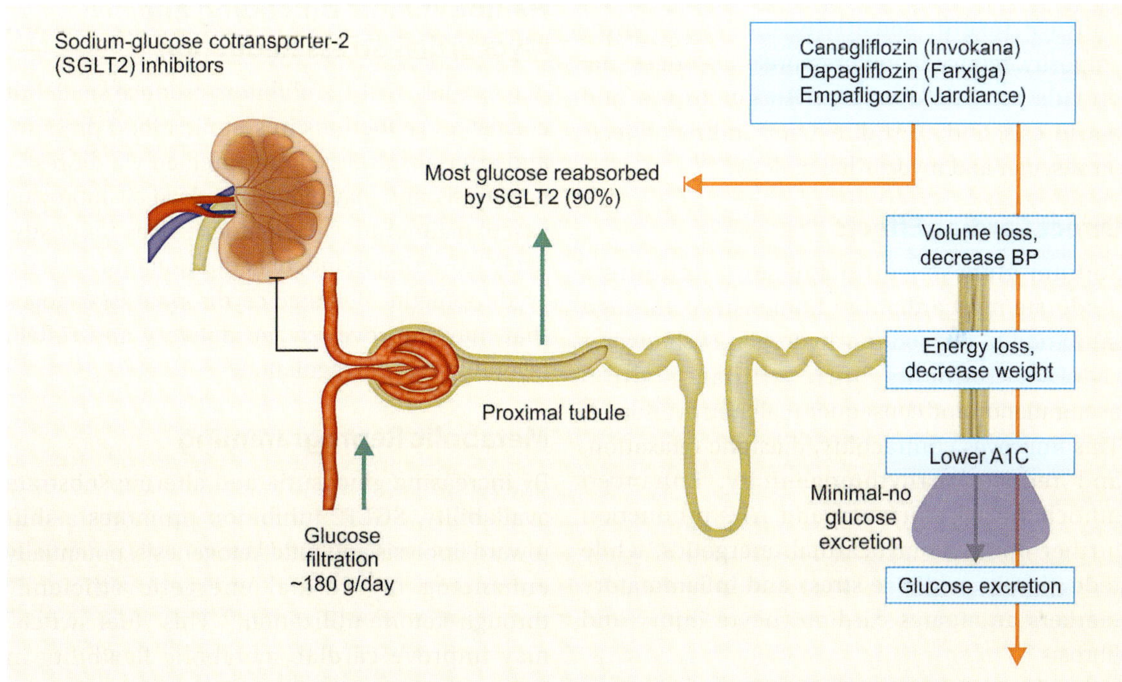

Fig. 1: Mechanism of action and systemic effects of sodium-glucose cotransporter-2 (SGLT2) inhibitors.
Source: Adapted from Lee YJ, Lee YJ, Han HJ. Regulatory mechanisms of $Na^{(+)}$/glucose cotransporters in renal proximal tubule cells. Kidney Int Suppl. 2007;(106):S27-35; Hummel CS, Lu C, Loo DD, Hirayama BA, Voss AA, Wright EM. Glucose transport by human renal Na^+/D-glucose cotransporters SGLT1 and SGLT2. Am J Physiol Cell Physiol. 2011;300(1):C14-21. Erratum in: Am J Physiol Cell Physiol. 2011;300(3):C721.

Pharmacokinetics and Dosing

Sodium-glucose cotransporter-2 inhibitors are administered once daily, reach steady-state concentrations rapidly, and require no dose titration for HF benefit. Importantly, CV and renal benefits persist even at reduced estimated glomerular filtration rate (eGFR), despite attenuated glycemic efficacy.[19]

Mechanisms of Cardiovascular and Renal Protection

Diabetes promotes HF through myocardial fibrosis, microvascular dysfunction, impaired energetics, renal sodium retention, and systemic inflammation, pathways that contribute to both HFrEF and HFpEF phenotypes.[3] SGLT2 inhibitors address several of these upstream drivers simultaneously: they reduce glucotoxicity, improve insulin sensitivity modestly, lower adiposity, reduce blood pressure and congestion, provide osmotic diuresis with glucosuria and natriuresis, and exert direct and indirect effects on vascular and myocardial biology.[20,21]

Direct Cardiac Effects

Sodium-glucose cotransporter-2 inhibitors modulate myocardial ion homeostasis through inhibition of the sodium-hydrogen exchanger-1 (NHE1), reducing intracellular sodium accumulation and consequent calcium overload.[22] This improves contractility, diastolic relaxation, and reduces arrhythmogenicity. Enhanced mitochondrial efficiency and ATP production further optimize myocardial energetics, while reduction in oxidative stress and inflammatory markers attenuates cardiomyocyte injury and fibrosis.[21,23]

Hemodynamic and Renal Mechanisms

Sodium-glucose cotransporter-2 transporters in the proximal convoluted tubule reabsorb the majority of filtered glucose alongside sodium. By blocking these transporters, SGLT2 inhibitors increase urinary glucose excretion with accompanying natriuresis and osmotic diuresis **(Fig. 1)**, thereby reducing intravascular volume and ventricular preload without neurohormonal activation typical of loop diuretics.[24]

Sodium-glucose cotransporter-2 inhibition also restores tubuloglomerular feedback. Increased distal sodium delivery constricts the afferent arteriole, lowering intraglomerular pressure and mitigating hyperfiltration—one plausible explanation for the characteristic early "dip" in eGFR followed by long-term preservation of kidney function.[25,26] These kidney-mediated effects are central to the cardiorenal benefits observed in both diabetic and nondiabetic populations.

Hemodynamic Unloading and Myocardial Stress Reduction

Across trials, SGLT2 inhibitors produce small but consistent reductions in systolic blood pressure and arterial stiffness, lower preload via diuresis/natriuresis, and may reduce afterload by improving vascular function.[27] Hematocrit rises modestly, likely reflecting hemoconcentration and, in part, erythropoietin-mediated erythropoiesis, changes that may improve oxygen delivery and reflect favorable volume regulation.[28]

Metabolic Reprogramming

By increasing glucosuria and altering substrate availability, SGLT2 inhibition promotes a shift toward lipolysis and mild ketogenesis, potentially enhancing myocardial energetic efficiency through ketone utilization.[29] This "fuel switch" may improve cardiac metabolic flexibility in HF, where impaired oxidative metabolism and mitochondrial dysfunction are common. Furthermore, metabolic flexibility, combined with modest weight reduction and improved insulin sensitivity, may activate cellular longevity pathways including AMPK and SIRT1, promoting autophagy and stress resistance.[21,30]

Anti-inflammatory and Endothelial Effects

A growing mechanistic literature supports reductions in inflammation, oxidative stress, and endothelial dysfunction with SGLT2 inhibition with downstream effects on microvascular perfusion and ventricular remodeling.[31,32] Reductions in circulating inflammatory markers [interleukin-6 (IL-6), tumor necrosis factor-α (TNF-α), and C-reactive protein (CRP)] and improved endothelial-dependent vasodilation through enhanced nitric oxide bioavailability contribute to improved microvascular function.[23,33]

Experimental data also suggest improvements in intracellular sodium and calcium homeostasis (including putative NHE1-related pathways), potentially stabilizing cardiomyocyte energetics and electrical function.[34] Additionally, sympathetic nervous system inhibition and favorable neurohormonal remodeling, evidenced by declining N-terminal pro-B-type natriuretic peptide (NT-proBNP) levels, further support CV actions.[35,36] While no single mechanism fully explains the rapid and consistent clinical benefits, their convergence offers a coherent biological rationale for early event curve separation (hemodynamic actions) and sustained protection.

EVIDENCE BASE ACROSS THE CARDIOMETABOLIC SPECTRUM

Cardiovascular Outcome Trials in Diabetes: Early HF Signals and a Class Effect

The SGLT2 inhibitor evidence base originated from four pivotal CVOTs enrolling over 40,000 patients with T2DM and high CV risk. EMPA-REG OUTCOME (n = 7,020) demonstrated that empagliflozin reduced the three-point major adverse cardiovascular events (3-point MACE) by 14%, driven by striking 38% and 32% reductions in CV and all-cause mortality, respectively, alongside 35% lower HHF.[8] CANVAS (n = 10,142) confirmed canagliflozin's CV benefits with similar MACE and HHF reductions, though safety concerns regarding lower-extremity amputations emerged.[6] A combined post-hoc analysis of CV outcomes from EMPA-REG OUTCOME and CANVAS demonstrated improvement in the composite of CV mortality and HHF along with renoprotective effects of the SGLT2 inhibitors as a drug class **(Fig. 2)**.

The DECLARE-TIMI 58 (n = 17,160) extended evidence to broader populations including primary prevention cohorts, with dapagliflozin achieving neutral MACE results but significant 17% reduction in CV death or HHF, predominantly through 27% fewer HF hospitalizations.[7] **Figure 3** illustrates the early separation of event curves for HHF across major trials, establishing this as a consistent class effect. Later, VERTIS-CV (n = 8,246) demonstrated ertugliflozin's noninferiority for MACE with consistent 30% HHF reduction.[37]

Collectively, these trials established that SGLT2 inhibitors prevent HF events independent of atherosclerotic risk profile, with minimal impact on myocardial infarction or stroke, highlighting reduced risk of hospitalization for HF and prevention of HF as the primary CV benefits.[38]

DEDICATED HEART FAILURE TRIALS: SGLT2 INHIBITORS AS FOUNDATIONAL THERAPY IN HFrEF

Following CVOT signals, dedicated HF trials revolutionized the field by demonstrating efficacy regardless of diabetes or EF status. DAPA-HF enrolled 4,744 patients with HFrEF [left ventricular ejection fraction (LVEF) ≤ 40%], approximately 45% without diabetes.[39] Dapagliflozin reduced the composite of CV death or worsening HF by 26%

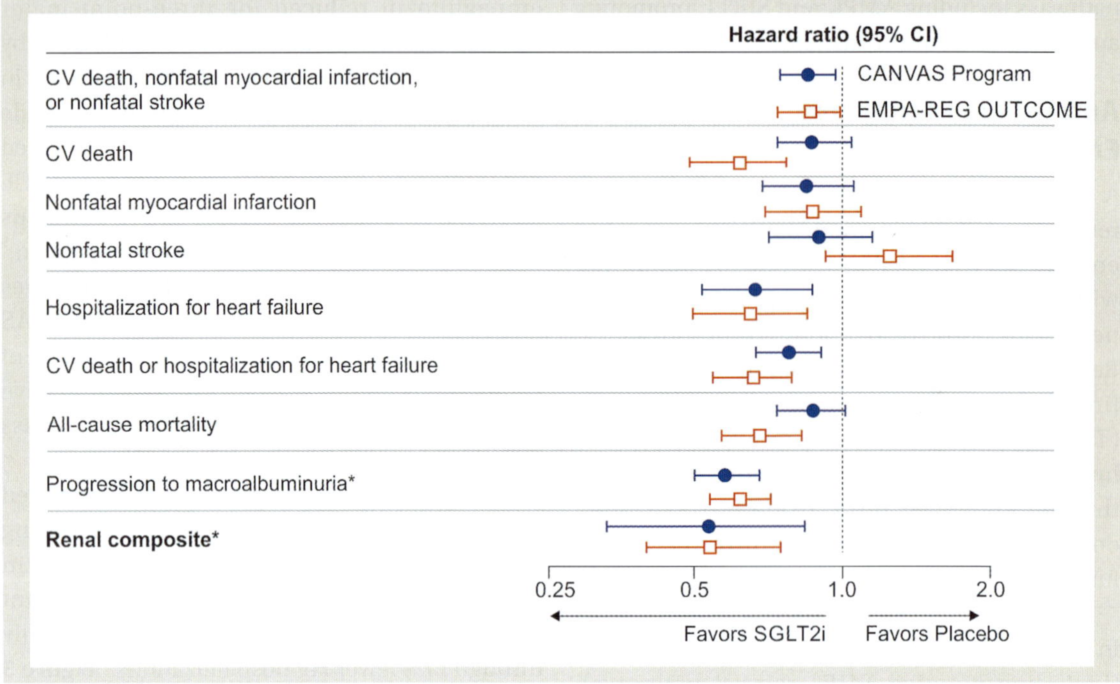

Fig. 2: Cardiovascular outcomes from EMPA-REG OUTCOME and CANVAS trials showing consistent heart failure benefits with neutral effects on myocardial infarction and stroke. (CI: confidence interval; CV: cardiovascular; SGLT2i: sodium-glucose cotransporter-2 inhibitor)

*CANVAS program endpoints comparable with EMPA-REG OUTCOME.

Source: Adapted from Zinman B, Wanner C, Lachin JM, Fitchett D, Bluhmki E, Hantel S, et al. Empagliflozin, Cardiovascular Outcomes, and Mortality in Type 2 Diabetes. N Engl J Med. 2015;373(22):2117-28; Wanner C, Inzucchi SE, Lachin JM, Fitchett D, von Eynatten M, Mattheus M, et al. Empagliflozin and Progression of Kidney Disease in Type 2 Diabetes. N Engl J Med. 2016;375(4):323-34.

[hazard ratio (HR): 0.74, 95% confidence interval (CI): 0.65–0.85, $p < 0.001$; **Fig. 4A**], with benefits appearing within weeks and consistent across diabetic subgroups. These benefits remained equivalent in patients with and without diabetes (**Fig. 4B**).

EMPEROR-Reduced (n = 3,730, ~50% nondiabetic patients) similarly demonstrated 25% reduction in CV death or HHF with empagliflozin, driven primarily by fewer hospitalizations for HF.[31] Both trials confirmed SGLT2 inhibitors as essential therapy for HFrEF, irrespective of glycemic status.

HFpEF/HFmrEF: Broadening Benefit Across LVEF

Heart failure with preserved ejection fraction is heterogeneous, encompassing multiple pathobiological phenotypes **(Fig. 5)**. Despite this complexity, SGLT2 inhibitors delivered reproducible benefits. EMPEROR-Preserved (n = 5,988, LVEF > 40%) was the first large HF with mildly reduced or preserved ejection fraction trial to significantly reduce the composite of CV death or HF hospitalization by 21%, predominantly through hospitalization prevention.[40] DELIVER subsequently confirmed dapagliflozin's efficacy in

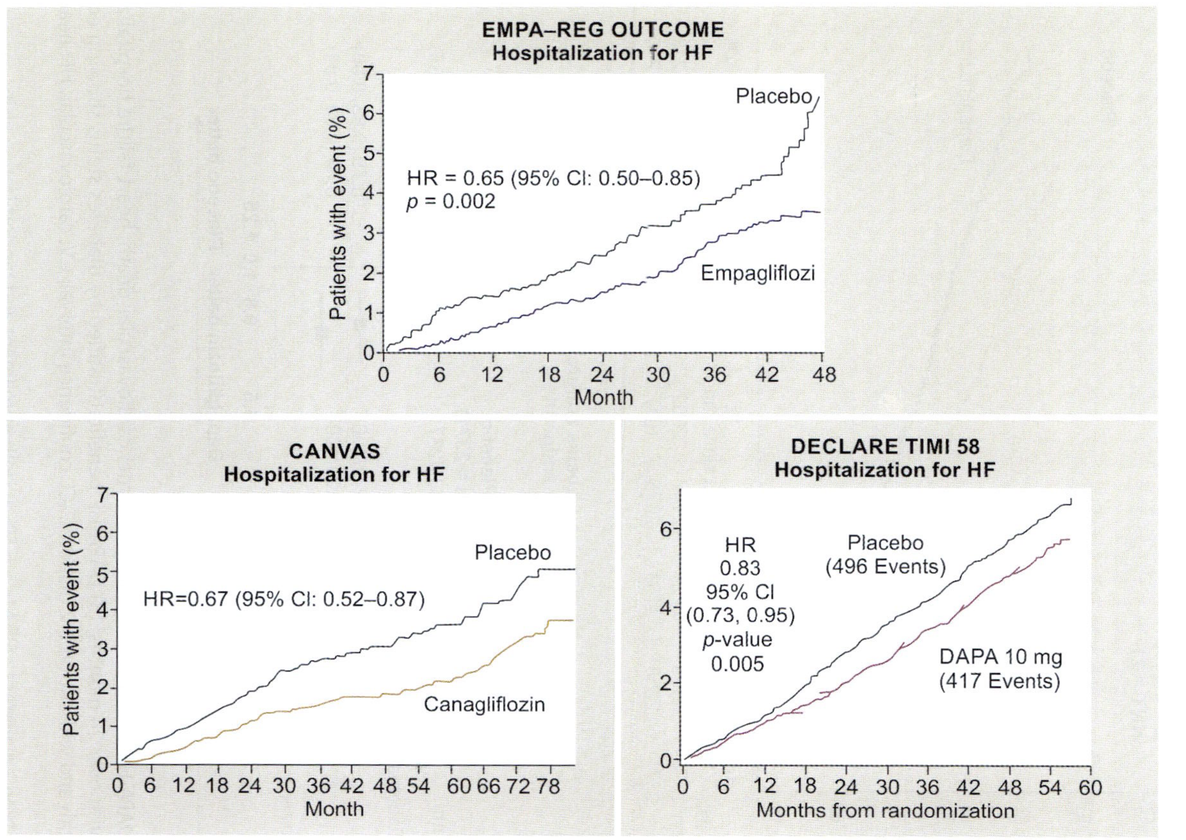

Fig. 3: Early separation of heart failure hospitalization curves across major sodium-glucose cotransporter-2 (SGLT2) inhibitor cardiovascular outcome trials (EMPA-REG OUTCOME, CANVAS, and DECLARE-TIMI 58).

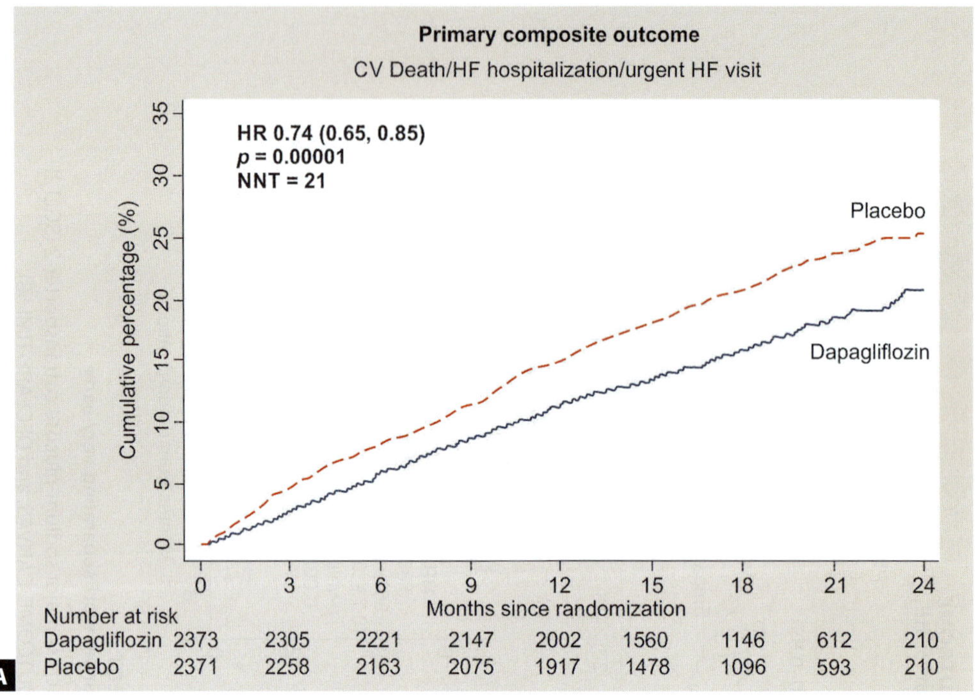

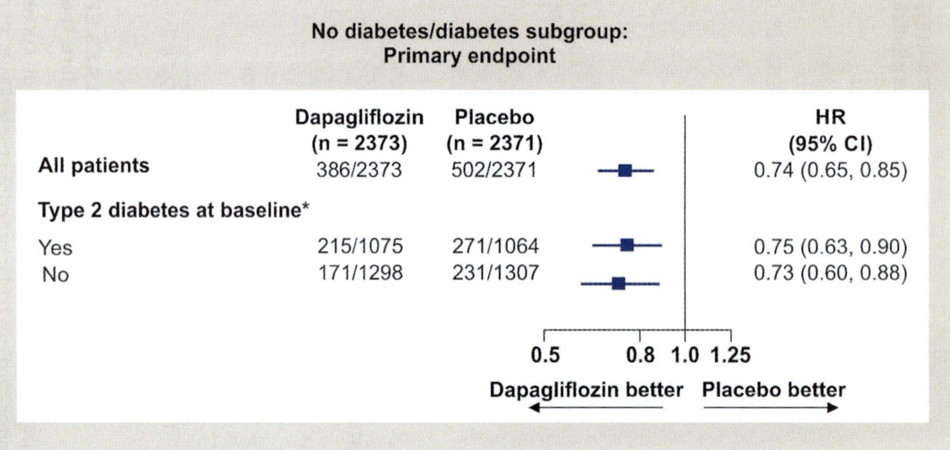

Figs. 4A and B: (A) DAPA-HF primary composite outcome: cardiovascular death, heart failure hospitalization, or urgent heart failure visit over 24 months; (B) DAPA-HF benefits stratified by diabetes status showing equivalent efficacy in patients with and without type 2 diabetes. (CI: confidence interval; CV: cardiovascular; HF: heart failure; HR: hazard ratio)

*Defined as history of type 2 diabetes or HbA1c ≥ 6.5% at both enrollment and randomization visits.

Source: Adapted from McMurray JJV, Solomon SD, Inzucchi SE, Køber L, Kosiborod MN, Martinez FA, et al. Dapagliflozin in Patients with Heart Failure and Reduced Ejection Fraction. N Engl J Med. 2019;381(21):1995-2008.

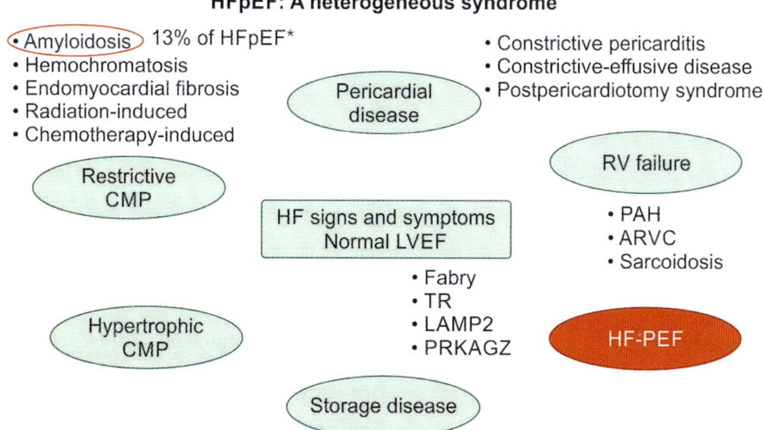

Fig. 5: Heart failure with preserved ejection fraction as a heterogeneous syndrome with multiple underlying etiologies. (HFpEF: heart failure with preserved ejection fraction; LVEF: left ventricular ejection fraction; RV: right ventricular)

*ATTRwt detected in 13.3% (16/120) of elderly HFpEF patients with LV hypertrophy (≥12 mm) screened by ^{99m}Tc-DPD scintigraphy

Source: Adapted from González-López E, Gallego-Delgado M, Guzzo-Merello G, de Haro-Del Moral FJ, Cobo-Marcos M, Robles C, et al. Wild-type transthyretin amyloidosis as a cause of heart failure with preserved ejection fraction. Eur Heart J. 2015;36(38):2585-94.

HFmrEF and HFpEF.[41] Pooled analyses reinforce consistent reductions in worsening HF events across ejection fraction (EF) categories, with less consistent effects on CV mortality.[5] Furthermore, a meta-analysis combining the DELIVER and EMPEROR-Preserved trials showed consistent benefit across the EF spectrum **(Fig. 6A)**, and maintained efficacy across LVEF ranges from <50 to ≥60% **(Fig. 6B)**.[42]

DUAL SGLT1/2 INHIBITION

Sotagliflozin's dual mechanism was evaluated in two pivotal trials. SOLOIST-WHF (*n* = 1,222) studied patients with T2DM and recent worsening HF, demonstrating 33% reduction in total CV death, HHF, and urgent visits for worsening HF, when initiated before or shortly after discharge.[15] SCORED (*n* = 10,584) enrolled patients with T2DM and CKD, showing favorable trends in HF outcomes and a notable 25% stroke reduction, an effect not observed with selective SGLT2 inhibitors, potentially reflecting SGLT1-mediated platelet or postprandial glycemic effects.[16] These findings suggest potential incremental benefits of dual inhibition, though definitive head-to-head comparisons are lacking. **Figure 7** displays key results from DAPA-HF, EMPEROR-Reduced, and SOLOIST-WHF, demonstrating consistent benefit across HF phenotypes while **Table 2** summarizes all major trials of SGLT2 inhibitors across HF phenotypes.[16,31,39]

REAL-WORLD EVIDENCE AND META-ANALYSES

Real-world studies corroborate trial findings. The CVD-REAL registries (>300,000 patients) demonstrated 39% lower HHF and 51% lower all-cause mortality with SGLT2 inhibitors versus other glucose-lowering agents in routine practice.[43,44] Later, a 2024 Danish cohort reported 25% mortality reduction with real-world SGLT2 inhibitor use.[45]

Comprehensive meta-analyses provide further evidence of class-wide benefits. The SMART-C

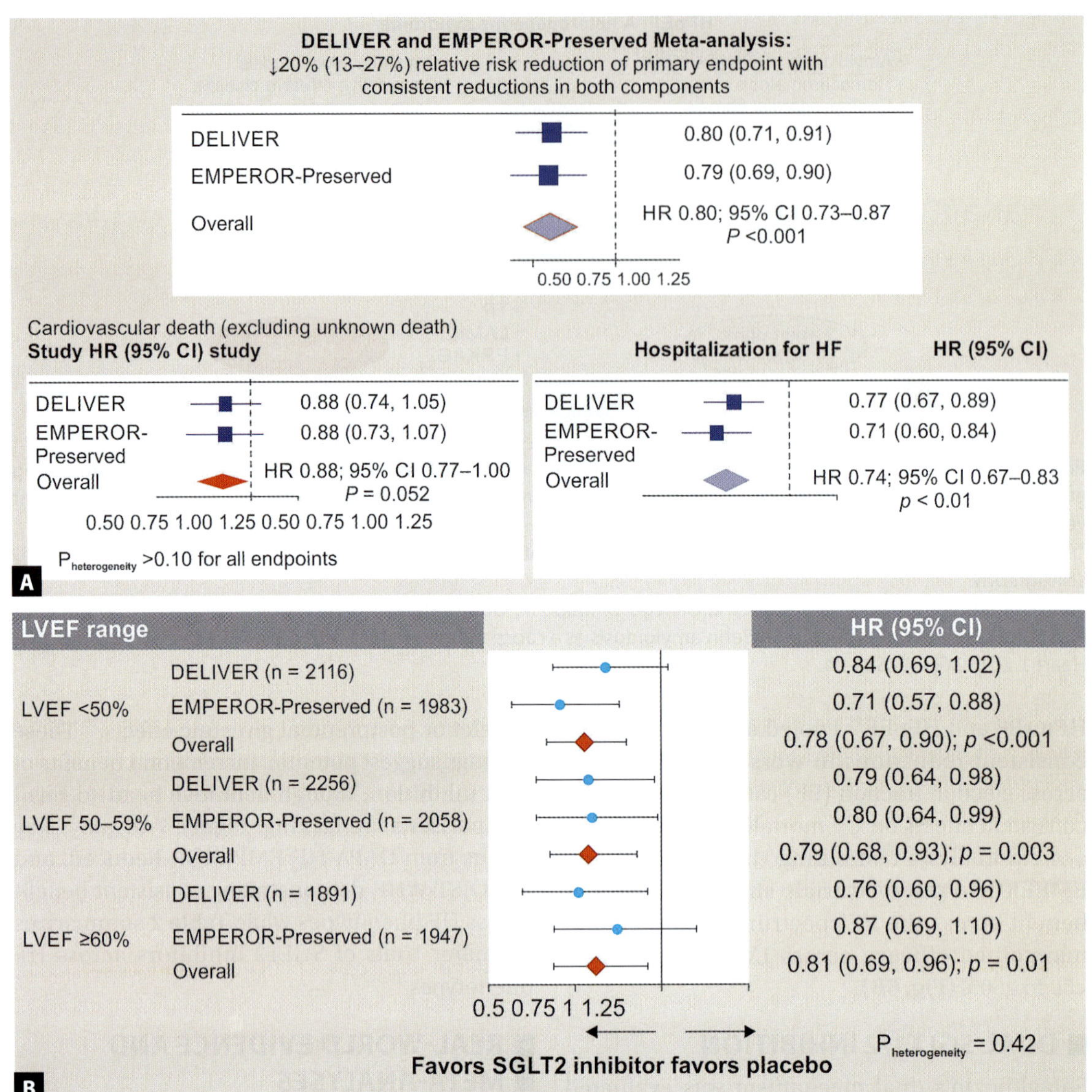

Figs. 6A and B: (A) Pooled analysis of DELIVER and EMPEROR-Preserved demonstrating reduced risk of the composite endpoint (cardiovascular death or worsening HF) with SGLT2 inhibitors across HFmrEF/HFpEF; (B) Treatment effect of SGLT2 inhibitors across left ventricular ejection fraction strata in HFmrEF/HFpEF, showing preserved efficacy across LVEF ranges.

Source: Adapted from Vaduganathan M, Docherty KF, Claggett BL, Jhund PS, de Boer RA, Hernandez AF, et al. SGLT-2 inhibitors in patients with heart failure: a comprehensive meta-analysis of five randomised controlled trials. Lancet. 2022;400(10354):757-67. Erratum in: Lancet. 2023;401(10371):104.

collaborative analysis (78,607 participants) showed 9% MACE reduction, 14% CV mortality reduction, and 32% HHF reduction.[46] Bhattarai et al. (71,553 participants) demonstrated 33% reduction in CV death or HHF and 16% all-cause mortality benefit.[38] Analyses of sotagliflozin trials

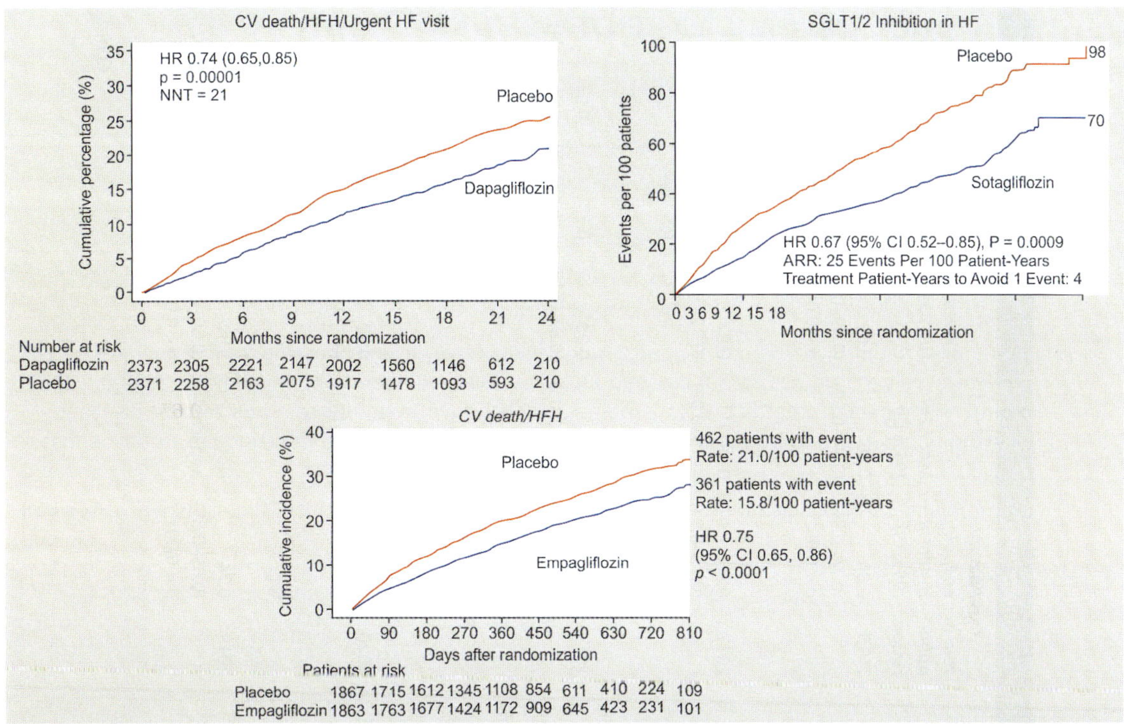

Fig. 7: Comparative effect sizes from key heart failure trials (DAPA-HF, EMPEROR-Reduced, and SOLOIST-WHF) demonstrating consistent reductions in worsening HF events with SGLT inhibition across populations and phenotypes.

Source: Adapted from McMurray JJV, Solomon SD, Inzucchi SE, Køber L, Kosiborod MN, Martinez FA, et al. Dapagliflozin in Patients with Heart Failure and Reduced Ejection Fraction. N Engl J Med. 2019;381(21):1995-2008; Packer M, Anker SD, Butler J, Filippatos G, Pocock SJ, Carson P, et al. Cardiovascular and Renal Outcomes with Empagliflozin in Heart Failure. N Engl J Med. 2020;383(15):1413-24; Bhatt DL, Szarek M, Steg PG, Cannon CP, Leiter LA, McGuire DK, et al. Sotagliflozin in Patients with Diabetes and Recent Worsening Heart Failure. N Engl J Med. 2021;384(2):117-28.

revealed 34% HHF reduction and 25% stroke reduction, supporting potential additive effects of SGLT1 inhibition.[47]

CLINICAL GUIDELINES AND RECOMMENDATIONS

Contemporary HF guidelines universally endorse SGLT2 inhibitors as foundational therapy. The 2022 AHA/ACC/HFSA guidelines assign class I, level A recommendations for dapagliflozin or empagliflozin in all HFrEF patients regardless of diabetes, positioning SGLT2 inhibitors as one of four therapeutic pillars alongside renin-angiotensin-aldosterone system (RAAS) inhibition, β-blockers, and mineralocorticoid receptor antagonists (**Flowchart 1A**).[10] For HFpEF and HF with mildly reduced ejection fraction (HFmrEF), class IIa recommendations reflect EMPEROR-Preserved and DELIVER evidence (**Flowchart 1B**).

The 2023 ESC guidelines provide class I indication for SGLT2 inhibitors across all HF phenotypes irrespective of EF, emphasizing early initiation including during hospitalization once hemodynamically stable.[17] Diabetes and kidney disease guidelines similarly prioritize

TABLE 2: Summary of major cardiovascular outcome and heart-failure trials of SGLT2 inhibitors.

Trial	*Agent*	*Study design*	*Population*	*N*	*Primary endpoint*	*Year of publication*	*Primary endpoint result HR (95% CI)*	*MACE HR (95% CI)*	*CV death HR (95% CI)*	*HF hospitalization HR (95% CI)*	*All-cause mortality HR (95% CI)*
EMPA-REG OUTCOME[8]	Empagliflozin 10/25 mg	Randomized, double-blind, placebo-controlled CVOT	T2DM + established CVD	7,020	3-point MACE (CV death, MI, stroke)	2015	0.86 (0.74–0.99), $p < 0.05$	0.86 (0.74–0.99)	0.62 (0.49–0.77), $p < 0.001$	0.65 (0.50–0.85), $p < 0.001$	0.68 (0.57–0.82), $p < 0.001$
CANVAS Program[6]	Canagliflozin 100/300 mg	Randomized, double-blind, placebo-controlled CVOT	T2DM + CVD or high CV risk	10,142	3-point MACE (CV death, MI, stroke)	2017	0.86 (0.75–0.97), $p < 0.05$	0.86 (0.75–0.97)	0.87 (0.72–1.06)	0.67 (0.52–0.87), $p < 0.001$	0.87 (0.74–1.01)
DECLARE-TIMI 58[7]	Dapagliflozin 10 mg	Randomized, double-blind, placebo-controlled CVOT	T2DM + multiple risk factors	17,160	Dual primary: MACE + CV death/HF hospitalization	2019	MACE: 0.93 (0.84–1.03); CV death/HF hospitalization: 0.83 (0.73–0.95), $p < 0.05$	0.93 (0.84–1.03)	0.98 (0.82–1.17)	0.73 (0.61–0.88), $p < 0.001$	0.93 (0.82–1.04)
VERTIS-CV[37]	Ertugliflozin 5/15 mg	Randomized, double-blind, placebo-controlled CVOT	T2DM + established ASCVD	8,246	3-point MACE (CV death, MI, stroke)	2020	0.97 (0.85–1.11)	0.97 (0.85–1.11)	0.92 (0.77–1.11)	0.70 (0.54–0.90), $p < 0.001$	0.93 (0.78–1.11)
DAPA-HF[39]	Dapagliflozin 10 mg	Randomized, double-blind, placebo-controlled	HFrEF (EF ≤ 40%) ± diabetes	4,744	CV death or worsening HF	2019	0.74 (0.65–0.85), $p < 0.001$	Not applicable	0.82 (0.69–0.98), $p < 0.05$	0.70 (0.59–0.83), $p < 0.001$	0.83 (0.71–0.97, $p < 0.001$

Contd...

Contd...

Trial	*Agent*	*Study design*	*Population*	*N*	*Primary endpoint*	*Year of publication*	*Primary endpoint result HR (95% CI)*	*MACE HR (95% CI)*	*CV death HR (95% CI)*	*HF hospitalization HR (95% CI)*	*All-cause mortality HR (95% CI)*
EMPEROR-Reduced[31]	Empagliflozin 10 mg	Randomized, double-blind, placebo-controlled	HFrEF (EF ≤ 40%) ± diabetes	3,730	CV death or HF hospitalization	2020	0.75 (0.65–0.86), $p < 0.001$	Not applicable	0.92 (0.75–1.12)	0.69 (0.59–0.81), $p < 0.001$	0.92 (0.77–1.10)
EMPEROR-Preserved[40]	Empagliflozin 10 mg	Randomized, double-blind, placebo-controlled	HFpEF (EF > 40%) ± diabetes	5,988	CV death or HF hospitalization	2021	0.79 (0.69–0.90), $p < 0.001$	Not applicable	1.00 (0.87–1.15)	0.71 (0.60–0.83), $p < 0.001$	1.00 (0.87–1.15)
DELIVER[41]	Dapagliflozin 10 mg	Randomized, double-blind, placebo-controlled	HF with mildly reduced or preserved EF (>40%) ± diabetes	6,263	Composite of worsening HF (HF hospitalization or urgent visit) or CV death	2022	0.82 (0.73–0.92) $p < 0.001$	Not applicable	0.88 (0.74–1.05)	0.79 (0.69–0.91)	0.94 (0.83–1.07)
SOLOIST-WHF[16]	Sotagliflozin 200 mg	Randomized, double-blind, placebo-controlled	T2DM + recent worsening HF	1,222	Total CV death, HF hospitalizations, urgent HF visits	2020	0.67 (0.52–0.85), $p < 0.05$	CV death: 0.84 (0.58–1.22)	0.43 (0.17–1.10)	0.66 (0.32–1.37)	0.64 (0.49–0.83), $p < 0.01$
SCORED[15]	Sotagliflozin 200 mg	Randomized, double-blind, placebo-controlled	T2DM + CKD/ CV risk	10,584	Total CV death, HF hospitalizations, urgent HF visits	2021	0.84 (0.72–0.99), $p < 0.05$	MACE: 0.84 (0.72–0.99), $p < 0.05$	0.66 (0.48–0.91), $p < 0.05$	0.74 (0.56–0.97), $p < 0.05$	0.67 (0.52–0.87), $p < 0.01$

(CKD: chronic kidney disease; CVD: cardiovascular disease; CVOT: cardiovascular outcome trial; EF: ejection fraction; HF: heart failure; SGLT2: sodium-glucose cotransporter-2; T2DM: type 2 diabetes mellitus)

Flowchart 1A and B: (A) 2022 AHA/ACC/HFSA guideline-directed medical therapy framework for HFrEF highlighting four foundational pillars, including sodium-glucose cotransporter-2 (SGLT2) inhibitors; (B) Guideline recommendations for SGLT2 inhibitor use in HFpEF and HFmrEF based on EMPEROR-Preserved and DELIVER evidence.

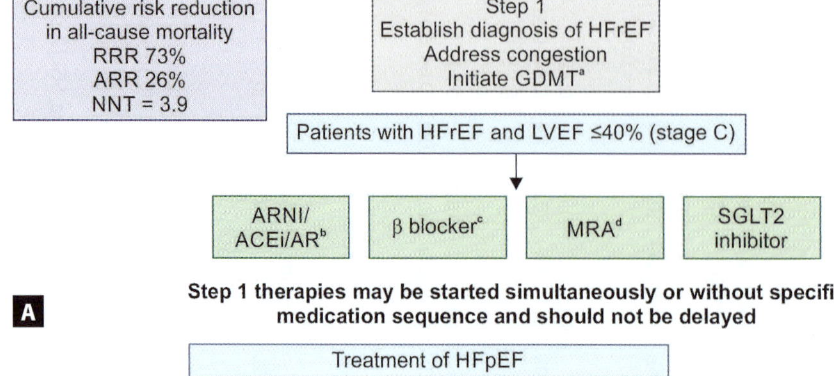

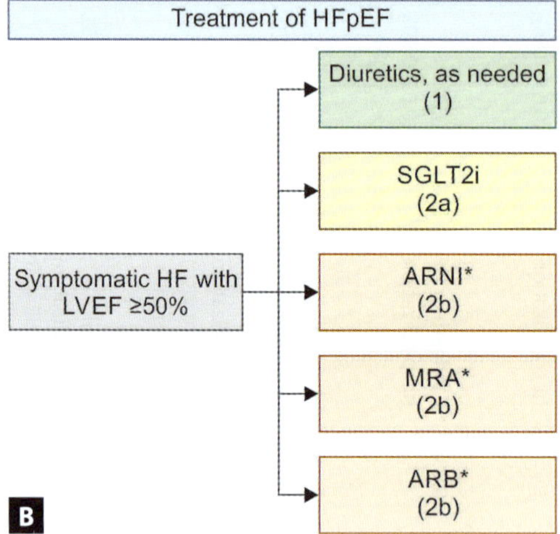

[a]Diuretics are also recommended as needed in patients with fluid retention

[b]ARNI is recommended as de novo treatment or to replace ACEi or ARB in patients with NYHA class II–III. In patients with NYHA class II–IV, ACEi (or ARB when intolerant to ACEi due to cough or angioedema) is recommended when ARNI use is not feasible

[c]One of the three β-blockers proven to reduce mortality

[d]estimated glomerular filtration rate >30 mL/min/1.73 m^2 and potassium <5.0 mEq/L

*Greater benefit expected in patients with LVEF on the lower end of the preserved spectrum (i.e., closer to 50%).

(ACC: American College of Cardiology; ACEi: angiotensin-converting enzyme inhibitor; AHA: American Heart Association; ARB: angiotensin receptor blocker; ARNI: angiotensin receptor neprilysin inhibitor; COR: class of recommendation; GDMT: guideline-directed medical therapy; HF: heart failure; HFrEF: heart failure with reduced ejection fraction; HFSA: Heart Failure Society of America; LOE: level of evidence; LVEF: left ventricular ejection fraction; MRA: mineralocorticoid receptor antagonist; NYHA: New York Heart Association; SGLT2: sodium-glucose co-transporter 2)

Source: Adapted from Heidenreich Paul A, Bozkurt B, Aguilar D, Allen Larry A, Byun Joni J, Colvin Monica M, et al. 2022 AHA/ACC/HFSA Guideline for the Management of Heart Failure. JACC. 2022;79(17):e263-e421.

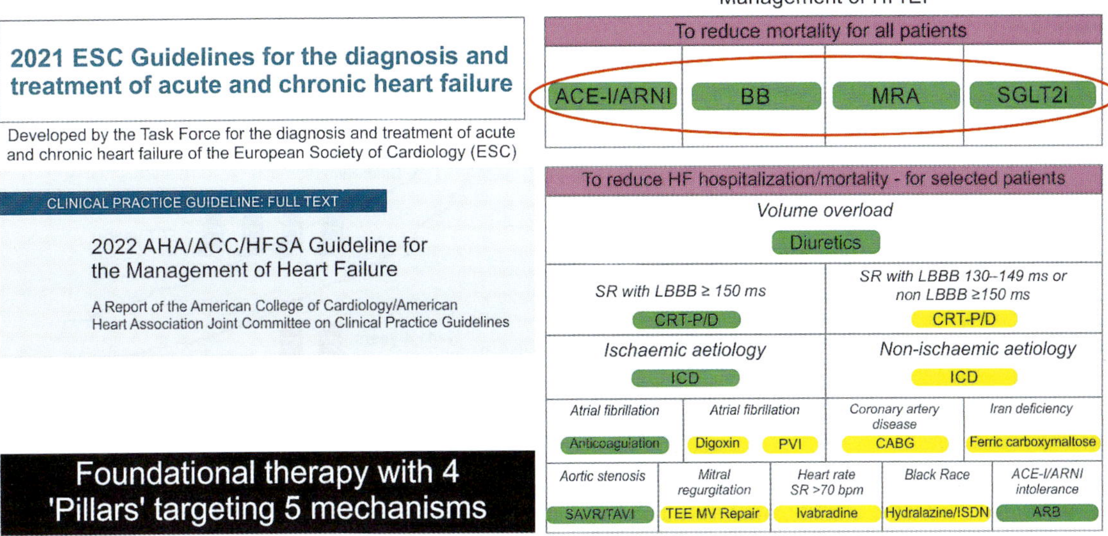

Fig. 8: Comparison of American and European heart failure guidelines regarding sodium-glucose cotransporter-2 (SGLT2) inhibitor initiation across heart failure (HF) phenotypes, including emphasis on early initiation once hemodynamically stable.

Sources: Adapted from McDonagh TA, Metra M, Adamo M, Gardner RS, Baumbach A, Böhm M, et al. 2021 ESC Guidelines for the diagnosis and treatment of acute and chronic heart failure. Eur Heart J. 2021;42(36):3599-726. Erratum in: Eur Heart J. 2021;42(48):4901; Heidenreich Paul A, Bozkurt B, Aguilar D, Allen Larry A, Byun Joni J, Colvin Monica M, et al. 2022 AHA/ACC/HFSA Guideline for the Management of Heart Failure. JACC. 2022;79(17):e263-e421.

SGLT2 inhibitors as first-line agents in T2DM with HF, atherosclerotic cardiovascular disease, or CKD, often superseding metformin in such populations.[48,49] **Figure 8** shows both American and European guideline recommendations for HF management.

The concept of early, near-simultaneous initiation of the four pillars is supported by modeling studies suggesting substantial survival gains with comprehensive four-pillar therapy, with addition of SGLT2 inhibitors contributing meaningfully to projected benefit compared to conventional approaches **(Fig. 9)**. However, despite strong evidence and guideline endorsements, real-world prescription rates remain suboptimal at below 50% among eligible patients, reflecting therapeutic inertia, misconceptions about initiating "diabetes drugs" in nondiabetics, and concerns about transient eGFR declines.[50,51] Implementation strategies incorporating electronic health record prompts, standardized order sets, and multidisciplinary education are improving uptake.[52]

SAFETY PROFILE AND ADVERSE EFFECTS

Sodium-glucose cotransporter-2 inhibitors demonstrate favorable overall safety with predictable class-related adverse events manageable through patient selection, patient education, and close monitoring.

Common Adverse Effects

Genital mycotic infections represent the most frequent adverse event, occurring in 3–6% of users versus 1–2% with placebo.[6,8] Episodes are typically mild, responsive to topical therapy, and rarely

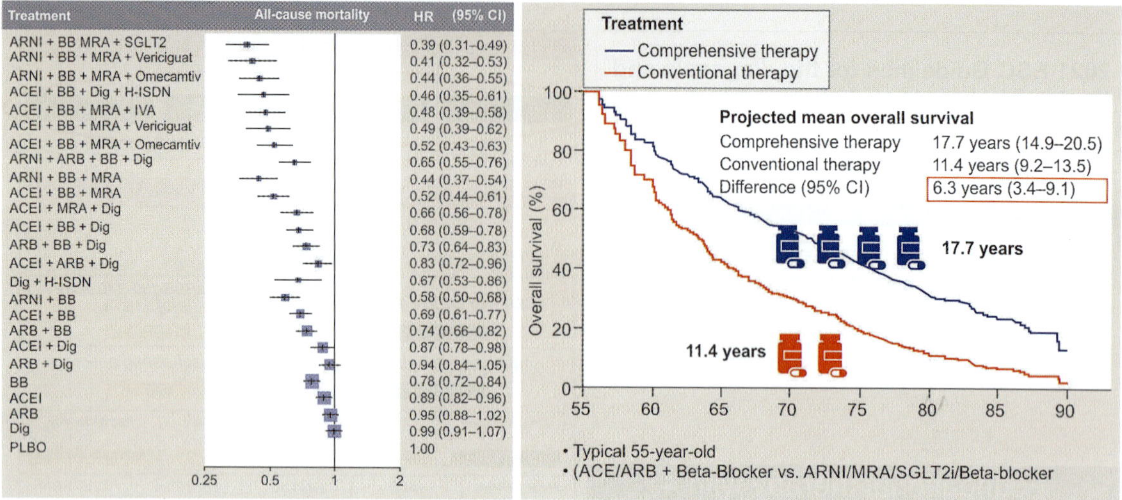

Fig. 9: Modeled benefits of early, near-simultaneous initiation of the four pillars of HFrEF therapy, illustrating projected survival gains with comprehensive therapy compared with sequential or delayed initiation.
Sources: Adapted from Tromp J, Ouwerkerk W, van Veldhuisen DJ, Hillege HL, Richards AM, van der Meer P, et al. A Systematic Review and Network Meta-Analysis of Pharmacological Treatment of Heart Failure With Reduced Ejection Fraction. JACC Heart Fail. 2022;10(2):73-84. Erratum in: JACC Heart Fail. 2022;10(4):295-96; Vaduganathan M, Docherty KF, Claggett BL, Jhund PS, de Boer RA, Hernandez AF, et al. SGLT-2 inhibitors in patients with heart failure: a comprehensive meta-analysis of five randomised controlled trials. Lancet. 2022;400(10354):757-67. Erratum in: Lancet. 2023;401(10371):104.

necessitate discontinuation. Proper hygiene counseling minimizes recurrence.

Urinary tract infections show modest increases in some analyses, though severe complications like pyelonephritis remain uncommon.[53] Importantly, urinary tract infection (UTI) occurrence does not mandate drug discontinuation; large registry data demonstrate that SGLT2 inhibitor cessation after UTI associates with 35% higher subsequent CV and renal events without reducing UTI recurrence.[54] Temporary interruption is appropriate only for severe infections.

Volume depletion and orthostatic symptoms affect 1–5% of users, are typically manageable with assessment of congestion, adjustment of loop diuretic dose, and counseling on hydration. Elderly patients and those on high-dose diuretics warrant diuretic dose adjustment and closer monitoring.[31]

Euglycemic diabetic ketoacidosis (DKA) is rare (<0.3 events per 1,000 patient-years) but clinically important.[7] Risk rises with prolonged fasting, acute illness, surgery, or inappropriate insulin reduction. SGLT2 inhibitors should be held during major illness and perioperatively, and patients should be taught "sick-day rules" and early symptom recognition. SGLT2 inhibitors are contraindicated in type 1 diabetes given elevated DKA risk.[55,56]

Agent-specific Considerations

Canagliflozin showed approximately twofold increased lower-extremity amputation risk in CANVAS (6.3 vs. 3.4 per 1,000 patient-years), though subsequent trials did not replicate this finding, suggesting patient selection and foot care practices as critical determinants.[6,57] Empagliflozin and dapagliflozin demonstrate no excess amputation or fracture risk across extensive trial programs.[7,8,39] Fournier's gangrene represents a rare but serious event (~1–2 per 100,000), warranting prompt recognition and drug cessation if suspected.[58]

Renal Considerations

Sodium-glucose cotransporter-2 inhibitors induce an acute, reversible eGFR decline of 3–5 mL/min/1.73 m^2 upon initiation, reflecting beneficial reduction in intraglomerular pressure analogous to RAAS inhibitors.[25] The early eGFR dip should be anticipated and contextualized as a hemodynamic reset rather than drug toxicity, provided volume status is appropriate, and the decline is within expected ranges.[25,26] Declines up to 20–30% from baseline are acceptable if stable; greater or progressive declines warrant evaluation for volume depletion or concurrent nephrotoxins. Long-term, SGLT2 inhibitors slow kidney function decline and reduce progression to end-stage renal disease.[26,59]

Chronic kidney disease strongly amplifies HF risk and worsens outcomes. SGLT2 inhibitors slow CKD progression and reduce renal endpoints across diabetic and, for some agents, nondiabetic CKD populations.[57] Kidney protection likely arises from reduced intraglomerular pressure (tubuloglomerular feedback restoration), improved renal oxygenation, and reduced inflammation and fibrosis.[25,26,32]

Current guidelines support use down to eGFR 20–25 mL/min/1.73 m^2, below which glycosuric effects diminish though cardiorenal benefits may persist.[49,60] Renal function monitoring at 1–2 weeks postinitiation with subsequent 3–6 months intervals is recommended.

Contraindications

Absolute contraindications include type 1 diabetes (DKA risk), severe renal impairment (eGFR <20–25 mL/min), active DKA, pregnancy/lactation (limited safety data), and active Fournier's gangrene. Relative precautions include active diabetic foot ulcers (particularly with canagliflozin), perioperative periods (hold 3–4 days presurgery), and acute illness with reduced oral intake.[61]

CLINICAL IMPLEMENTATION

Patient Selection and Initiation

Sodium-glucose cotransporter-2 inhibitors should be initiated in virtually all patients with HFrEF (LVEF ≤ 40%) without contraindications, alongside other foundational therapies.[10] For HFpEF/HFmrEF, evidence supports early use particularly following recent decompensation.[40,41] In T2DM, SGLT2 inhibitors are first-line for patients with HF, CKD, or atherosclerotic CV disease.[48]

Standard therapeutic doses require no titration: empagliflozin 10 mg daily, dapagliflozin 10 mg daily, canagliflozin 100 mg daily, and ertugliflozin 5 mg daily.[14] Baseline assessment includes blood pressure, eGFR, and infection screening. Patient education should address transient polyuria, genital hygiene, hydration, and sick-day medication holds. Insulin or sulfonylurea doses may require reduction to prevent hypoglycemia.

Follow-up at 2–4 weeks with serum creatinine and electrolytes is advised; mild creatinine elevation (≤20–30%) is acceptable. Thereafter, monitoring every 3–6 months suffices. SGLT2 inhibitors combine safely with all guideline-directed HF therapies; judicious diuretic down-titration may prevent excessive volume loss once euvolemia is achieved. Their mild kaliuretic effect may mitigate RAAS inhibitor-associated hyperkalemia.[62]

SPECIAL POPULATIONS

Elderly patients derive equivalent relative risk reductions with maintained functional improvements and no excess falls or volume-related complications.[63] Morning dosing may minimize nocturia. In atrial fibrillation, SGLT2 inhibitors are safe without drug interactions with anticoagulants or rate/rhythm agents, though definitive AF prevention data are lacking.[64] Post-myocardial infarction initiation after stabilization appears safe and may limit subsequent HF development, though recent data show no impact on composite mortality or HHF in nondiabetic, non-HF post-MI patients.[65,66]

FUTURE DIRECTIONS AND KNOWLEDGE GAPS

Several critical questions remain. The mechanistic basis and clinical significance of potential stroke reduction with dual SGLT1/2 inhibition require dedicated randomized controlled trials (RCTs) for confirmation.[67] No head-to-head trials compare individual SGLT2 inhibitors; current comparative assessments rely on network meta-analyses suggesting broadly similar efficacy.[71] Combination strategies with GLP-1 receptor agonists show promise for additive cardiometabolic benefits, though definitive outcome trials are needed.[68]

Mechanistic research continues elucidating nonglycemic pathways including myocardial sodium handling, mitochondrial biogenesis, and endothelial signaling. Cardiac imaging and omics-based studies may identify predictive biomarkers enabling precision therapy. Emerging applications include pediatric cardiomyopathy, chemotherapy-induced HF, and post-transplant cardiorenal syndrome.

Implementation science addressing adoption barriers through pragmatic trials, cost-effectiveness analyses, and health system interventions will be essential to achieving near-universal use and realizing population-level benefits comparable to other foundational HF therapies.[69,70]

CONCLUSION

Sodium-glucose cotransporter-2 inhibitors represent a transformative advance in cardiometabolic medicine, providing consistent reductions in HFH, CV mortality, and renal disease progression across diverse patient populations. Current evidence demonstrates benefits independent of diabetes status, EF, or baseline glycemic control, reflecting multifaceted mechanisms encompassing hemodynamic optimization, metabolic reprogramming, direct myocardial protection, and renal preservation that transcend glucose lowering. Dual SGLT1/2 inhibition offers potential incremental cerebrovascular benefits requiring further validation. As one of four foundational pillars of contemporary HF therapy, SGLT2 inhibitors should be initiated early alongside RAAS inhibition, β-blockers, and mineralocorticoid receptor antagonists, with continued long-term use barring intolerance. Their favorable safety profile, with manageable adverse effects preventable through appropriate patient selection and education, supports broad applicability.

Disclaimer: This chapter reflects contemporary scientific evidence and clinical practice as of early 2026. Medical knowledge evolves continuously; readers should consult current guidelines, product labeling, and institutional protocols when making clinical decisions. The authors have synthesized published literature to provide educational content; individual patient management requires personalized assessment by qualified healthcare professionals. The opinions expressed represent the authors' interpretation of available evidence and do not constitute official recommendations from any professional society or regulatory body.

REFERENCES

1. Abdul-Ghani MA, Norton L, DeFronzo RA. Role of Sodium-Glucose Cotransporter 2 (SGLT 2)

Inhibitors in the Treatment of Type 2 Diabetes. Endocrine Reviews. 2011;32(4):515-31.
2. Deedwania P, Acharya T. Cardiovascular Protection with Anti-hyperglycemic Agents. Am J Cardiovasc Drugs. 2019;19(3):249-57.
3. Heerspink HJL, Perkins BA, Fitchett DH, Husain M, Cherney DZI. Sodium Glucose Cotransporter 2 Inhibitors in the Treatment of Diabetes Mellitus. Circulation. 2016;134(10):752-72.
4. Deedwania P. SGLT2 Inhibitors: The Dawn of a New Era in Cardio-Metabolic Therapeutics. Am J Cardiovasc Drugs. 2022;22(1):1-4.
5. Vaduganathan M, Docherty KF, Claggett BL, Jhund PS, de Boer RA, Hernandez AF, et al. SGLT2 inhibitors in patients with heart failure: a comprehensive meta-analysis of five randomised controlled trials. Lancet. 2022;400(10354):757-67.
6. Neal B, Perkovic V, Mahaffey KW, De Zeeuw D, Fulcher G, Erondu N, et al. Canagliflozin and Cardiovascular and Renal Events in Type 2 Diabetes. N England Journal of Medicine. 2017;377(7):644-57.
7. Wiviott SD, Raz I, Bonaca MP, Mosenzon O, Kato ET, Cahn A, et al. Dapagliflozin and Cardiovascular Outcomes in Type 2 Diabetes. New Engl J Med. 2019;380(4):347-57.
8. Zinman B, Wanner C, Lachin JM, Fitchett D, Bluhmki E, Hantel S, et al. Empagliflozin, Cardiovascular Outcomes, and Mortality in Type 2 Diabetes. N Engl J Med. 2015;373(22):2117-28.
9. Docherty KF, Bayes-Genis A, Butler J, Coats AJS, Drazner MH, Joyce E, et al. The four pillars of HFrEF therapy: is it time to treat heart failure regardless of ejection fraction? Eur Heart J Suppl. 2022;24(Suppl L):L10-l9.
10. Heidenreich Paul A, Bozkurt B, Aguilar D, Allen Larry A, Byun Joni J, Colvin Monica M, et al. 2022 AHA/ACC/HFSA Guideline for the Management of Heart Failure. JACC. 2022;79(17):e263-e421.
11. Bays H. Sodium Glucose Co-transporter Type 2 (SGLT2) Inhibitors: Targeting the Kidney to Improve Glycemic Control in Diabetes Mellitus. Diabetes Ther. 2013;4(2):195-220.
12. Song P, Onishi A, Koepsell H, Vallon V. Sodium glucose cotransporter SGLT1 as a therapeutic target in diabetes mellitus. Expert Opin Ther Targets. 2016;20(9):1109-25.
13. Sano R, Shinozaki Y, Ohta T. Sodium-glucose cotransporters: Functional properties and pharmaceutical potential. J Diabetes Investig. 2020;11(4):770-82.
14. Scheen AJ. Pharmacokinetics, Pharmacodynamics and Clinical Use of SGLT2 Inhibitors in Patients with Type 2 Diabetes Mellitus and Chronic Kidney Disease. Clin Pharmacokinet. 2015;54(7):691-708.
15. Bhatt DL, Szarek M, Pitt B, Cannon CP, Leiter LA, McGuire DK, et al. Sotagliflozin in Patients with Diabetes and Chronic Kidney Disease. N Engl J Med. 2021;384(2):129-39.
16. Bhatt DL, Szarek M, Steg PG, Cannon CP, Leiter LA, McGuire DK, et al. Sotagliflozin in Patients with Diabetes and Recent Worsening Heart Failure. N Engl J Med. 2021;384(2):117-28.
17. McDonagh TA, Metra M, Adamo M, Gardner RS, Baumbach A, Böhm M, et al. 2023 Focused Update of the 2021 ESC Guidelines for the diagnosis and treatment of acute and chronic heart failure. Eur Heart J. 2023;44(37):3627-39.
18. Ostrominski JW, Defilippis EM, Bansal K, Riello RJ, Bozkurt B, Heidenreich PA, et al. Contemporary American and European Guidelines for Heart Failure Management. JACC Heart Fail. 2024;12(5):810-25.
19. Cherney DZI, Perkins BA, Soleymanlou N, Maione M, Lai V, Lee A, et al. Renal Hemodynamic Effect of Sodium-Glucose Cotransporter 2 Inhibition in Patients With Type 1 Diabetes Mellitus. Circulation. 2014;129(5):587-97.
20. Chen YR, Zhu FY, Zhou R. SGLT2 inhibitors for alleviating heart failure through non-hypoglycemic mechanisms. Front Cardiovasc Med. 2024;11:1494882.
21. Karakasis P, Theofilis P, Vlachakis PK, Apostolos A, Milaras N, Ktenopoulos N, et al. SGLT2 inhibitors and cardiac fibrosis: A comprehensive review. Curr Probl Cardiol. 2025;50(10):103149.
22. Piperis C, Marathonitis A, Anastasiou A, Theofilis P, Mourouzis K, Giannakodimos A, et al. Multifaceted Impact of SGLT2 Inhibitors in Heart Failure Patients: Exploring Diverse Mechanisms of Action. Biomedicines. 2024;12(10):2314.
23. La Grotta R, De Candia P, Olivieri F, Matacchione G, Giuliani A, Rippo MR, et al. Anti-inflammatory effect of SGLT-2 inhibitors via uric acid and insulin. Cell Mol Life Sci. 2022;79(5).

24. Upadhyay A. SGLT2 Inhibitors and Kidney Protection: Mechanisms Beyond Tubuloglomerular Feedback. Kidney360. 2024;5(5):771-82.
25. Meraz-Muñoz AY, Weinstein J, Wald R. eGFR Decline after SGLT2 Inhibitor Initiation: The Tortoise and the Hare Reimagined. Kidney360. 2021;2(6):1042-7.
26. Umanath K, Testani JM, Lewis JB. "Dip" in eGFR: Stay the Course With SGLT-2 Inhibition. Circulation. 2022;146(6):463-5.
27. Verma S, McMurray JJV. SGLT2 inhibitors and mechanisms of cardiovascular benefit: a state-of-the-art review. Diabetologia. 2018;61(10):2108-17.
28. Mazer CD, Hare GMT, Connelly PW, Gilbert RE, Shehata N, Quan A, et al. Effect of Empagliflozin on Erythropoietin Levels, Iron Stores, and Red Blood Cell Morphology in Patients With Type 2 Diabetes Mellitus and Coronary Artery Disease. Circulation. 2020;141(8):704-7.
29. Wen X, Zhang B, Wu B, Xiao H, Li Z, Li R, et al. Signaling pathways in obesity: mechanisms and therapeutic interventions. Signal Transduct Target Ther. 2022;7(1):298. Erratum in: Signal Transduct Target Ther. 2022;7(1):369.
30. de Boer RA, Núñez J, Kozlovski P, Wang Y, Proot P, Keefe D. Effects of the dual sodium–glucose linked transporter inhibitor, licogliflozin vs placebo or empagliflozin in patients with type 2 diabetes and heart failure. Br J Clin Pharmacol. 2020;86(7):1346-56.
31. Packer M, Anker SD, Butler J, Filippatos G, Pocock SJ, Carson P, et al. Cardiovascular and Renal Outcomes with Empagliflozin in Heart Failure. N Engl J Med. 2020;383(15):1413-24.
32. Tsimihodimos V, Filippatos TD, Elisaf MS. SGLT2 inhibitors and the kidney: Effects and mechanisms. Diabetes Metab Syndr. 2018;12(6):1117-23.
33. Göpel SO, Adingupu D, Wang J, Semenova E, Behrendt M, Jansson-Löfmark R, et al. SGLT2 inhibition improves coronary flow velocity reserve and contractility: role of glucagon signaling. Cardiovasc Diabetol. 2024;23(1):408.
34. Baartscheer A, Schumacher CA, Wüst RCI, Fiolet JWT, Stienen GJM, Coronel R, et al. Empagliflozin decreases myocardial cytoplasmic Na+ through inhibition of the cardiac Na+/H+ exchanger in rats and rabbits. Diabetologia. 2017;60(3):568-73.
35. Herat LY, Magno AL, Rudnicka C, Hricova J, Carnagarin R, Ward NC, et al. SGLT2 Inhibitor-Induced Sympathoinhibition: A Novel Mechanism for Cardiorenal Protection. JACC Basic Transl Sci. 2020;5(2):169-79.
36. Manolis AA, Manolis TA, Manolis AS. Neurohumoral Activation in Heart Failure. Int J Mol Sci. 2023;24(20):15472.
37. Cannon CP, Pratley R, Dagogo-Jack S, Mancuso J, Huyck S, Masiukiewicz U, et al. Cardiovascular Outcomes with Ertugliflozin in Type 2 Diabetes. N Engl J Med. 2020;383(15):1425-35.
38. Bhattarai M, Salih M, Regmi M, Al-Akchar M, Deshpande R, Niaz Z, et al. Association of Sodium-Glucose Cotransporter 2 Inhibitors With Cardiovascular Outcomes in Patients With Type 2 Diabetes and Other Risk Factors for Cardiovascular Disease. JAMA Network Open. 2022;5(1):e2142078.
39. McMurray JJV, Solomon SD, Inzucchi SE, Køber L, Kosiborod MN, Martinez FA, et al. Dapagliflozin in Patients with Heart Failure and Reduced Ejection Fraction. N Engl J Med. 2019;381(21):1995-2008.
40. Anker SD, Butler J, Filippatos G, Ferreira JP, Bocchi E, Böhm M, et al. Empagliflozin in Heart Failure with a Preserved Ejection Fraction. N Engl J Med. 2021;385(16):1451-61.
41. Solomon SD, McMurray JJV, Claggett B, De Boer RA, Demets D, Hernandez AF, et al. Dapagliflozin in Heart Failure with Mildly Reduced or Preserved Ejection Fraction. N Engl J Med. 2022;387(12):1089-98.
42. Sattar N, Butler J, Lee MMY, Harrington J, Sharma A, Zannad F, et al. Body mass index and cardiorenal outcomes in the EMPEROR-Preserved trial: Principal findings and meta-analysis with the DELIVER trial. Eur J Heart Fail. 2024;26(4):900-9.
43. Cavender Matthew A, Norhammar A, Birkeland Kåre I, Jørgensen Marit E, Wilding John P, Khunti K, et al. SGLT-2 Inhibitors and Cardiovascular Risk. JACC. 2018;71(22):2497-506.
44. Kosiborod M, Cavender MA, Fu AZ, Wilding JP, Khunti K, Holl RW, et al. Lower Risk of Heart Failure and Death in Patients Initiated on Sodium-Glucose Cotransporter-2 Inhibitors Versus Other Glucose-Lowering Drugs. Circulation. 2017;136(3):249-59.

45. Svanström H, Mkoma GF, Hviid A, Pasternak B. SGLT-2 inhibitors and mortality among patients with heart failure with reduced ejection fraction: linked database study. BMJ. 2024;387:e080925.
46. Patel SM, Kang YM, Im K, Neuen BL, Anker SD, Bhatt DL, et al. Sodium-Glucose Cotransporter-2 Inhibitors and Major Adverse Cardiovascular Outcomes: A SMART-C Collaborative Meta-Analysis. Circulation. 2024;149(23):1789-801.
47. Bantounou MA, Sardellis P, Plascevic J, Awaes-Mahmood R, Kaczmarek J, Black Boada D, et al. Meta-analysis of sotagliflozin, a dual sodium-glucose-cotransporter 1/2 inhibitor, for heart failure in type 2 diabetes. ESC Heart Fail. 2025;12(2):968-79.
48. Davies MJ, Aroda VR, Collins BS, Gabbay RA, Green J, Maruthur NM, et al. Management of Hyperglycemia in Type 2 Diabetes, 2022. A Consensus Report by the American Diabetes Association (ADA) and the European Association for the Study of Diabetes (EASD). Diabetes Care. 2022;45(11):2753-86.
49. Rossing P, Caramori ML, Chan JCN, Heerspink HJL, Hurst C, Khunti K, et al. KDIGO 2022 Clinical Practice Guideline for Diabetes Management in Chronic Kidney Disease. Kidney Int. 2022;102(5):S1-S127.
50. Greene SJ, Butler J, Albert NM, Devore AD, Sharma PP, Duffy CI, et al. Medical Therapy for Heart Failure With Reduced Ejection Fraction. J Am Coll Cardiol. 2018;72(4):351-66.
51. Pierce JB, Vaduganathan M, Fonarow GC, Ikeaba U, Chiswell K, Butler J, et al. Contemporary Use of Sodium-Glucose Cotransporter-2 Inhibitor Therapy Among Patients Hospitalized for Heart Failure With Reduced Ejection Fraction in the US: The Get With The Guidelines-Heart Failure Registry. JAMA Cardiol. 2023;8(7):652-61.
52. Elmegaard M, Køber L, Ersbøll MK, Lange T, Tuxen CD, Mouridsen MR, et al. Digital implementation strategy to increase SGLT2 inhibitor uptake in heart failure: Study design of EMAIL-HF. ESC Heart Fail. 2025;12(6):3953-65.
53. Li D, Wang T, Shen S, Fang Z, Dong Y, Tang H. Urinary tract and genital infections in patients with type 2 diabetes treated with sodium-glucose co-transporter 2 inhibitors: A meta-analysis of randomized controlled trials. Diabetes Obes Metab. 2017;19(3):348-55.
54. Wu MZ, Guo R, Chandramouli C, Liu L, Tung AMO, Tsang CTW, et al. Urinary tract infection and continuation of sodium-glucose cotransporter-2 inhibitors in diabetic patients. Eur Heart J; 2025.
55. Chow E, Clement S, Garg R. Euglycemic diabetic ketoacidosis in the era of SGLT-2 inhibitors. BMJ Open Diabetes Res Care. 2023;11(5):e003666.
56. Oosterom-Eijmael MJP, Hermanides J, van Raalte DH, Hulst AH. Risk of perioperative discontinuation of SGLT2 inhibitors. Br J Anaesth. 2024;133(2):239-40.
57. Perkovic V, Jardine MJ, Neal B, Bompoint S, Heerspink HJL, Charytan DM, et al. Canagliflozin and Renal Outcomes in Type 2 Diabetes and Nephropathy. N Engl J Med. 2019;380(24):2295-306.
58. Patorno E, Pawar A, Wexler DJ, Glynn RJ, Bessette LG, Paik JM, et al. Effectiveness and safety of empagliflozin in routine care patients: Results from the EMPagliflozin compaRative effectIveness and SafEty (EMPRISE) study. Diabetes Obes Metabol. 2022;24(3):442-54.
59. Heerspink HJL, Stefánsson BV, Correa-Rotter R, Chertow GM, Greene T, Hou FF, et al. Dapagliflozin in Patients with Chronic Kidney Disease. N Engl J Med. 2020;383(15):1436-46.
60. Awdishu L, Maxson R, Gratt C, Rubenzik T, Battistella M. KDIGO 2024 clinical practice guideline on evaluation and management of chronic kidney disease: A primer on what pharmacists need to know. Am J Health Syst Pharm. 2025;82(12):660-71.
61. Yau K, Dharia A, Alrowiyti I, Cherney DZI. Prescribing SGLT2 Inhibitors in Patients With CKD: Expanding Indications and Practical Considerations. Kidney Int Rep. 2022;7(7):1463-76.
62. Madero M, Chertow GM, Mark PB. SGLT2 Inhibitor Use in Chronic Kidney Disease: Supporting Cardiovascular, Kidney, and Metabolic Health. Kidney Med. 2024;6(8):100851.
63. Minami K, Terashima R, Freeman L, Yamada Y, Vest AR, Yano Y, et al. SGLT2 Inhibitors in Older Adults With Cardiovascular Disease: A Systematic Review and Meta-Analysis. J Am Geriatrics Society. 2025;73(12):3708-18.
64. Ouyang X, Wang J, Chen Q, Peng L, Li S, Tang X. Sodium-glucose cotransporter 2 inhibitor may not prevent atrial fibrillation in patients with heart

failure: a systematic review. Cardiovasc Diabetol. 2023;22(1):124.

65. James S, Erlinge D, Storey Robert F, McGuire Darren K, de Belder M, Eriksson N, et al. Dapagliflozin in Myocardial Infarction without Diabetes or Heart Failure. NEJM Evidence. 2024;3(2):EVIDoa2300286.
66. Semirani-Nezhad D, Soleimani H, Taebi M, Roozbehi K, Jahangiri S, Sattartabar B, et al. Early initiation of SGLT2 inhibitors in acute myocardial infarction and cardiovascular outcomes, an updated systematic review and meta-analysis. BMC Cardiovasc Disord. 2025;25(1):527.
67. Requena-Ibáñez JA, Zafar MU, Ferrandez-Escarabajal M, Escolar G, Santos-Gallego C, Lam D, et al. Rationale and Design of the SOTA-THROMBOSIS Trial (ATRU-VI): Antithrombotic Activities of Sotagliflozin Compared With Empagliflozin. J Cardiovasc Pharmacol. 2025;86(5):458-62.
68. Shokravi A, Seth J, Mancini GBJ. Cardiovascular and renal outcomes of dual combination therapies with glucagon-like peptide-1 receptor agonists and sodium-glucose transport protein 2 inhibitors: a systematic review and meta-analysis. Cardiovasc Diabetol. 2025;24(1):370.
69. Svanström H, Mkoma GF, Hviid A, Pasternak B. Initiation of SGLT2 inhibitors versus mineralocorticoid receptor antagonists as third-line therapy in heart failure with reduced ejection fraction: a nationwide cohort study. Lancet Reg Health Eur. 2026;60:101510.
70. Zhang X, Davison B, Adamo M, Arrigo M, Biegus J, Chioncel O, et al. Guideline-Directed Medical Therapy Use in the STRONG-HF Trial. Circ Heart Fail. 2025;18(9):e012716.

CHAPTER 16

New Drugs for Hypertension: Status 2025

Narsingh Verma, Shivam Verma, Manish Kumar Verma

ABSTRACT

Hypertension remains a major cause of cardiovascular morbidity and mortality worldwide, with many patients achieving inadequate blood pressure control despite existing therapies. Recent advances have introduced novel antihypertensive drugs targeting new neurohormonal and vascular pathways. These emerging agents offer improved treatment options, particularly for resistant hypertension, and may enhance cardiovascular and renal outcomes.

Keywords: Hypertension, novel antihypertensive drugs, resistant hypertension, emerging therapies.

INTRODUCTION

Hypertension, a chronic medical condition characterized by persistently elevated arterial blood pressure (BP), remains a leading modifiable risk factor for cardiovascular, cerebrovascular, and renal diseases. It is implicated in >10 million deaths annually worldwide, with ischemic heart disease and stroke being the principal consequences.[1]

As per the World Health Organization (WHO) 2023 hypertension report, over 1.28 billion adults aged 30–79 years are estimated to be living with hypertension globally, with two-thirds residing in low- and middle-income countries (LMICs). Alarmingly, nearly 46% of adults with hypertension are unaware of their condition, and only about 42% receive treatment, with merely 21% achieving optimal BP control.[2]

INDIAN SCENARIO

India mirrors this global trend with a rapidly rising burden. According to the National Family Health Survey (NFHS-5, 2019–21), 24% of men and 21% of women aged 15 and above were found to have elevated BP or were on antihypertensive medication.[3]

Urbanization, sedentary lifestyles, dietary sodium excess, and increasing obesity have driven prevalence rates in urban India to 30–35%, while rural areas are catching up with rates between 12 and 17%.[4] Moreover, awareness treatment, and control rates in India remain dismally low at approximately 50%, 30%, and 12% respectively.[5]

UNMET NEEDS AND NOVEL THERAPIES

Despite the availability of Decal drug classes—such as diuretics, β-blockers, calcium channel blockers (CCBs), angiotensin-converting enzyme inhibitors (ACEIs), and angiotensin receptor blockers (ARBs) on a pressure control remains suboptimal in a significant portion of patients. This is especially evident in cases of resistant hypertension, defined as uncontrolled BP despite the use of at least three antihypertensives of different classes including a diuretic.[6]

Recent advancements in hypertension pharmacotherapy are driven by an enhanced understanding of renal, neurohormonal, and vascular mechanisms, as well as genetic and metabolic factors influencing BP regulation. Novel therapeutic targets are being explored to address limitations such as adverse effects, pharmacoresistance, and comorbidity interactions.

Novel Mineralocorticoid Receptor Antagonists

Finerenone is a nonsteroidal, selective mineralocorticoid receptor antagonist (MRA) that represents a significant advancement over traditional steroidal MRAs such as spironolactone and eplerenone. Unlike its predecessors, finerenone exhibits higher receptor selectivity and tighter binding affinity, which translates into reduced off-target hormonal side effects such as gynecomastia and menstrual irregularities commonly seen with spironolactone.

Importantly, finerenone has been shown to minimize the risk of hyperkalemia, a major limiting factor in the long-term use of MRAs, particularly in patients with chronic kidney disease (CKD) and type 2 diabetes mellitus (T2DM). Through its anti-inflammatory and antifibrotic properties, finerenone not only lowers BP modestly but more significantly improves cardiovascular and renal outcomes, even in patients with relatively preserved eGFR.

Evidence from pivotal trials such as FIDELIO-DKD and FIGARO-DKD has firmly established finerenone's role in reducing progression of CKD and major adverse cardiovascular events (MACE) in patients with diabetic kidney disease, independent of glycemic control or background use of renin-angiotensin system inhibitors.[7]

Endothelin Receptor Antagonists

Endothelin-1 (ET-1) is one of the most potent endogenous vasoconstrictors and plays a key role in the pathophysiology of resistant hypertension. It promotes vascular smooth muscle contraction, inflammation, fibrosis, and sodium retention, primarily through its action on endothelin receptor antagonists (ETA) and ETB receptors located in the vasculature, heart, and kidneys. Overactivity of the ET-1 system is associated with endothelial dysfunction and sustained BP elevation, particularly in patients with treatment-resistant hypertension.

Aprocitentan, a novel dual ERA that blocks both ETA and ETB receptors, has emerged as a promising oral antihypertensive agent for this challenging patient population. By inhibiting the deleterious effects of ET-1 on vascular tone and fluid homeostasis, aprocitentan offers a new mechanistic pathway beyond the conventional renin-angiotensin-aldosterone system (RAAS) and sympathetic nervous system blockers.

The PRECISION trial (2023)—a multicenter, phase 3 randomized controlled trial—demonstrated that aprocitentan, when added to standard triple therapy [a diuretic, a calcium channel blocker, and a renin-angiotensin system (RAS) blocker], led to a significant and sustained reduction in office and ambulatory systolic BP in patients with resistant hypertension. Importantly, the drug was generally well tolerated, with mild fluid retention being the most commonly reported side effect, manageable with diuretics. Given its novel mechanism and favorable efficacy profile, aprocitentan may soon become an important adjunct in managing resistant hypertension, particularly in patients unresponsive to current standard therapies.[8]

Angiotensin Receptor Neprilysin Inhibitors

Angiotensin receptor-neprilysin inhibitors (ARNIs) represent a novel class of antihypertensive agents that combine the blockade angiotensin II type 1 (AT1) receptors with inhibition of neprilysin, an enzyme responsible for degrading natriuretic peptides, bradykinin, and other vasodilatory substances. This dual action leads to vasodilation, natriuresis, diuresis, and reduced sympathetic tone, offering a comprehensive approach to BP control.

Sacubitril/valsartan, the first-in-class ARNI, was originally approved for patients with heart failure with reduced ejection fraction (HFrEF). However, subsequent studies have demonstrated its potent BP-lowering effects, particularly in individuals with isolated systolic hypertension and heart failure with preserved ejection fraction (HFpEF).

Clinical trials such as PARAMETER have shown that sacubitril/valsartan reduces central aortic systolic pressure and brachial systolic BP more effectively than ARBs alone, especially in elderly patients with stiff arteries—a hallmark of isolated systolic hypertension. These findings have sparked growing interest in the use of ARNIs in the management of primary hypertension, particularly in patients with concomitant metabolic or cardiovascular comorbidities.

With its dual mechanism offering benefits beyond traditional RAAS blockade, sacubitril/valsartan is being increasingly recognized as a next-generation antihypertensive agent, though further large-scale trials are needed to establish its routine use in uncomplicated hypertension.[9]

Soluble Guanylate Cyclase Stimulators

Soluble guanylate cyclase (sGC) stimulators represent a novel class of agents that enhance the nitric oxide (NO)-sGC—cyclic guanosine monophosphate (cGMP) signaling pathway, a key mediator of vascular relaxation, inhibition of smooth muscle proliferation, and endothelial function. By directly stimulating sGC independently of NO and also sensitizing it to endogenous NO, these agents offer a promising approach to restoring vasodilation in conditions characterized by endothelial dysfunction, such as hypertension and heart failure.

Vericiguat, a second-generation sGC stimulator, has been approved for use in chronic HFrEF in patients at high risk of hospitalization. While its primary indication is heart failure, vericiguat has demonstrated modest BP-lowering effects, particularly in patients with hypertensive heart disease or those with stiff vasculature and impaired NO signaling.

Emerging data suggest that vericiguat may help reverse maladaptive cardiac remodeling and improve vascular compliance, making it an attractive candidate for further investigation in resistant or difficult-to-control hypertension, especially where standard vasodilators are inadequate or poorly tolerated.

Though its antihypertensive effects are less pronounced than other dedicated BP-lowering agents, the dual benefit on both vascular tone and cardiac function underscores the therapeutic potential of sGC stimulators in complex cardiovascular diseases with anunderlying hypertensive component.

Praliciguat is another oral sGC stimulator with antihypertensive and metabolic benefits, showing promise in early clinical studies, especially in patients with metabolic syndrome.[10,11]

Dual-acting Renin-angiotensin System Blockers

Firibastat is a first-in-class brain aminopeptidase A (APA) inhibitor, representing a novel approach in antihypertensive therapy by selectively targeting the central (brain) RAS. Unlike conventional RAS inhibitors that act peripherally, firibastat penetrates the blood–brain barrier and inhibits APA, the enzyme responsible for converting angiotensin II to angiotensin III within the brain. Angiotensin III is a potent stimulator of vasopressin release, sympathetic nervous system activation, and BP elevation.

By reducing central angiotensin III levels, firibastat attenuates neurogenic hypertension pathways, resulting in reduced sympathetic tone and lower systemic BP. This mechanism offers a promising strategy for patients with treatment-resistant or neurogenic hypertension, particularly those with obesity or metabolic syndrome, where central RAS overactivity is often implicated.

In Phase II trials, including the NEW-HOPE study, firibastat demonstrated a significant reduction in systolic BP, particularly in overweight and obese hypertensive patients, with a favorable safety and tolerability profile. Notably, the BP reduction was consistent across ethnicities and comorbidity profiles, supporting its broad applicability. As research progresses into phase III, firibastat is being positioned as a first-in-class central RAS modulator for future hypertension management, especially in populations not well-served by conventional therapies.[12]

Sodium-glucose Cotransporter 2 Inhibitors

While originally developed as oral antidiabetic agents, sodium-glucose co-transporter 2 (SGLT2) inhibitors—including empagliflozin, dapagliflozin, and canagliflozin—have demonstrated modest but clinically meaningful BP-lowering effects, independent of their glucose-lowering properties. These drugs inhibit glucose and sodium reabsorption in the proximal renal tubules, leading to osmotic diuresis, natriuresis, and mild volume depletion, which contribute to their diuretic-like antihypertensive effect.

In addition to volume reduction, SGLT2 inhibitors promote weight loss, reduce visceral adiposity, and improve arterial compliance and vascular stiffness, further enhancing BP control. Meta-analyses of clinical trials have consistently shown reductions in systolic BP by 3–5 mm Hg and diastolic pressure by 1–2 mm Hg, even in nondiabetic individuals with hypertension or heart failure.

Moreover, these agents confer cardiorenal protection, making them particularly valuable in patients with coexisting hypertension, type 2 diabetes, heart failure, or chronic kidney disease. Their pleiotropic effects make SGLT2 inhibitors attractive as adjuncts to conventional antihypertensive therapy, especially in patients with metabolic comorbidities. As clinical evidence continues to expand, SGLT2 inhibitors are emerging as an integral part of comprehensive cardiovascular risk management, including in those with suboptimal BP control.[13]

Aldosterone Synthase Inhibitors

Baxdrostat is a novel, selective aldosterone synthase inhibitor designed to target aldosterone biosynthesis without interfering with cortisol production—a key limitation seen in earlier, nonselective agents. By inhibiting CYP11B2 (aldosterone synthase) and sparing CYP11B1 (responsible for cortisol synthesis), baxdrostat achieves precise suppression of aldosterone, a hormone central to sodium retention, vascular stiffness, and hypertension, especially in resistant forms of the disease.

The importance of targeting aldosterone lies in its significant role in promoting volume expansion, sympathetic activation, and end-organ damage. In patients with resistant hypertension, characterized by uncontrolled BP despite the use of three or more antihypertensive agents including a diuretic, excess aldosterone activity is often a key contributor.

The BrigHTN trial, a phase II randomized, double-blind, placebo-controlled study, demonstrated that baxdrostat significantly reduced systolic BP in patients with treatment-resistant hypertension, without significant adverse effects on cortisol levels or electrolyte balance. The drug was well tolerated, with a safety profile comparable to placebo, and no cases of adrenal insufficiency were reported.

Baxdrostat represents a next-generation approach to precision antihypertensive therapy, offering targeted endocrine modulation in a population with limited therapeutic options.

Its unique mechanism positions it as a promising candidate for broader use in primary aldosteronism and high-risk hypertensive populations.[14]

Other Emerging Therapies

Antisense Oligonucleotides

IONIS-AGT-LRx is an innovative antisense oligonucleotide (ASO) that specifically targets the mRNA of hepatic angiotensinogen, the precursor of angiotensin I, thereby inhibiting the upstream component of the RAAS. Unlike traditional RAAS inhibitors that block downstream receptors or enzymes, this approach reduces the synthesis of angiotensinogen itself, offering a novel and highly selective method of BP control.

Early-phase clinical trials have demonstrated that IONIS-AGT LRx leads to significant and sustained reductions in systolic and diastolic BP in patients with hypertension, with a favorable safety profile and minimal off-target effects. By leveraging GalNAc conjugation technology, the drug achieves liver-specific delivery, thereby improving potency and reducing systemic exposure.

This gene-silencing approach represents a promising frontier in precision medicine, potentially useful in patients with resistant or genetically driven hypertension, and may complement or even replace conventional pharmacologic agents in the future.[15]

Gut Microbiota-based Therapies

Recent scientific advances have highlighted the gut microbiome as a key player in BP regulation through complex interactions involving immune modulation, metabolic signaling, and neurohormonal pathways. Although still largely in the preclinical or early clinical stages, microbiota-targeted therapies are being investigated as potential adjuncts in hypertension management.

Certain probiotics, postbiotics, and microbial metabolites—particularly short-chain fatty acids (SCFAs) such as acetate, propionate, and butyrate—have been shown to lower systemic inflammation, improve endothelial function, and modulate sympathetic activity, all of which contribute to BP reduction in animal models. Additionally, dysbiosis an imbalance in gut microbiota) has been associated with elevated BP and increased cardiovascular risk.

Therapeutic strategies under investigation include targeted probiotic formulations, prebiotics, fecal microbiota transplantation (FMT), and dietary interventions aimed at reshaping the gut microbial composition. While robust clinical data in humans are still pending, this emerging area holds promise for individualized, nonpharmacological approaches to hypertension management.[16]

Clinical Implications and Future Perspectives

The introduction of these novel agents expands the therapeutic armamentarium for clinicians managing hypertension, particularly in complex and resistant cases. Future research should focus on long-term cardiovascular outcomes, combination strategies, and personalized medicine approaches. Moreover, affordability and accessibility will determine the real-world impact of these therapies, especially in LMICs.

CONCLUSION

New antihypertensive drugs represent a significant advancement in hypertension management. These therapies offer diverse mechanisms of action and the potential for greater BP control, improved patient outcomes, and reduced side effects. As clinical experience and data grow, these drugs may shift current treatment paradigms and offer hope for patients inadequately managed with conventional therapies.

REFERENCES

1. GBD 2021 Risk Factors Collaborators. Global burden of 87 risk factors in 204 countries and territories, 1990-2021: a systematic analysis for the Global Burden of Disease Study 2021. Lancet. 2023;402(10397):1806-32.
2. World Health Organization. The WHO World Report on Hypertension 2023. [Online] Available from https://www.who.int/publications/i/item/978924008 1492 [Last accessed March, 2026].
3. International Institute for Population Sciences (IIPS). National Family Health Survey-J (NFHS-5), India, 2019-21. Mumbai: IIPS; 2021.
4. Prabhakaran D, Jeemon P, Roy A. Cardiovascular diseases in India: current epidemiology and future directions. Circulation. 2021;144(19): 1601-8.
5. Geldsetzer P, Manne-Goehler J, Theilmann M, Davies JI, Awasthi A, Vollmer S, et al. Diabetes and hypertension in India: a nationally representative study of 1.3 million adults. JAMA Intern Med. 2022;182(5):463-72.
6. Carey RM, Calhoun DA, Bakris GL, Brook RD, Daugherty SL, Dennison-Himmelfarb C, et al. Resistant Hypertension: Detection, Evaluation, and Management. Hypertension. 2023;80(1):e14-e32.
7. Bakris GL, Agarwal R, Anker SD, Pitt B, Ruilope LM, Rossing P, et al. Effect of finerenone on chronic kidney disease outcomes in type 2 diabetes. N Engl J Med. 2020;383(23):2219-29.
8. Verweij N, Jones A, Wirtz H, Menard J, B6nner G, Bohm M, et al. Aprocitentan for resistant hypertension: PRECISION trial results. Lancet. 2023;401(10377):1113-23.
9. Schmieder RE, Wagner F, Mayr M, Delles C, Ott C. The effect of sacubitril/valsartan on ambulatory blood pressure in patients with hypertension: a randomized, double- blind study. J Hypertens. 2021;39(2):387-95.
10. Armstrong PW, Lam CSP, Anstrom KJ, Ezekowitz J, Hernandez AF, O'Connor CM, et al. Vericiguat in patients with heart failure and reduced ejection fraction. N Engl J Med. 2020;382(20):1883-93.
11. Hanrahan JP, Stasch JP, Lipicky RJ. Praliciguat: a novel sGC stimulator with therapeutic potential for metabolic diseases. Curr Hypertens Rep. 2022;24(3):171-9.
12. Azizi M, Jover B, Flamenbaum W, Persu A, Ménard J. Efficacy of the first-in-class brain aminopeptidase A inhibitor firibastat in hypertension: the NEW-HOPE study. Hypertension. 2020;75(4):927-35.
13. Wanner C, Inzucchi SE, Lachin JM, Fitchett D, Mattheus M, George JT, et al. Empagliflozin and progression of kidney disease in type 2 diabetes. N Engl J Med. 2020;383(2):171-81.
14. Doberer D, Domenig O, Lercher A, Plank J, Schmid A, Pilz R, et al. Baxdrostat for treatment of resistant hypertension: the BrigHTN trial. N Engl J Med. 2023;389(13):1172-83.
15. Thamilarasan M, Patel R, Ruff C, Triscari J, Krueger J, Min J, et al. Angiotensinogen inhibition by antisense oligonucleotides reduces blood pressure: a phase | trial. Hypertension. 2021;77(1):26-34.
16. Li J, Zhao F, Wang Y, Chen J, Tao J, Tian G, et al. Gut microbiota and hypertension: a new perspective. Clin Sci (Lond). 2021;135(2):129-45.

SECTION 10

Future of Diabetes

CHAPTER 17

Digital Twin Technology and Personalized Diabetes Management

Mala Dharmalingam, Mohamed Thajudeen

ABSTRACT

Type 2 diabetes (T2D) is a complex, chronic disorder influenced by heterogeneous factors such as metabolic, behavioral, and environmental. Traditional care models rely on episodic measurements and treatment algorithms which may fail to achieve sustained disease control. This chapter explores the clinical potential of digital twin (DT) technology, an artificial intelligence (AI)-powered, real-time modeling framework that enables dynamic simulation of individual physiology to guide precision lifestyle and therapeutic interventions in T2D management.

Digital twin technology continuously integrates multimodal data from wearable sensors, laboratory tests, diet, physical activity, sleep, and psychosocial inputs. Using machine learning, DT platforms simulate glycemic dynamics, predict response to interventions, and provide personalized, real-time recommendations. These closed-loop systems adaptively guide nutrition, exercise, stress management, and medication adjustments to restore metabolic balance.

In a randomized controlled trial, 72.7% of individuals with T2D achieved remission at 1 year, with 94% discontinuing all diabetes medications. At 3 years, 53.6% sustained remission. Significant improvements were observed across glycated hemoglobin (HbA1c; from 9.0% to 6.1% at 1 year), blood pressure, lipid profiles, liver fat, renal function, neuropathy, and mental health. In a large real-world cohort (n = 1,853), 89.0% of participants achieved HbA1c <7% by the end of 1 year. These outcomes underscore the multisystem benefits and scalability of DT-guided care.

Digital twin technology marks a transformative shift in diabetes management—from reactive disease control to proactive, individualized metabolic restoration. Digital twin stimulates the physiological impact of lifestyle and therapeutic changes; DT platforms enable sustainable remission of T2D and broader improvements in cardiometabolic health.

Keywords: Digital twin, type 2 diabetes remission, AI in healthcare, metabolic dysfunction, personalized therapy, continuous glucose monitoring.

INTRODUCTION

Diabetes has emerged as a major global health challenge. The International Diabetes Federation (IDF) Diabetes Atlas 2025 estimates that 589 million adults (1 in 9 adults) are having diabetes. This number is projected to rise to 853 million by 2050.[1] In 2024, diabetes was responsible for an estimated 3.4 million deaths globally—equivalent to one life lost every 9 seconds. The associated health expenditure exceeded USD 1 trillion, a 338% increase compared to 2007.[1] Moreover, diabetes is a leading cause of mortality and disability worldwide, with vascular complications contributing to 26.8% of the burden.[2]

The UK Prospective Diabetes Study (UKPDS) established the benefits of intensive glycemic control.[3] In routine clinical practice, glycemic targets remain difficult to achieve—only about 23.4–38% of individuals with diabetes are within guideline-recommended thresholds.[4] Current guidelines continue to advocate for strict glycemic control as a cornerstone strategy to delay or prevent diabetes-related complications, and professional societies increasingly highlight the value of digital tools, continuous glucose monitoring (CGM), and telemedicine in facilitating real-time decision-making and personalized care.[5,6]

Despite these advances, a fundamental gap remains: Standardized care pathways often fail to address the profound interindividual variability in metabolic responses, behavioral context, genetic predisposition, and psychosocial determinants.[7] Moreover, the conventional model of care—centered around infrequent assessments [such as quarterly glycated hemoglobin (HbA1c) checks], retrospective data collection remains largely reactive, offering limited scope for real-time adaptation or prevention of disease progression.[7]

Amid the digital transformation of healthcare, digital twin (DT) technology has emerged as a novel paradigm, offering an opportunity to revolutionize the personalized management of chronic metabolic diseases such as type 2 diabetes (T2D)[8] by enabling continuous physiological monitoring, real-time simulation of therapeutic outcomes, and adaptive treatment guidance, DTs aim to suppress the root cause—the resolution of metabolic dysfunction. DT has shown promising potential in addressing core metabolic impairments such as insulin resistance, oxidative stress, and mitochondrial dysfunction—factors often inadequately targeted by traditional care. These platforms unify behavioral data, biomarker trends, and AI-driven analytics to deliver precision care that evolves dynamically with the individual.

DIGITAL TWIN TECHNOLOGY

Introduction to Digital Twin Technology

Digital twin technology represents an advanced application of AI-enabled simulation in clinical medicine.[9-12] Unlike traditional disease management models that respond to static biomarkers or symptomatic thresholds, DT technology continuously simulates a person's physiological and behavioral processes to detect early signs of metabolic dysfunction and deliver personalized interventions.[13] The primary objective extends beyond disease control toward correcting underlying physiological imbalances driving chronic conditions such as T2D, obesity, and cardiovascular risk.[13]

Artificial Intelligence-First Design and Data Infrastructure

Digital twin technology is designed around an artificial intelligence (AI)-first infrastructure, where AI is not an auxiliary analytical tool but the primary driver of data collection, decision-making, and system learning.[13]

The platform leverages:

- Rule-based expert systems to encode clinical knowledge
- Supervised learning algorithms to classify health states
- Unsupervised clustering to discover latent patterns
- Reinforcement learning to continuously optimize intervention strategies
- Deep neural networks and LSTM models to forecast glycemic dynamics based on temporal data

The system collects and processes over 3,000 unique variables per user, including:

- *Cardiometabolic biomarkers:* HbA1c, CGM-based glucose, lipids, blood pressure, insulin sensitivity, liver and renal function, hormones, and cardiac risk profile
- *Behavioral data:* Macronutrient, micro-nutrient, probiotics, prebiotics intake, timing and frequency of meals, and types and duration of exercise
- *Psychosocial metrics:* Mood fluctuations, energy levels, stress levels, and subjective well-being
- *Sensor-derived metrics:* Step count, sedentary minutes, sleep staging, heart rate variation, respiration rate, and resting heart rate

These data are ingested via wearables, medical devices (e.g., CGMs), mobile applications, and cloud-connected labs, creating a real-time, living model of the user's internal physiology.

Core System Capabilities

The DT technology offers several clinical and computational capabilities:

- *Predictive simulation* of metabolic responses to food, medication, and activity
- *Intervention modeling* that tests how changes in diet or exercise will affect future glycemic control
- *Personalized behavioral coaching* using dynamically generated "action cards"
- *Medication titration support* based on predicted need and real-world response.

Critically, these recommendations are not static but adapt in real-time as new data emerge, enabling fully closed-loop digital therapeutic management.

PERSONALIZED LIFESTYLE INTERVENTIONS USING DIGITAL TWIN TECHNOLOGY

Personalized Lifestyle Interventions Using Digital Twin Technology

Digital twin-powered precision treatment addresses the root cause of chronic metabolic diseases—dysfunctional metabolism—by modeling the body as an integrated physiological system **(Fig. 1)**, rather than managing downstream symptoms such as hyperglycemia or hypertension, DT platforms focus on upstream drivers, including mitochondrial dysfunction, oxidative stress, inflammation, and metabolic inflexibility. This systems-based approach aims to restore homeostatic balance and prevent both microvascular (e.g., nephropathy and retinopathy) and macrovascular (e.g., myocardial infarction and stroke) complications, redefining chronic disease care as metabolic restoration rather than symptom suppression.

Digital twin technology enables precision lifestyle interventions across four domains: Medication, nutrition, activity, and sleep/stress, by continuously integrating physiological, behavioral, and environmental data. These interventions operate as a closed-loop system, dynamically adapting in response to the individual's metabolic status to support sustained healing and disease remission.

Precision Medication

Digital twin-enabled precision medication begins with a review of the individual's pre-twin pharmacologic regimen. As metabolic parameters evolve, the DT platform simulates and recommends personalized medication adjustments—either tapering or intensification—based on glycemic trends, organ function, and therapeutic response. These recommendations are, however, to be ratified by a qualified physician.

Precision Nutrition

Digital twin-guided nutrition applies real-time modeling of dietary intake, metabolic biomarkers, and behavioral variables to deliver individualized meal plans. Moving beyond fixed macronutrient ratios, DT platforms integrate data on macronutrients, micronutrient density, fiber content, and food-derived metabolic load, in relation to activity, sleep, medications, and glucose dynamics.

Foods are categorized into green (metabolic boosters), orange (moderately tolerated), and red (healing disruptors) based on their impact on insulin sensitivity, mitochondrial function, oxidative stress, gut microbiota, and fat metabolism. These categories are dynamic, reflecting metabolic improvements over time.[13-19] Initial guidance emphasizes low-glycemic, fiber-rich foods, functional superfoods, and

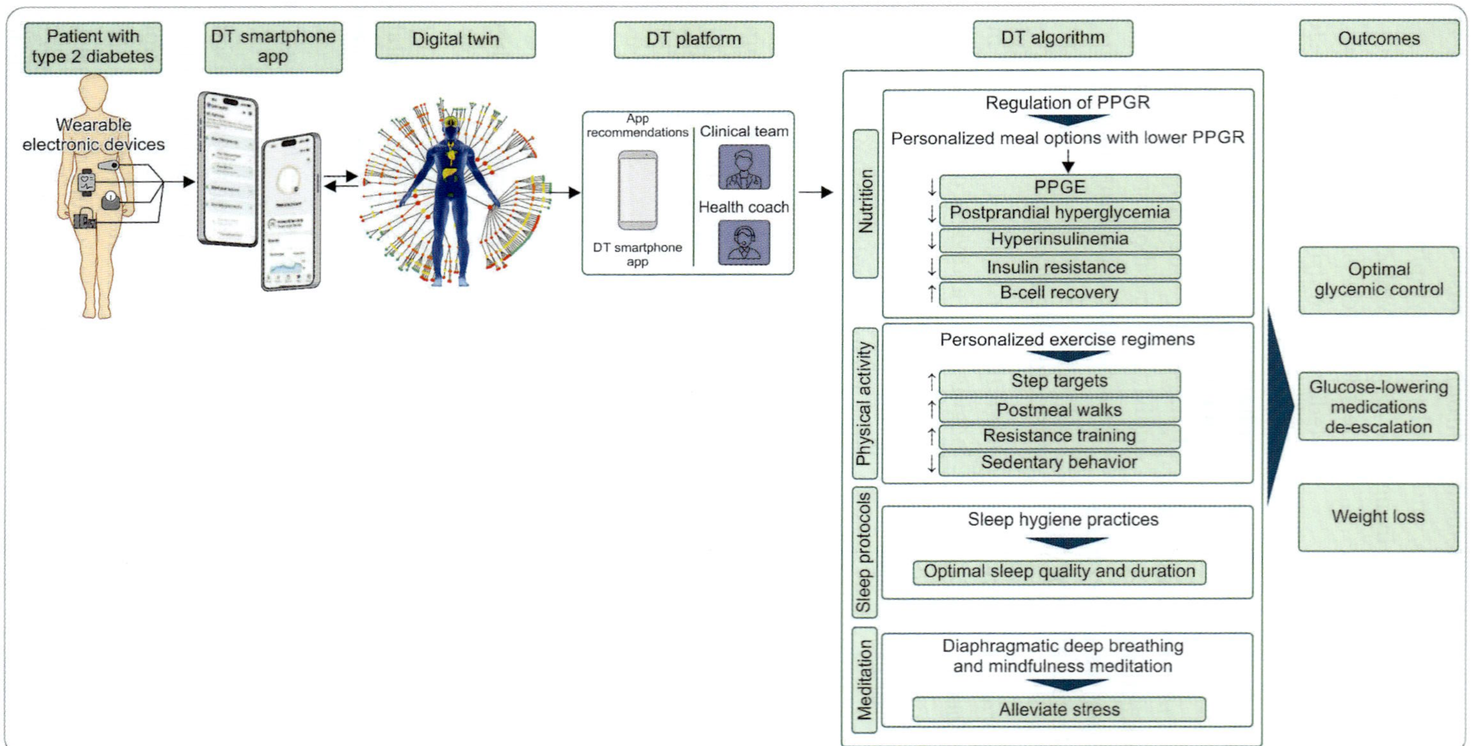

Fig. 1: Workflow of personalized lifestyle interventions enabled by digital twin technology in type 2 diabetes management. The digital twin ecosystem integrates continuous data from wearable devices, smartphone applications, and patient-reported inputs to simulate individual physiology. Personalized recommendations for nutrition, physical activity, sleep, and stress management are generated through AI-driven algorithms. These interventions are designed to regulate postprandial glucose response (PPGR), reduce insulin resistance, improve β-cell function, and support metabolic recovery. Clinical outcomes include optimal glycemic control, glucose-lowering medication de-escalation, and weight loss. (DT: digital twin; PPGE: postprandial glucose excursion; PPGR: postprandial glucose response; T2D: type 2 diabetes)

supplementation of mitochondrial cofactors such as magnesium, B vitamins, zinc, and others to support adenosine triphosphate (ATP) production and redox homeostasis. Microbiome profiling and short-chain fatty acid (SCFA) modeling further refine personalized recommendations for prebiotics, probiotics, and fermentable fibers, enhancing β-oxidation and reducing systemic inflammation.[13,19]

Precision Activity

Digital twin-guided activity interventions target visceral adiposity, inflammation, and poor metabolic flexibility—key contributors to insulin resistance. By stabilizing insulin metabolism and restoring energy regulation, DT supports fat loss without compromising muscle mass. Recommendations are generated through continuous integration of data on basal metabolic rate (BMR), thermic effect of food, nonexercise activity thermogenesis (NEAT), and structured physical activity. Personalized regimens align with circadian rhythms, mitochondrial thresholds, and ROS dynamics, incorporating aerobic, resistance, and high-intensity interval training (HIIT) tailored to individual recovery needs, VO_2 max, and insulin sensitivity.[13,19]

Sleep and Stress Optimization

Digital twin technology models sleep architecture and simulates the effects of targeted interventions such as melatonin, blue light therapy, and nutritional cofactors to support mitochondrial repair during rest. Stress modulation is guided by metrics such as cortisol levels, heart rate variability (HRV), and oxidative stress markers, informing individualized recommendations for paced breathing, progressive relaxation, and mindfulness practices. These strategies enhance autonomic recovery, promote mitochondrial biogenesis, and mitigate stress-induced metabolic dysfunction.[19,20]

Real-time Feedback Loop

A core strength of DT technology lies in its ability to deliver continuous, real-time feedback, allowing interventions to be adjusted dynamically in response to metabolic changes. This closed-loop system enables adaptive refinement of nutrition, activity, sleep, and medication strategies to promote mitochondrial health, glycemic control, and whole-body metabolic recovery. Through this personalized, systems-based approach, DT technology supports sustainable remission of type 2 diabetes and related metabolic conditions by addressing their root cause—metabolic dysfunction—rather than just their clinical manifestations.[13,19,20]

CLINICAL OUTCOMES OF DIGITAL TWIN TECHNOLOGY (TABLE 1)

Randomized Controlled Trial Outcomes

An open-label randomized controlled trial (RCT) titled "Randomized Controlled Trial of Twin Precision Treatment (TPT): A Novel Digital Twin-Based Precision Approach for Reversing Diabetes" was registered with the Clinical Trials Registry-India (CTRI/2020/08/027072) and approved by the Medisys Ethics Review Board (MCERB/2020/07). Designed as a 5-year study (2-year primary endpoint with a 3-year extension), it evaluates the effectiveness of DT technology in managing T2D.

Type 2 Diabetes Outcomes

The trial enrolled 319 participants: 233 in the DT group and 86 in the standard care (SC) group at 1 year. Dropout rates were comparable (15.9% in DT and 18.6% in SC), indicating no group-specific attrition. The digital twin group showed a significant HbA1c reduction from 9.0 (±1.9) to 6.1 (±0.7) ($p < 0.001$), while the SC group experienced a nonsignificant change from 8.5 (±1.9) to 8.2 (±1.6) ($p = 0.051$). By 1 year, 94% of patients in the

TABLE 1: Clinical outcomes of digital twin technology.

Application	*Key clinical outcomes*
T2D Management	HbA1c reduced by 2.9%, 94% off all T2D medications, 72.7% achieved T2D remission at 1 year,[20] and 53.6% sustained T2D remission at 3 years[21]
MASLD	Liver fat reduced to 5.5% (MRI-PDFF), 83.2% reached <6% threshold; NAFLD-LFS normalized in 67.4%[20]
Hypertension	Systolic BP reduced by 7.6 mm Hg, diastolic BP reduced by 4.3 mm Hg; 68.2% off antihypertensives, 50% achieved hypertension remission[22]
Dyslipidemia	HDL increased by 8.5 mg/dL, TG reduced by 94.8 mg/dL, LDL decreased by 12.3 mg/dL, TG/HDL ratio decreased by 3.9[23]
CVD Risk	ASCVD risk score reduced from 7.9 to 3.5%; 76.6% moved to low-risk category[24]
Diabetic neuropathy and retinopathy	96.4% improved touch sensitivity, 63.0% improved vibration perception;[25] 43.75% retinopathy resolution[26]
Obesity	Mean weight loss of 7.4 kg, BMI reduced by 2.7, waist circumference reduced by 9.5 cm[20]
Mental health	67% of mild and 94% of moderate depression improved; PHQ-9 correlated with T2D medication reduction[27]

(ASCVD: atherosclerotic cardiovascular disease; BMI: body mass index; BP: blood pressure; HbA1c: hemoglobin A1c; HDL: high-density lipoprotein; LDL: low-density lipoprotein; MASLD: metabolic dysfunction-associated steatotic liver disease; MRI-PDFF: magnetic resonance imaging–proton density fat fraction; NAFLD-LFS: nonalcoholic fatty liver disease–liver fat score; PHQ-9: patient health questionnaire-9; T2D: type 2 diabetes; TG: triglycerides; TG/HDL: triglycerides-to-HDL ratio)

DT arm had discontinued all T2D medications, and 72.7% achieved T2DM remission compared to none in SC.[20,28]

Liver Health and Metabolic Dysfunction-associated Fatty Liver Disease

Participants in the DT group exhibited marked improvements in hepatic markers. Normal NAFLD-LFS increased from 11.8 to 67.4% (vs. 16 to 9.9% in SC; $p < .00001$). FLI improved from 13.6 to 54.3% in DT and declined from 15.9 to 13.4% in SC ($p = 0.0003$). FSI improved from 13.1 to 61.1% in DT but remained stable in SC ($p = 0.0008$). NFS scores normalized in 94.4% (from 77.6%) in DT, compared to 65.5% (from 60.7%) in SC ($p = 0.58$). MRI-PDFF liver fat dropped significantly to 5.5 ± 4.7% in DT versus 10.9 ± 6.8% in SC ($p < .001$), with 83.2% of DT participants achieving <6% liver fat versus 34% in SC.[20]

Cardiovascular, Lipid, and Renal Outcomes

In 1 year, the DT group experienced greater reductions in systolic BP (–7.6 vs. –3.2; $p < 0.007$) and diastolic BP (–4.3 vs. –2.2; $p = 0.046$) compared with SC. Among those with hypertension, 68.2% in the DT group remained off antihypertensive medications compared to none in SC. The DT subgroup also achieved higher rates of normotension (40.9% vs. 6.7%; $p = 0.0009$) and hypertension remission (50 vs. 0%; $p < 0.0001$).[22]

Substantial improvements were also observed in lipid parameters at 6 months. HDL-C increased by 8.5 (±8.2) mg/dL, reaching 43.3 (±8.9) mg/dL ($p < 0.001$). The triglycerides/HDL ratio decreased from 7.1 (±7.5) to 3.2 (±2.1), a change of –3.9 (±7) ($p < 0.001$). Triglyceride levels reduced from 223.5 (±181.5) mg/dL to 128.7 (±72.3) mg/dL ($p < 0.001$), while sdLDL decreased from 49.8 (±24.1) mg/dL to 37.5 (±15.5) mg/dL ($p < 0.001$).[23]

The DT group demonstrated a marked shift toward a lower ASCVD risk profile at day 360, with 76.6% ($n = 170$) of participants categorized as low risk compared to 49.1% ($n = 109$) at baseline. High-risk category reductions were more pronounced in the DT group, decreasing from 8.1% ($n = 18$) to 0.9% ($n = 2$). The mean 10-year ASCVD risk score in the DT group declined significantly, from 7.9 ± 7.8% (95% CI: 6.8–8.9) at baseline to 3.5 ± 3.9% (95% CI: 3.0–4.0) at 1 year ($p < 0.0001$).[24]

Renal function also improved, as microalbuminuria normalized in 92.4% of the DT group. Macroalbuminuria declined from 4 to 1%, and mean albuminuria levels improved from 36.5 mg/g to 17 mg/g ($p = 0.0166$). Levels rose in the SC group.[29]

Diabetic Neuropathy and Retinopathy

Touch sensitivity improved in 96.4% and vibration perception in 63.0% of the DT group.[25] Among patients with diabetic retinopathy at baseline, 43.75% showed complete resolution.[26]

Weight and Metabolic Parameters

In 1 year, 73.8% of participants in the DT group achieved ≥5% weight loss, and 41.6% achieved ≥10% reduction. Mean weight declined by 7.4 ± 5.9 kg versus 0.4 ± 3.6 kg ($p < 0.001$), BMI by 2.7 ± 2.3 versus 0.1 ± 1.8 kg/m^2 ($p < 0.001$), and waist circumference by 9.5 ± 7.7 versus 1.2 ± 10.8 cm ($p < 0.001$).[20]

Durability and Sustainability

In a long-term follow-up at 3 years, 53.6% (112 out of 209) of participants in the DT group achieved sustained remission compared to 0% in the standard care group ($p < 0.001$). Statistically significant improvements were also observed in HbA1c, which decreased from 9.0 ± 1.9% at baseline to 6.8 ± 1.2% at 3 years ($p < 0.0001$).[21]

Mental Health Outcomes

In a separate analysis, 96 individuals with T2D and coexisting depression were assessed. At baseline, 54.1% had depressive symptoms, categorized as mild (28%), moderate (18%), moderate-to-severe (5%), and severe (3%). Postintervention, 67% of those with mild, 94% with moderate, and all with more severe categories improved, with no participants remaining in the higher severity groups.[27]

Real-World Evidence

A 90-day study conducted in India and the United States showed significant reductions in HbA1c, HOMA-IR, triglyceride- glucose index (TyG index), and Framingham Risk Score in both cohorts. Results demonstrated the model's generalizability across different populations.[30] In another real-world study, 1985 enrollees, 132 (6.6%) were lost to follow-up, leaving 1,853 participants who completed 1 year of the program. A significant mean HbA1c reduction of −1.8 ± 1.7% ($p < 0.0001$) was observed at the end of 1 year, 1,650 individuals (89.0%) achieved HbA1c levels below 7%, indicating good glycemic improvement.[31] In a U.S.-based 1-year follow-up, HbA1c improved from 7.73 ± 1.38 to 6.22 ± 0.62, with 71.9% achieving HbA1c <6.5%, and 55.5% meeting reversal criteria (HbA1c <6.5% on metformin only).[32]

These outcomes underscore the multisystem impact of metabolic restoration, achieved through integrated physiological and behavioral modeling.

IMPLEMENTATION CHALLENGES: ETHICAL, REGULATORY, AND CLINICAL INTEGRATION

Navigating Evolving Regulatory Pathways

Digital twin technology holds promise for proactive, personalized care but challenges existing regulatory models. While agencies such as the FDA and EMA have advanced standards for software as a medical device (SaMD), the adaptive, learning nature of DT systems requires clearer guidelines.

Key regulatory concerns include:

- Validating real-time adaptive algorithms without limiting innovation
- Defining update thresholds that require re-evaluation
- Correctly classifying DT platforms as decision-support, diagnostic, or therapeutic tools

Regulators increasingly support flexible, risk-based frameworks. As DT platforms prove safety and efficacy via real-world data and trials, they can align with and shape emerging standards.

Advancing Data Privacy and Responsible Governance

Digital twin platforms rely on continuous biometric, behavioral, and psychosocial data inputs, demanding strong privacy frameworks to protect autonomy and build trust.

Best practices include:

- Compliance with HIPAA, GDPR, India's DPDP Act, and similar global laws
- Clear, user-friendly informed consent sovereign data storage and localization
- Use of anonymization, federated learning, and secure access protocols

By employing encryption, distributed data models, and role-based controls, DT developers embed privacy into platform architecture.

Promoting Equity and Inclusive Access

To maximize impact, DT technology must be accessible across socioeconomic and demographic boundaries. Developers are increasingly focused on ensuring that DT interventions are not confined to urban or tech-savvy populations.

Strategies for equity include:

- Development of multilingual and culturally adaptive interfaces
- Use of voice-enabled assistants and community health worker tools
- Partnerships with public health institutions to distribute affordable or subsidized wearable devices.

With conscious design and policy collaboration, DT platforms can bridge rather than widen health disparities. Their scalability, real-time adaptability, and remote monitoring capabilities make them uniquely suited for deployment in both urban and underserved settings.

CONCLUSION

With increasing prevalence of diabetes and its complications, it becomes imperative for us to get more people into target control. With the conventional treatment regimes, the number of people in control remains small in spite of the advent of multiple treatment modalities. DT offers a technology which is redefining the landscape of T2D management by moving beyond reactive care toward a predictive, personalized, and precision-based paradigm. DTs enable clinicians and patients to proactively reverse metabolic dysfunction, rather than merely managing its symptoms. The clinical evidence demonstrates significant improvements across glycemic control, cardiovascular risk, liver health, renal markers, weight management, and even mental well-being. Despite the inherent challenges in regulation, data privacy, clinical integration, and equitable access, DTs offer a powerful, scalable solution for achieving sustainable T2D remission. As the field advances, collaborative efforts among technologists, clinicians, regulators, and policymakers will be essential to realize the full potential of this transformative innovation. With careful implementation and ongoing research, DT technology is poised to become the cornerstone of future-ready, patient-centered diabetes care.

REFERENCES

1. International Diabetes Federation. IDF Diabetes Atlas, 11th edition. Brussels, Belgium: International Diabetes Federation; 2025.
2. Lu Y, Wang W, Liu J, Xie M, Liu Q, Li S. Vascular complications of diabetes: A narrative review. Medicine. 2023;102(40):e35285.
3. Holman R, For the UKPDS Group. A brief history of the UK Prospective Diabetes Study. Br J Diabetes. 2022;22(Suppl 1):S32-5.
4. Borgharkar SS, Das SS. Real-world evidence of glycemic control among patients with type 2 diabetes mellitus in India: the TIGHT study. BMJ Open Diabet Res Care. 2019;7(1):e000654.
5. American Diabetes Association Professional Practice Committee. Glycemic Goals and Hypoglycemia: Standards of Care in Diabetes—2024. Diabetes Care. 2024;47(Suppl_1): S111-25.
6. American Diabetes Association Professional Practice Committee. Diabetes Technology: Standards of Care in Diabetes—2024. Diabetes Care. 2024;47 (Suppl_1): S126-44.
7. Sugandh FN, Chandio M, Raveena FN, Kumar L, Karishma FN, Khuwaja S, et al. Advances in the management of diabetes mellitus: a focus on personalized medicine. Cureus. 2023;15(8).
8. Mosquera-Lopez C, Jacobs PG. Digital twins and artificial intelligence in metabolic disease research. Trends Endocrinol Metab. 2024;35(6):549-57.
9. Singh M, Fuenmayor E, Hinchy EP, Qiao Y, Murray N, Devine D. Digital twin: Origin to future. Appl Syst Innov. 2021;4(2):36.
10. Subasi A, Subasi ME. Digital twins in healthcare and biomedicine. In: De Pablos PO, Zhang X (Eds.). Artificial Intelligence, Big Data, Blockchain and 5G for the Digital Transformation of the Healthcare Industry. Academic Press; 2024. pp. 365-401.
11. Chu Y, Li S, Tang J, Wu H. The potential of the Medical Digital Twin in diabetes management: a review. Front Med. 2023;10:1178912.
12. Rajamurugu N, Karthik MK. Introduction, History, and Concept of Digital Twin. In: Vohra M (Ed). Digital Twin Technology: Fundamentals and Applications. Scrivener Publishing LLC; 2023. pp. 19-32.
13. Shamanna P, Joshi S, Thajudeen M, Shah L, Poon T, Mohamed M,et al. Personalized nutrition in type 2 diabetes remission: application of digital twin technology for predictive glycemic control. Front Endocrinol. 2024;15:1485464.
14. Hadley F, Wilson J, Poon TCY, Mohammed J. Precision treatment with machine learning and digital twin technology for optimal metabolic outcomes. US patent US11723595B2; 2021.
15. Mohammed J, Poon TCY, Mohamed MA, Shah LM. Precision treatment platform enabled by Whole Body Digital Twin technology. US patent 11,957,484 B2;2024.
16. Clemente-Suárez VJ, Martín-Rodríguez A, Redondo-Flórez L, López-Mora C, Yáñez-Sepúlveda R, Tornero-Aguilera JF. New insights and potential therapeutic interventions in metabolic diseases. Int J Mol Sci. 2023;24(13): 10672.
17. Yousef H, Khandoker AH, Feng SF, Helf C, Jelinek HF. Inflammation, oxidative stress and mitochondrial dysfunction in the progression of type II diabetes mellitus with coexisting hypertension. Front Endocrinol. 2023;14:1173402.
18. Cortés-Rojo C, Vargas-Vargas MA. Don't give up on mitochondria as a target for the treatment of diabetes and its complications. World J Diabet. 2024;15(10):2015.
19. Mohamed M, Thajudeen M, Damodharan S, Raza JA, Erukulapati RS, Joshi SR, et al. Digital Twin Technology for Management of Chronic Metabolic Disease. In: Mechanick JI, Kushner RF (Eds). Lifestyle Medicine: Closing Research, Practice, and Knowledge Gaps. Cham: Springer Nature Switzerland; 2025. pp. 651-70.
20. Joshi S, Shamanna P, Dharmalingam M, Vadavi A, Keshavamurthy A, Shah L, et al. Digital Twin-Enabled Personalized Nutrition Improves Metabolic Dysfunction-Associated Fatty Liver Disease in Type 2 Diabetes: Results of a 1-Year Randomized Controlled Study. Endocr Pract. 2023;29(12):960-70.
21. Joshi S, Dharmalingam M, Vadavi A, Shamanna P, Keshavamurthy A, Shah L, et al. 1913-LB: Digital Twin Technology in Type 2 Diabetes Remission and Glycemic Improvement—Three-Year Results from a Randomized Controlled Trial. Diabetes. 2025;74(Suppl_1):1913-LB.

22. Shamanna P, Joshi S, Dharmalingam M, Vadavi A, Keshavamurthy A, Shah L, et al. Digital twin in managing hypertension among people with type 2 diabetes: 1-year randomized controlled trial. JACC: Adva. 2024;3(9_Part_2):101172.
23. Joshi Sr, Shah L, Mohamed M, Mohammed J, Poon T, Dharmalingam M, et al. 26-Or: Metabolic Benefits Beyond Glycemic Control With Artificial Intelligence, Internet Of Things, And Whole-Body Digital Twin: Initial Six Months Results of a Randomized Control Trial. Diabetes. 2022;71(Suppl_1).
24. Shamanna P, Dharmalingam M, Vadavi A, Keshavamurthy A, Thajudeen M, Bhonsley S, et al. The Impact of Digital Twin Technology on HbA1c Reduction and ASCVD Risk in Participants Enrolled for Type 2 Diabetes Remission: Outcomes of RCCT At 1 Year. Endocrine Pract. 2024;30(5):S78.
25. Shamanna P, Dharmalingam M, Vadavi A, Keshavamurthy A, Bhonsley S, Mohamed M, et al. 1806-LB: Improvement in Sensory Function and Achieving Remission of Type 2 Diabetes Mellitus through Digital Twin Technology—A One-Year Intervention Study. Diabetes. 2024;73(Suppl_1).
26. Joshi S, Dharmalingam M, Vadavi A, Keshavamurthy A, Bhonsley S, Mohamed M, et al. 1811-LB: improvement in diabetic retinopathy and achieving remission of type 2 diabetes mellitus through digital twin technology—A one-year intervention study. Diabetes. 2024;73:1811-LB.
27. Shashank J, Mohammed J, Mohamed M, Poon T, Dharmalingam M, Saboo B, et al. Bhonsley S. LBSUN149 Effectiveness of Digital Twin Technology For The Improvement In Depression Among Patients Undergoing Remission of Diabetes. J Endocr Soc. 2022;6(Suppl 1):A279.
28. Joshi SR, Shamanna P, Dharmalingam M, Vadavi A, Keshavamurthy A, Shah L, et al. Digital Twin Intervention for Type 2 Diabetes: One-Year Outcomes of a Randomized Trial. Preprint available at SSRN: http://dx.doi.org/10.2139/ssrn.4499693
29. Shamanna P, Joshi S, Dharmalingam M, Vadavi A, Keshavamurthy A, Thajudeen M, et al. Impact of Digital Twin Intervention on Microalbuminuria Progression in Participants Enrolled for Type 2 Diabetes Remission: Outcomes of RCCT At 1 Year. Endocrine Pract. 2024;30(5):S50-1.
30. Shah L, Joshi S, Dharmalingam M, Shamanna P, Damodaran S, Mohammed J, et al. IDF21-0598 Remission of T2DM by digital twin technology across Indian and American cohorts–Initial insights from real-world study. Diabetes Res Clin Pract. 2022;186:109579.
31. Shamanna P, Erukulapati RS, Shukla A, Shah L, Willis B, Thajudeen M, et al. One-year outcomes of a digital twin intervention for type 2 diabetes: a retrospective real-world study. Sci Rep. 2024;14(1):25478.
32. Shah L, Joshi SR, Mohammed J, Mohamed M, Thajudeen M, Kaufman FR, et al. 851-P: whole body digital twin (WBDT) enabled diabetes reversal—US real-world findings. Diabetes. 2024;73(Suppl 1):851-P.

CHAPTER 18

Artificial Intelligence in Diabetes Care: Current Status and Future Prospects

Rakesh M Parikh, Alok Modi, Avani Verma

ABSTRACT

Artificial intelligence (AI) is transforming diabetes care by enabling data-driven diagnosis, monitoring, treatment optimization, and predictive analytics. AI techniques such as machine learning (ML) and deep learning (DL) facilitate personalized treatment planning, improved glycemic monitoring through continuous glucose monitoring (CGM) systems, and early detection of complications including retinopathy and diabetic foot disease. AI-based predictive models also support proactive management by identifying patients at risk of complications. Despite promising advancements, challenges related to data privacy, algorithmic bias, and clinical integration remain. AI is expected to play an increasingly important role in advancing precision medicine and improving outcomes in diabetes management.

Keywords: Artificial intelligence, diabetes management, machine learning, continuous glucose monitoring, predictive analytics, precision medicine

INTRODUCTION

Diabetes mellitus, a chronic metabolic disorder, poses a significant public health challenge due to its chronic complications such as cardiovascular disease, neuropathy, retinopathy, and nephropathy. The diversity and complexity of diabetes, characterized by its multifactorial etiology and heterogeneous clinical presentation, complicate its management. Effective diabetes care necessitates continuous monitoring and individualized treatment strategies aimed at preventing development of complications. The advent of artificial intelligence (AI) has revolutionized the landscape of diabetes management, offering advanced tools for data analysis, predictive modeling, and personalized medicine.[1]

Artificial intelligence technologies such as machine learning (ML) and deep learning (DL) have the capability to analyze vast and complex datasets, identifying patterns and correlations.[2] These technologies enable the clustering of patient data to identify different diabetes phenotypes, facilitating a more nuanced understanding of the disease.[3] This, in turn, allows for the provision of precision care tailored to the unique needs of individual patients. AI-driven approaches can predict disease onset, progression, and response to treatment, enhancing clinical decision-making and optimizing patient outcomes.[4]

Moreover, AI's ability to integrate and analyze data from diverse sources—including electronic health records (EHRs), continuous glucose monitoring (CGM) systems, and wearable devices—provides a comprehensive view of a patient's health status.[5] This holistic approach supports the development of personalized treatment plans and proactive management strategies, improving glycemic control and reducing the risk of complications.

This chapter aims to critically examine the role of AI in diabetes management, focusing on its applications in diagnosis, treatment, monitoring, and predictive analytics. Additionally, it explores the potential of AI to advance personalized and precision medicine in diabetes care, addressing the current challenges and future prospects of integrating AI technologies into clinical practice.

ARTIFICIAL INTELLIGENCE IN DIAGNOSIS

Diabetes can be easily diagnosed by measuring venous plasma glucose or hemoglobin A1C (HbA1C) limiting the role of AI in diagnosis. Although some AI-based models have been developed for mass screening of diabetes. AI has further been explored in revising the classification of diabetes. With the use of data driven cluster analysis novel subgroups of adult-onset diabetes have been identified.[6] New and unique clusters of type 2 diabetes have been identified with clustering by using six clinical parameters in Indian population.[7] AI and ML is being used for developing models that can predict the risk of developing diabetes over next few years. The area under the curve (AUC) for predicting new-onset diabetes within 5 years for hospitalized patients from ML-based logistic regression was reported to 0.78.[8] In another study with ML model using administration health data the AUC for predicting development of diabetes within 5 years was 0.8.[9]

Early Diagnosis of Complications

- *Diabetic retinopathy:* Diabetic retinopathy, a leading cause of blindness, can be detected early using AI-enabled fundus cameras. These devices analyze retinal images to identify signs of retinopathy often before symptoms appear. Studies have shown that AI-based fundus cameras can achieve diagnostic accuracy comparable to ophthalmologists, facilitating timely intervention, and preventing vision loss.[10] Such AI-based fundus cameras can be easily deployed in diabetes clinics for regular screening among diabetic patients.[11]
- *Diabetic foot infections:* Diabetic foot infections, particularly those complicated by ulcers, pose a significant risk of amputation. AI-enabled spectrometric cameras can diagnose the type of infection (gram positive or gram negative) by analyzing images of diabetic foot wounds. This rapid diagnostic capability allows for targeted antibiotic therapy, improving patient outcomes.[12] AI-based models have also been found to be useful in grading of diabetic foot.
- *Predictive foot care:* AI-enabled insoles and socks are designed to monitor foot health continuously. These devices can predict the risk of developing diabetic foot ulcers by analyzing pressure distribution, temperature changes, and gait patterns. Early detection of at-risk feet enables preventative measures, reducing the incidence of severe complications.[13]

ARTIFICIAL INTELLIGENCE IN TREATMENT

Artificial intelligence has transformed diabetes treatment by enabling personalized care and optimizing therapeutic strategies. AI algorithms analyze patient data to tailor treatment plans, predict responses to therapies, and manage lifestyle interventions effectively.

Personalized Treatment Plans

Artificial intelligence leverages patient-specific data, including genetic, clinical, and lifestyle factors, to develop personalized treatment plans. These plans consider individual variability in drug metabolism, disease progression, and treatment adherence, leading to more effective management of diabetes. For example, AI algorithms can predict patient responses to various oral antidiabetic drugs, based on genetic markers and clinical data, allowing for personalized drug regimens.[14]

Optimization of Insulin Therapy

Artificial intelligence-driven systems optimize insulin therapy by predicting glucose levels and recommending precise insulin dosages. Closed-loop insulin delivery systems, also known as artificial pancreas systems, use real-time data from continuous glucose monitors (CGMs) and AI algorithms to adjust insulin delivery automatically. Studies have demonstrated that these systems improve glycemic control and reduce the risk of hypoglycemia compared to traditional insulin therapy.[15] DreaMed Advisor Pro is the first Food and Drug Administration (FDA) approved AI platform that assists healthcare providers in optimizing insulin therapy by analyzing CGM and insulin pump data. Clinical trials have shown its effectiveness in improving glycemic control in patients with type 1 diabetes.[16]

Management of Lifestyle Interventions

Artificial intelligence supports the management of lifestyle interventions such as diet, exercise, and weight management. By analyzing data from wearable devices and mobile apps, AI provides personalized recommendations and real-time feedback, enhancing patient engagement and adherence to lifestyle modifications. A systematic review of 25 studies concluded that technology-enabled self-management solutions significantly improve HbA1C.[17]

ARTIFICIAL INTELLIGENCE IN MONITORING

Artificial intelligence has revolutionized diabetes monitoring by integrating advanced data analytics with real-time health tracking systems. This section explores the role of AI in CGM, self-monitoring of blood glucose (SMBG) data analysis, and other innovative monitoring tools.

Integration of Continuous Glucose Monitoring Systems

Continuous glucose monitoring systems provide real-time glucose data, allowing for continuous monitoring without the need for frequent finger-pricks. These systems use sensors to measure interstitial glucose levels and transmit the data. AI algorithms with multimodal DL architecture can analyze glucose trends and predict future glucose levels.[18] The integration of AI with CGM systems enhances the accuracy and reliability of glucose measurements, enabling timely adjustments to therapy and diet.[19]

Real-time Data Analytics for Patient Compliance

Artificial intelligence algorithms analyze data from CGM systems and wearable devices to provide personalized feedback and actionable insights. For instance, AI-driven platforms can detect patterns in glucose fluctuations and suggest modifications to insulin dosages, diet, and physical activity. This real-time data analytics supports patient adherence to treatment plans and improves overall diabetes management.[20] Mobile applications equipped with AI can send reminders and alerts to patients, helping them stay compliant with their medication and lifestyle regimens.[21]

Enhancements in Glycemic Control

Artificial intelligence technology plays a crucial role in enhancing glycemic control by predicting hyperglycemic and hypoglycemic events before they occur. Predictive models analyze historical glucose data along with factors such as meal intake and physical activity to forecast potential glucose excursions. This proactive approach allows patients and healthcare providers to take preventive measures, reducing the risk of complications associated with poor glycemic control.

Artificial Intelligence in Self-monitoring of Blood Glucose Data

Artificial intelligence is also used to analyze SMBG data from glucometers. Smartphone applications such as Glucose Buddy and Diabetes Buddy help patients log and analyze their blood glucose readings, providing insights into patterns and trends. AI algorithms can process these data to offer personalized recommendations and predictive insights, improving daily glucose management.[21]

ARTIFICIAL INTELLIGENCE IN PREDICTIVE ANALYTICS

Artificial intelligence has shown significant potential in predictive analytics for diabetes management, enabling proactive measures and personalized care plans. This section explores how AI predicts diabetes complications and supports proactive management strategies.

Predicting Diabetes Complications

Artificial intelligence algorithms can predict various complications associated with diabetes, such as cardiovascular diseases, neuropathy, and nephropathy, by analyzing a wide range of patient data. These predictive models utilize historical health records, genetic information, lifestyle factors, and real-time data from monitoring devices. For instance, AI can analyze CGM data to forecast potential hyperglycemic or hypoglycemic events, allowing patients and healthcare providers to take preventive measures.[22]

- *Cardiovascular complications:* AI systems can predict the risk of cardiovascular diseases in diabetic patients by analyzing electrocardiogram (ECG) data and other relevant health parameters. Studies have demonstrated the efficacy of ML models in identifying early signs of cardiovascular issues such as arrhythmias and ischemic changes, thereby enabling timely interventions.[23,24]
- *Neuropathy:* By evaluating nerve conduction studies and other neurological assessments, AI can predict the onset and progression of diabetic neuropathy. Predictive models help in identifying patients at high risk, allowing for early therapeutic interventions to prevent severe neuropathic complications.[25]
- *Nephropathy:* AI-driven predictive analytics can assess the risk of diabetic nephropathy by analyzing renal function tests, including serum creatinine levels and glomerular filtration rate (GFR). These models facilitate early detection and management of renal impairment in diabetic patients.[26]

Proactive Management Strategies

Predictive analytics enable healthcare providers to adopt proactive management strategies for diabetes care. By identifying high-risk patients and potential complications early, AI supports the implementation of personalized care plans tailored to individual patient needs.

- *Personalized care plans:* AI algorithms analyze patient data to create personalized care plans that address specific health risks and treatment responses. These plans include tailored medication regimens, lifestyle modifications, and monitoring schedules designed to optimize diabetes management.[27]
- *Preventive measures:* Predictive models inform patients and healthcare providers about imminent risks, allowing for timely preventive measures. For example, AI can predict the likelihood of hypoglycemia during specific activities, prompting patients to adjust their insulin doses or carbohydrate intake accordingly.[28]
- *Enhanced patient engagement:* AI-driven predictive analytics foster patient engagement by providing actionable insights and real-time feedback.[29] Mobile applications equipped with predictive models offer personalized

recommendations, encouraging patients to adhere to their treatment plans and make informed decisions about their health.

FUTURE PROSPECTS

The future of diabetes management holds promising advancements with the continued development of AI technologies. This section discusses several studies and products under development that utilize AI for diabetes care, highlighting their potential impact on personalized medicine, and remote patient monitoring.

Artificial Intelligence-driven Innovations in Diabetes Care

- *Advanced predictive models:* Future AI systems are expected to incorporate even more sophisticated predictive models. These models will leverage vast datasets, including genomic, proteomic, and metabolomic information, to predict disease progression and treatment responses with unprecedented accuracy.
- *AI-enhanced insulin delivery systems:* Research is underway to improve closed-loop insulin delivery systems, also known as artificial pancreas systems. These next-generation devices aim to integrate more advanced AI algorithms to enhance the precision of insulin dosing, further reducing the risk of hypoglycemia and hyperglycemia.
- *AI-based nutritional and lifestyle coaching:* AI-powered applications are being developed to provide real-time nutritional and lifestyle advice tailored to individual patients. These tools will analyze CGM data, dietary logs, and physical activity patterns to offer personalized recommendations that can significantly improve glycemic control and overall health outcomes.
- *Remote patient monitoring platforms:* AI-driven remote monitoring platforms are being designed to integrate data from various sources, including CGM systems, glucometers, and wearable devices. These platforms will enable continuous monitoring of patients' health status, allowing healthcare providers to make informed decisions and adjust treatment plans remotely.

Potential Advancements in Artificial Intelligence Technology

- *Integration with EHRs:* Future AI systems will seamlessly integrate with EHRs to provide a comprehensive view of a patient's health. This integration will enhance the accuracy of predictive models and support the development of more personalized treatment plans.
- *Real-time data processing and analytics:* Advances in AI technology will enable real-time processing and analysis of vast amounts of data. This capability will support immediate decision-making and timely interventions, improving patient outcomes and reducing the burden on healthcare systems.
- *AI in personalized medicine:* The future of AI in diabetes care lies in its potential to advance personalized medicine. By analyzing individual patient data, AI will enable the customization of treatment strategies to meet the unique needs of each patient, optimizing therapeutic outcomes and enhancing quality of life.

ETHICAL AND PRACTICAL CONSIDERATIONS

The integration of AI in diabetes management presents significant ethical and practical challenges. This section discusses the primary ethical concerns, including data privacy, algorithmic bias, and the transparency of AI models, as well as practical challenges related to implementation and regulation.

Data Privacy and Security Concerns

Artificial intelligence systems in healthcare rely on vast amounts of personal health data, raising concerns about data privacy and security. Ensuring that patient data is stored and transmitted securely is paramount to maintaining patient trust and compliance. Health data breaches can lead to significant personal and financial repercussions for patients. Robust encryption methods, strict access controls, and comprehensive data protection policies are essential to safeguard sensitive patient information.

Algorithmic Bias and Fairness

Artificial intelligence algorithms can inadvertently perpetuate or even exacerbate existing biases in healthcare. These biases can arise from unrepresentative training datasets or flawed algorithm design, potentially leading to disparities in healthcare outcomes. For instance, if an AI system is trained predominantly on data from a particular demographic group, its predictions may be less accurate for individuals from other groups. Addressing algorithmic bias requires careful dataset curation, regular auditing of AI models, and the inclusion of diverse patient populations in training datasets.

Transparency and Explainability of Artificial Intelligence Models

The complexity of AI algorithms often results in "black-box" models where the decision-making process is not easily interpretable. This lack of transparency can hinder the trust and acceptance of AI systems by healthcare providers and patients. Ensuring the explainability of AI models is crucial for their integration into clinical practice. Techniques such as model interpretability tools and transparent reporting of AI model performance can help in understanding and validating AI decisions.

Regulatory and Implementation Challenges

The implementation of AI in healthcare is subject to regulatory scrutiny to ensure safety and efficacy. Regulatory bodies such as the US FDA and the European Medicines Agency (EMA) have developed frameworks for evaluating AI-based medical devices and systems. However, the rapidly evolving nature of AI technology poses challenges for regulatory processes, which must balance innovation with patient safety. Additionally, the integration of AI systems into existing healthcare infrastructure requires substantial investment in technology and training for healthcare professionals.

Ethical Use of Artificial Intelligence in Patient Care

Ethical considerations extend beyond technical and regulatory aspects to the ethical use of AI in patient care. This includes obtaining informed consent from patients for the use of AI tools, ensuring that AI recommendations align with patients' values and preferences, and maintaining the physician-patient relationship. AI should complement, not replace, the clinical judgment of healthcare providers, supporting them in delivering high-quality and patient-centered care. Studies on AI in diabetes management have also emphasized the need for transparent and explainable AI models to foster trust among healthcare providers and patients.

CONCLUSION

The integration of AI in diabetes management has brought about significant advancements in the diagnosis, treatment, monitoring, and predictive analytics of the disease. AI technologies such as

ML and DL have revolutionized the approach to diabetes care by enabling personalized and precision medicine. Through the analysis of vast and complex datasets, AI systems can provide tailored treatment plans, optimize insulin therapy, and support lifestyle interventions, ultimately improving patient outcomes.

Artificial intelligence-driven CGM systems and SMBG data analysis have enhanced patient compliance and glycemic control by offering real-time feedback and predictive insights. Additionally, AI-enabled tools such as smart insoles and fundus cameras have shown promise in early detection and proactive management of diabetic complications such as retinopathy and foot ulcers.

The future of AI in diabetes management is bright with ongoing research and development focused on advancing predictive models, enhancing insulin delivery systems, and improving remote patient monitoring platforms. The potential for AI to integrate seamlessly with EHRs and process real-time data will further support the implementation of personalized treatment strategies and timely interventions.

However, the ethical and practical challenges associated with AI in healthcare must not be overlooked. Ensuring data privacy and security, addressing algorithmic bias, and maintaining the transparency and explainability of AI models are critical to fostering trust and acceptance among healthcare providers and patients. Regulatory frameworks must evolve to keep pace with technological advancements, balancing innovation with patient safety.

In conclusion, AI has the potential to transform diabetes management by providing individualized care and enhancing the overall quality of life for patients. Continued research, ethical considerations, and thoughtful implementation will be key to unlocking the full potential of AI in this field.

REFERENCES

1. Topol EJ. High-performance medicine: the convergence of human and artificial intelligence. Nat Med. 2019;25(1):44-56.
2. Chen JH, Asch SM. Machine learning and prediction in medicine—beyond the peak of inflated expectations. N Engl J Med. 2017;376(26):2507-9.
3. Li Q, Zhao H, Shi Y, Li J, Tian Z. Application of machine learning-based models in the prediction and classification of clinical outcomes of type 2 diabetes mellitus: a review. Diabetes Ther. 2020;11(6):1163-73.
4. Beam AL, Kohane IS. Big data and machine learning in health care. JAMA. 2018;319(13):1317-8.
5. Jacobs PG, Resalat N, Hilts W, Young GM, Leitschuh J, Pinsonault J, et al. Integrating metabolic expenditure information from wearable fitness sensors into an AI-augmented automated insulin delivery system: a randomised clinical trial. Lancet Digit Health. 2023;5(9):e607-17.
6. Ahlqvist E, Storm P, Käräjämäki A, Martinell M, Dorkhan M, Carlsson A, et al. Novel subgroups of adult-onset diabetes and their association with outcomes: a data-driven cluster analysis of six variables. Lancet Diabetes Endocrinol. 2018;6:361-9.
7. Anjana RM, Pradeepa R, Unnikrishnan R, Tiwaskar M, Aravind SR, Saboo B, et al. New and Unique Clusters of Type 2 Diabetes Identified in Indians. J Assoc Physicians India. 2021;69(2):58-61.
8. Choi BG, Rha SW, Kim SW, Kang JH, Park JY, Noh YK. Machine learning for the prediction of new-onset diabetes mellitus during 5-year follow-up in non-diabetic patients with cardiovascular risks. Yonsei Med J. 2019;60:191-9.
9. Ravaut M, Harish V, Sadeghi H, Leung KK, Volkovs M, Kornas K, et al. Development and validation of a machine learning model using administrative health data to predict onset of type 2 diabetes. JAMA Netw Open. 2021;4: e2111315.
10. Ting DSW, Cheung CY, Lim G, Tan GSW, Quang ND, Gan A, et al. Development and validation of a deep learning system for diabetic retinopathy and related eye diseases using retinal images from multiethnic populations with diabetes. JAMA. 2017;318(22):2211-23.

11. Abràmoff MD, Lavin PT, Birch M, Shah N, Folk JC. Pivotal trial of an autonomous AI-based diagnostic system for detection of diabetic retinopathy in primary care offices. NPJ Digit Med. 2018;1:39.
12. Kesavan R, Sasikumar CS. Clinical significance of a novel imaging device to evaluate infection on wounds: performance comparison with culture method and metagenome sequencing. J Wound Manag. 2023;23(3):182-92.
13. Najafi B, Crews RT, Wrobel JS. Importance of time spent standing for those at risk of diabetic foot ulceration. Diabetes Care. 2010;33(11):2448-50.
14. Pearson ER. Personalized medicine in diabetes: the role of 'omics' and biomarkers. Diabet Med. 2016;33(6):712-7.
15. Dovc K, Battelino T. Closed-loop insulin delivery systems in children and adolescents with type 1 diabetes. Horm Res Paediatr. 2019;91(2):116-25.
16. Ziegler C, Liberman A, Nimri R, Muller I, Klemenčič S, Bratina N, et al. Reduced worries of hypoglycaemia, high satisfaction, and increased perceived ease of use after experiencing four nights of md-logic artificial pancreas at home (DREAM4). J Diabetes Res. 2015;2015:590308.
17. Greenwood DA, Gee PM, Fatkin KJ, Peeples MA. A systematic review of reviews evaluating technology-enabled diabetes self-management education and support. J Diabetes Sci Technol. 2017;11(5):1015-27.
18. Haleem MS, Rajan R, Mandal M, Bhattacharya S, Chakraborty C. A multimodal deep learning architecture for predicting blood glucose in type 2 diabetes. Sci Rep. 2025;15(1):14723.
19. Vettoretti M, Facchinetti A, Sparacino G, Cobelli C. Advanced decision support tools for type 1 diabetes management using continuous glucose monitoring sensors: a review of real-time applications. Sensors (Basel). 2020;20(14):3870.
20. Wang T, Wu Y, Li D, Zhang X, Liu Q. Effectiveness and safety of AI-based closed-loop systems for glycemic control in type 1 diabetes: a systematic review and meta-analysis. Diabetes Technol Ther. 2025;27(2):113-21.
21. Tahir M, Farhan M. Exploring the progress of artificial intelligence in managing Type 2 diabetes mellitus: a comprehensive review. Front Clin Diabetes Healthc. 2023;4:1316111.
22. Herrero P, Andorrà M, Babion N, Bos H, Koehler M, Klopfenstein Y, et al. Enhancing the Capabilities of Continuous Glucose Monitoring With a Predictive App. J Diabetes Sci Technol. 2024;18(5):1014-26.
23. Dinh A, Miertschin S, Young A, Mohanty SD. A data-driven approach to predicting diabetes and cardiovascular disease with machine learning. BMC Med Inform Decis Mak. 2019;19(1):211.
24. Lin CH, Liu Z, Chu PH, Chang YJ, Hung CL, Huang CM, et al. A multitask deep learning model utilizing electrocardiograms for major cardiovascular adverse events prediction. NPJ Digit Med. 2025;8(1):1
25. Toderean R, Cobuz M, Dimian M, Cobuz C. From evaluation to prediction: analysis of diabetic autonomic neuropathy using Sudoscan and artificial intelligence. Appl Sci (Basel). 2024;14(16):7406.
26. Dholariya S, Dutta S, Sonagra A, Kaliya M, Singh R, Parchwani D, et al. Unveiling the utility of artificial intelligence for prediction, diagnosis, and progression of diabetic kidney disease: an evidence-based systematic review and meta-analysis. Current Medical Research and Opinion. 2024;40(12);2025-55. https://doi.org/10.1080/03007995.2024.2423737
27. Zargoush M, Ghazalbash S, Madani Hosseini M, Alemi F, Perri D. Machine learning driven diabetes care using predictive-prescriptive analytics for personalized medication prescription. Sci Rep. 2025;15:26811.
28. Faruqui SH, Alaeddini A, Du Y, Li S, Sharma K, Wang J. (2024). Nurse-in-the-Loop Artificial Intelligence for Precision Management of Type 2 Diabetes in a Clinical Trial Utilizing Transfer-Learned Predictive Digital Twin. [online] Available from https://arxiv.org/abs/2401.02661. [Last accessed March, 2026].
29. Ying Z, Fan Y, Chen C, Liu Y, Tang Q, Chen Z, et al. Real-Time AI-Assisted Insulin Titration System for Glucose Control in Patients With Type 2 Diabetes: A Randomized Clinical Trial. JAMA Netw Open. 2025;8(5):e258910.

CHAPTER

19

Digital Diabetes Care: Innovations, Impact, and Future Directions

Ranjit Mohan Anjana, Sharma Nitika, Harish Ranjani

ABSTRACT

Digital health (DH) has undergone a significant transformation over the past decade, driven by advancements in technology and internet access. In the context of diabetes, the shift from irregular, clinic-based care to continuous, remote, and patient-driven management has been a major change. By leveraging telemedicine, mobile applications, wearables, and artificial intelligence (AI), DH has enabled personalized and timely care for individuals with diabetes. Telemedicine has emerged as a powerful component of digital diabetes care, improving access to expert care, especially in remote and underserved regions. Wearable health devices such as smartwatches and fitness bands provide continuous data on physical activity, heart rate, sleep patterns, and more, contributing to a holistic understanding of an individual's lifestyle. Continuous glucose monitoring systems offer real-time, dynamic glucose data, helping prevent both hypoglycemia and hyperglycemia. Mobile health applications serve as a one-stop platform for blood glucose logging, medication tracking, nutrition planning, physical activity monitoring, appointment scheduling, virtual coaching, and educational content. The future of digital diabetes care in India lies in personalized, predictive, and preventive care, integrated digital ecosystems, public-private partnerships, and a focus on equity and digital literacy.

Keywords: Digital health, telemedicine, continuous glucose monitoring systems, insulin pump, wearables, mHealth applications.

INTRODUCTION

India is experiencing a staggering rise in the burden of diabetes, with 101 million individuals currently living with diabetes, and an additional 136 million having prediabetes.[1] In 2024, the total diabetes-related expenditure in India amounted to approximately ₹84,502 crore, with a per-person cost of ₹9,408.[2] This data highlights a dire public health emergency, as a large section of the population is at risk of developing serious complications from the disease.

Traditional healthcare delivery systems in India are already stretched, with disparities in access, affordability, and continuity of care prevalent across both urban and rural regions.[3] The chronic nature of diabetes requires frequent monitoring, behavior modification, timely treatment adjustments, and coordinated care. These demands are difficult to meet with in-person visits alone.[4] Thus, the complexities of managing diabetes in a country with diverse sociocultural and economic backgrounds necessitate scalable, accessible, and cost-effective healthcare solutions.

Healthcare digitization has witnessed exponential growth globally in recent years, with a range of emerging and innovative technologies coming together to shape the future of digital health (DH) in diabetes care.[5] The global DH market is projected to reach USD 946.04 billion by 2030.[6] In India, the DH sector currently accounts for approximately 3%[7] of the overall healthcare market and is expected to grow to USD 9.90 billion by 2029.[8] Against this backdrop, DH interventions have emerged as promising tools to bridge the care gap.[5] Digital diabetes care refers to the integration of digital tools and technologies into the prevention, diagnosis, monitoring, treatment, and management of diabetes.[9,10]

KEY COMPONENTS OF DIGITAL DIABETES CARE

Evolution of Digital Health and its Relevance to Diabetes Care

Digital health has undergone a significant transformation over the past decade. The evolution of DH has been shaped by the convergence of mobile technology, internet access, cloud computing, artificial intelligence (AI), and big data analytics.[5,9,10] In India, this transformation began with digitization of hospital information systems and expanded through national health portals, electronic health records, telemedicine platforms, and more recently, AI-integrated health tools.[5,9,10] The field has grown in parallel with advancements in mobile and internet penetration across India. The initial phase involved basic telecommunication-based services, such as telephone counselling and SMS alerts. This has evolved into more sophisticated solutions as digital platforms are now used not only for delivering care but also for continuous patient engagement, education, and remote monitoring.[9] DH is now integrated into national health frameworks to support large-scale chronic disease management.[10]

In the context of diabetes, the move from irregular, clinic-based care to continuous, remote, and patient-driven management has been a major shift. Early models of diabetes education via text messaging[11] evolved into mobile applications with interactive behavior change modules, virtual coaching, and real-time data tracking.[12,13] By leveraging telemedicine, mobile applications, wearables, and AI, DH has enabled personalized and timely care for individuals with diabetes **(Fig. 1)**.

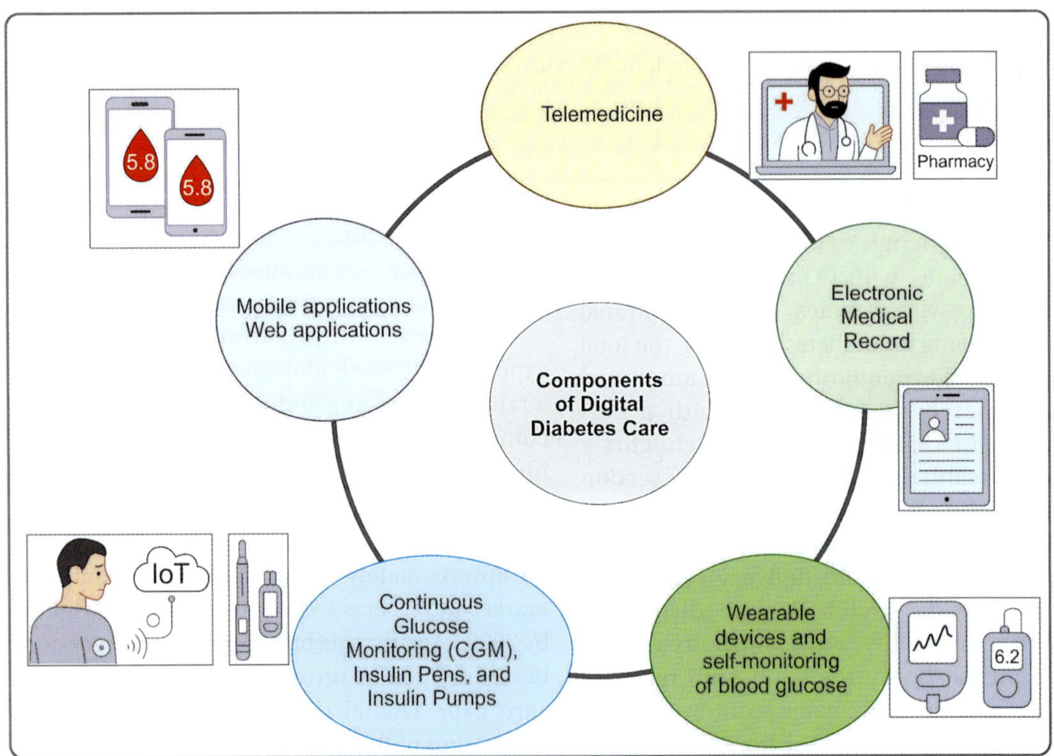

Fig. 1: Components of digital diabetes care.

Telemedicine

Telemedicine has emerged as a powerful component of digital diabetes care.[9,10] By enabling remote consultations between patients and healthcare providers, telemedicine platforms improve access to expert care, especially in remote and underserved regions.[3] A notable example is the Chunampet Rural Diabetes Prevention Project (CRDPP)[14] (2006–2010) in Tamil Nadu, which combined telemedicine with individualized care to screen over 27,000 adults across 42 villages. Using a mobile telemedicine van equipped for retinal photography, Doppler imaging, and other tests, the project successfully delivered comprehensive diabetes services and established a rural diabetes center.[14] Widely recognized as a scalable model, CRDPP highlights how telemedicine can enhance reach, cost-effectiveness, and glycemic control when integrated into routine care.

In last few years, India witnessed a rapid scale-up of teleconsultation services,[5] with diabetologists conducting follow-ups, adjusting medications, and offering counseling through secure digital platforms. This transformation was significantly accelerated by the COVID-19 pandemic, which necessitated remote healthcare delivery due to movement restrictions and fear of infection. As a result, both patients and providers were compelled to adopt virtual care models. What began as a temporary response has now evolved into an accepted and trusted mode of care, even among populations that were previously hesitant to engage with DH platforms.[5,9,10]

Wearable Devices and Self-Monitoring of Blood Glucose

Wearable health devices such as smartwatches, fitness bands, and activity trackers provide users with continuous data on physical activity, heart rate, sleep patterns, and more.[15] When integrated into diabetes applications or patient records, these wearables contribute to a holistic understanding of the individual's lifestyle, which is critical in managing type 2 diabetes.[15] Beyond general wellness tracking, wearable devices play a significant role in the prevention and management of diabetes by helping individuals with diabetes monitor their glucose levels, receive alerts for hypo- or hyperglycemia, and make timely lifestyle adjustments.[16] These devices also support self-management by tracking progress, setting personalized goals, and sending reminders, thereby keeping users engaged and motivated in their care plan.[15,16] By empowering users with real-time health insights and promoting adherence to treatment goals, wearables serve as valuable tools for long-term diabetes control and prevention.

Self-monitoring of blood glucose (SMBG) remains a cornerstone of diabetes self-care. With the advent of Bluetooth-enabled glucose meters, data from SMBG can now be synced with mobile applications or provider dashboards, allowing for trend analysis, automated alerts, and informed decision-making.[17] SMBG tools have become more compact, user-friendly, and affordable, making them more accessible for Indian users.

Continuous Glucose Monitoring, Insulin Pens, and Insulin Pumps

Advanced technologies such as continuous glucose monitoring (CGM) systems provide real-time, dynamic glucose data over several days or weeks, revealing patterns missed by traditional finger-prick testing.[9] These insights are helpful for individuals on insulin therapy, helping prevent both hypoglycemia and hyperglycemia. Current evidence indicates that individuals with diabetes using CGM devices experience a significant reduction in glycated hemoglobin (HbA1c) levels.[18]

Similarly, smart insulin pens and insulin pumps allow for precise and timely insulin delivery, often integrated with CGM data to inform dosing. While these tools are more prevalent in urban India and among higher-income groups, ongoing innovations and price reductions could improve their accessibility over time.[9]

However, cost remains a significant barrier—the price of CGM systems can range from ₹3,000 to ₹6,000 per sensor (lasting 7–14 days),[19] and insulin pumps typically cost between ₹1.5 and ₹6 lakh upfront,[20] with additional recurring expenses for consumables. Broader adoption will depend heavily on affordability, insurance coverage, and government support.

Mobile Health Applications

Mobile health (mHealth) applications form the most widespread and user-accessible tool for digital diabetes care. These applications often serve as a one-stop platform for blood glucose logging, medication tracking, nutrition planning, physical activity monitoring, appointment scheduling, virtual coaching, and educational content.[9,10]

India has seen a surge in diabetes-focused appicaltions,[9,21] but few have been tailored to the country's sociocultural context. A systematic review of mHealth applications for diabetes prevention among Asian Indians identified nearly 1,000 applications available on the Play Store, while a similar search for diabetes management applications revealed around 500 options. The Indian market hosts a wide range of such applications, offering single or multiple features focused on diabetes screening, monitoring, and control.[21] Evidence-based, research-driven interventions stand out in this space.

mDiab is among India's first evidence-based mHealth application focused on diabetes prevention and self-management.[22] Designed using behavior change theories, the application offers video-based educational sessions, activity tracking, automated SMS reminders, and virtual coaching, making it a low-cost, scalable model suitable for low- and middle-income countries.[22] In a 12-week randomized trial targeting individuals with prediabetes and/or obesity, participants in the intervention group used the mDiab application alongside weekly virtual coaching sessions, while the control group received standard care. The application enabled users to track weight, physical activity, and dietary habits, and provided 12 video lessons on type 2 diabetes prevention. There was a greater reduction in weight in the intervention group (average 1 kg loss vs. 0.3 kg in the control group), with a higher proportion achieving the 5% weight loss target. Notably, participants who engaged with the video content lost more weight than those who did not.[12] The study demonstrated that a mHealth intervention combined with human coaching could effectively reduce cardiometabolic risk factors in high-risk individuals.[13]

Similarly, a randomized controlled study evaluated the effectiveness of mHealth applications for cardiometabolic risk reduction among adults in urban and rural India.[23] Participants in the intervention group received lifestyle support through a mHealth applications featuring educational content, gamification, activity tracking, and virtual coaching, while the control group received usual care. The study demonstrated promising outcomes, with significant reductions in body mass index, waist circumference, blood pressure, fasting blood glucose and total serum cholesterol, and a positive effect on dietary and physical activity behaviors in the intervention group compared with controls.[23] These findings suggest that culturally tailored mHealth tools can be effective in promoting lifestyle changes across diverse Indian settings.

At the clinic level, a scalable 3D Digital Diabetes Delivery model comprising DIA, DIALA (DIAbetes Lifestyle Assistant Application), and

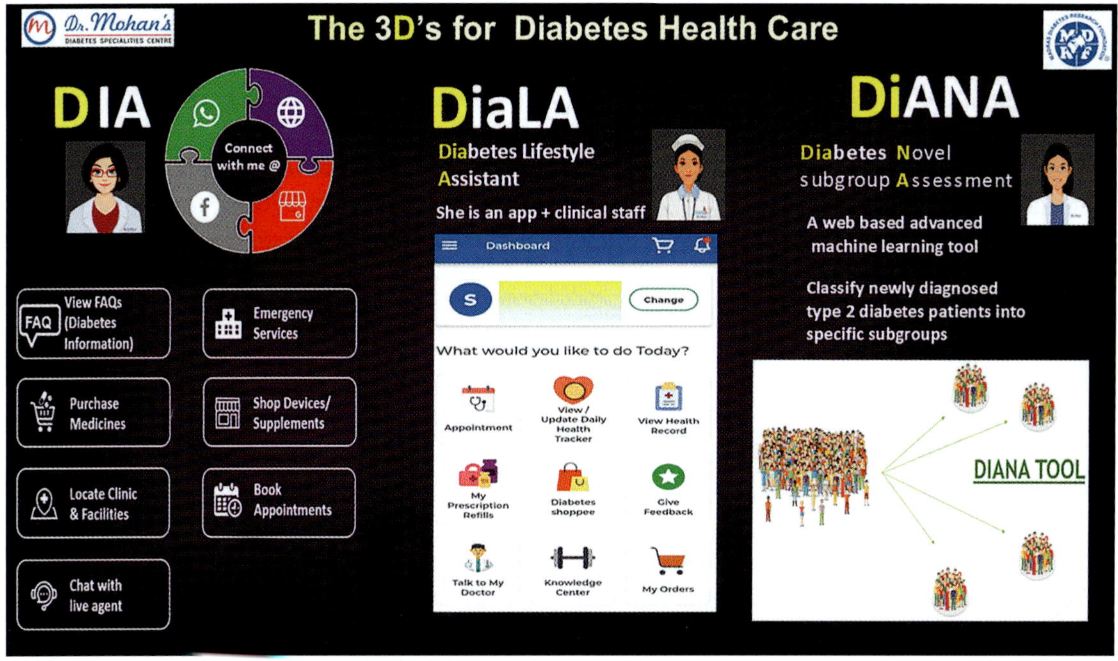

Fig. 2: The 3Ds-digital diabetes delivery model at Dr Mohan's Diabetes Specialties Center.

DIANA (DIAbetes Novel Subgroup Assessment) was launched by a tertiary diabetes care center in Chennai to enhance outcomes and bridge gaps between patients and healthcare providers.[24,25] DIA is an AI-powered chatbot that offers 24/7 information on diabetes and other noncommunicable diseases (NCDs), addressing lifestyle-related queries around diet, activity, stress, sleep, obesity, and more. It operates across platforms such as WhatsApp, Google Business Message, Facebook Messenger, and the web, using conversational AI technology to provide personalized guidance in English, notify users with updates, and enhance engagement through automated digital conversations. DIALA is a patient-friendly mobile application designed to support individuals with diabetes by enabling appointment bookings, prescription refills, glucose monitoring, and emergency provider access. It also helps track weight, step count, calories, and test reports, adjust diet plans, set reminders, and offer access to a diabetes-specific shop, thereby serving as a vital link between patients and healthcare providers. DIANA is a web-based precision medicine tool used by clinicians to classify newly diagnosed type 2 diabetes patients into specific subgroups—such as insulin-deficient or insulin-resistant types—assess their risk for microvascular complications and guide personalized treatment approaches based on likely therapeutic response. Together, this 3D approach offers a comprehensive, tech-enabled model of diabetes care delivery at the clinic level, as an effort to improve patient outcomes through seamless, integrated, and round-the-clock support **(Fig. 2)**.[24,25]

FUTURE DIRECTIONS

The digital transformation of diabetes care in India is still evolving, but the foundations are strong. Moving forward, several directions can shape its future.

Personalized, Predictive, and Preventive Care

Advancements in AI and machine learning will enable applications and provider platforms to deliver personalized care plans based on real-time data and historical patterns.[26] Predictive analytics can flag individuals at risk of poor outcomes, enabling preemptive interventions. Integration of genomics, sociodemographic data, and behavioral insights can further fine-tune prevention strategies.[27]

Integrated Digital Ecosystems

Future efforts in DH must focus on interoperability, enabling seamless data exchange between wearables, mobile applications, electronic medical records (EMRs), and national health portals such as Ayushman Bharat Digital Mission (ABDM).[5,15] Integration across platforms will support continuity of care and reduce duplication.

Public-Private Partnerships and Policy Support

Strong government leadership combined with industry and academic collaboration is essential for scale. Programs such as the National Digital Health Mission (NDHM), Ayushman Bharat, and Digital Health India must actively include diabetes-focused digital strategies. Incentives for startups, research grants for evidence generation, and subsidies for digital tools will further strengthen the ecosystem.[15]

Focus on Equity and Digital Literacy

While urban populations may adopt new technologies rapidly, rural and vulnerable communities need inclusive design, training and support. Digital literacy campaigns, vernacular content, and offline-compatible tools can extend reach.[15,27]

Strengthening Evidence and Evaluation

While pilot projects and application launches are abundant, robust implementation science and evaluation are often missing. Future interventions should include long-term studies on effectiveness, cost-benefit, user engagement, and health outcomes, especially across different socioeconomic strata.[23]

CONCLUSION

India's diabetes epidemic demands innovative, scalable, and patient-centric solutions; qualities that DH technologies are well-positioned to deliver. As we transition from reactive care to proactive prevention and empowerment, digital diabetes care offers a transformative pathway. Digital interventions grounded in evidence, designed for context, and supported by policy are the need of the hour. However, technology alone is not the panacea. The success of digital diabetes care in India will depend on human-centered design, stakeholder collaboration, ethical use of data, and a relentless focus on equity. If these elements align, India can not only manage its diabetes burden but also lead global innovation in digital chronic disease care.

REFERENCES

1. Anjana RM, Unnikrishnan R, Deepa M, Pradeepa R, Tandon N, Das AK, et al. Metabolic non-communicable disease health report of India: the ICMR-INDIAB national cross-sectional study (ICMR-INDIAB-17). Lancet Diabetes Endocrinol. 2023;11(7):474-89.
2. International Diabetes Federation. (2025). South-East Asia—Diabetes regional report 2000–2050. [online] Available from https://diabetesatlas.org/data-by-location/region/south-east-asia/ [Last accessed February, 2026].
3. Das AK, Saboo B, Maheshwari A, Nair M V, Banerjee S, C J, et al. Health care delivery model in India with relevance to diabetes care. Heliyon. 2022;8(10):e10904.

4. Nikpour S, Mehrdad N, Sanjari M, Aalaa M, Heshmat R, Khabaz Mafinejad M, et al. Challenges of type 2 diabetes mellitus management from the perspective of patients: Conventional content analysis. Interact J Med Res. 2022;11(2): e41933.
5. Ministry of Health and Family Welfare. (2025). From Data to Diagnosis. [online] Available from https://www.pib.gov.in/PressReleaseIframePage.aspx?PRID=2094604 [Last accessed February, 2026].
6. Grand View Research. (2025). Digital health market (2025–2030). [online] Available from https://www.grandviewresearch.com/industry-analysis/digital-health-market [Last accessed February, 2026].
7. Tata Capital Healthcare Fund. (2025). TCHF Industry Spotlight Series Digital Health—Where We Are. [online] Available from: https://tatacapitalhealthcarefund.com/content/dam/tata-capital/health-care-funds/pdf-file/DigitalHealth-Thematic. [Last accessed February, 2026].
8. Statista. (2025). Digital Health—India. [online] Available from https://www.statista.com/outlook/hmo/digital-health/india [Last accessed February, 2026].
9. Kesavadev J, Krishnan G, Mohan V. Digital health and diabetes: experience from India. Ther Adv Endocrinol Metab. 2021;12:20420188211054676.
10. Ranjani H, Nitika S, Pradeepa R, Anjana RM, Mohan V. The role of digital health in tackling India's diabetes epidemic. In: Klonoff DC, Kerr D, Espinoza J (Eds). Diabetes Digital Health, Telehealth, and Artificial Intelligence. Philadelphia: Elsevier; 2024. pp. 109-20.
11. Pfammatter A, Spring B, Saligram N, Davé R, Gowda A, Blais L, et al. MHealth intervention to improve diabetes risk behaviors in India: A prospective, parallel group cohort study. J Med Internet Res. 2016;18(8):e207.
12. Muralidharan S, Ranjani H, Mohan Anjana R, Jena S, Tandon N, Gupta Y, et al. Engagement and weight loss: Results from the mobile health and diabetes trial. Diabetes Technol Ther. 2019;21(9):507-13.
13. Muralidharan S, Ranjani H, Anjana RM, Gupta Y, Ambekar S, Koppikar V, et al. Change in cardiometabolic risk factors among Asian Indian adults recruited in a mHealth-based diabetes prevention trial. Digit Health. 2021; 7:20552076211039032.
14. Mohan V, Deepa M, Pradeepa R, Prathiba V, Datta M, Sethuraman R, et al. Prevention of diabetes in rural India with a telemedicine intervention. J Diabetes Sci Technol. 2012;6(6):1355-64.
15. Hazra S, Bora KS. Capitalization of digital healthcare: The cornerstone of emerging medical practices. Intelligent Pharmacy. 2025;14(3). 621-2.
16. Jafleh EA, Alnaqbi FA, Almaeeni HA, Faqeeh S, Alzaabi MA, Al Zaman K. The role of wearable devices in chronic disease monitoring and patient care: A comprehensive review. Cureus. 2024;16(9):e68921.
17. Rinzo L. (2024). Self-monitoring blood glucose: A vital tool for effective diabetes management. [online] Available from https://www.openaccessjournals.com/articles/selfmonitoring-blood-glucose-a-vital-tool-for-effective-diabetes-management-17853.html [Last accessed February, 2026].
18. Anjana RM, Kesavadev J, Neeta D, Tiwaskar M, Pradeepa R, Jebarani S, et al. A multicenter real-life study on the effect of flash glucose monitoring on glycemic control in patients with type 1 and type 2 diabetes. Diabetes Technol Ther. 2017;19(9):533-40.
19. Kalyanikar E; Times of India. (2025). No more affordable sugar monitor as pharma pulls back product. [online] Available from https://timesofindia.indiatimes.com/city/mumbai/no-more-affordable-sugar-monitor-as-pharma-pulls-back-product/articleshow/118689928.cms [Last accessed February, 2026].
20. Hospital Store. (2025). Insulin Pump price in India. [online]. Available from http://Hospitalstore.com [Last accessed February, 2026].
21. Ranjani H, Nitika S, Hariharan R, Charumeena H, Oliver N, Pradeepa R, et al. Systematic review and scientific rating of commercial apps available in India for diabetes prevention. J Diabetol. 2021;12(3):285-92.
22. Muralidharan S, Mohan V, Anjana RM, Jena S, Tandon N, Allender S, et al. Mobile health technology (mDiab) for the prevention of type 2

diabetes: Protocol for a randomized controlled trial. JMIR Res Protoc. 2017;6(12):e242.

23. Ranjani H, Avari P, Nitika S, Jagannathan N, Oliver N, Valabhji J, et al. Effectiveness of mobile health applications for cardiometabolic risk reduction in urban and rural India: A pilot, randomized controlled study. J Diabetes Sci Technol. 2025;19322968241310861.
24. BioSpectrumindia. (2022). Dr. Mohan's Diabetes launches AI enabled platforms for next gen diabetes care. [online] Available from https://www.biospectrumindia.com/news/98/22077/dr-mohans-diabetes-launches-ai-enabled-platforms-for-next-gen-diabetes-care.html [Last accessed February, 2026].
25. Jenkins AJ, Kodani N, Anjana RM, Ranjani H, Chow E, Cho YM, et al. Towards equitable access of innovative technologies such as continuous glucose monitoring and artificial intelligence for diabetes management. Diabetes Res Clin Pract. 2025;223(112157):112157.
26. Sanofi. (2023). The digital future of diabetes care. [online] Available from https://www.sanofi.com/en/magazine/your-health/the-digital-future-of-diabetes-care [Last accessed February, 2026].
27. Rana RK, Kapoor N, Kumar D, Verma M, Taneja G. Digital health revolution in India: Transforming health and medicine. Indian J Community Med. 2024;49(Suppl 2):S205-9.

CHAPTER 20

New Diabetes Care 2025

Anuj Maheshwari

ABSTRACT

The prevalence and complexity of diabetes mellitus are rising in both high- and low-income countries, making it a significant global health concern. A paradigm shift away from glucose-centric models and toward comprehensive, patient-centered care is highlighted by the New Diabetes Care 2025 framework. Pharmacotherapy advancements such as once-weekly basal insulins, glucagon-like peptide 1 receptor agonists (GLP-1 RAs), dual incretin therapies, and early sodium–glucose co-transporter 2 (SGLT-2) inhibitor initiation now target weight, cardiovascular, renal, and hepatic outcomes in addition to glycemia. Continuous glucose monitoring (CGM), hybrid closed-loop systems, telemedicine, and mobile health platforms are examples of digital technologies that have revolutionized self-management by improving glycemic stability and patient engagement. Personalized care is further supported by artificial intelligence (AI) through risk stratification for complications, integration of multimodal health data, and predictive models. Accessibility, affordability, infrastructure, and digital literacy issues still exist, though, especially in low- and middle-income (LMIC) nations, which emphasizes the need for solutions that prioritize equity. Though they need to be validated, standardized, and ethically protected, emerging fields like digital ecosystems, gene editing, and regenerative medicine have promise. In order to guarantee fair, efficient, and long-lasting management strategies, the future of diabetes care hinges on coordinating innovation with global systems-level initiatives.

Keywords: Diabetes care, continuous glucose monitoring, artificial intelligence, pharmacological innovation, digital health.

INTRODUCTION

Diabetes mellitus continues to be a crippling global epidemic, with a steadily rising prevalence in both developed and low- and middle-income (LMIC) nations. According to the International Diabetes Federation (IDF) Diabetes Atlas (2025), India has an estimated 89.8 million adults (20–79 years) living with diabetes, representing a prevalence of 9.5% (age-adjusted comparative prevalence: 10.5%). Alarmingly, around 43% of these cases remain undiagnosed, which equates to nearly 38.6 million people who are unaware of their condition.[1] Because of urbanization, changes in lifestyle, and socioeconomic transitions, India is experiencing the fastest increases in the burden **(Table 1)**. According to a systematic

TABLE 1: Risk factors for diabetes in India.

Category	*Key factors*
Genetic	Family history of T2DM, Asian Indian ethnicity (higher visceral adiposity at lower BMI)
Lifestyle	Sedentary behavior, unhealthy diet (refined carbohydrates, high glycemic load, processed foods)
Clinical	Obesity, central adiposity, hypertension, dyslipidemia, PCOS, history of GDM
Social determinants	Urbanization, low literacy, food insecurity, limited healthcare access

(BMI: body mass index; GDM: gestational diabetes; PCOS: polycystic ovary syndrome; T2DM: type 2 diabetes mellitus)

review by Deshpande et al. that analyzed 40 studies, the annual direct medical cost of diabetes care in India was estimated at ₹13,466.34, while the overall average annual cost per patient was ₹12,391.84. These findings underscore the significant economic burden of type 2 diabetes mellitus (T2DM) in India, with medications and hospitalization emerging as the primary cost drivers.[2]

Diabetes care has become more complicated in addition to being more common. In order to avoid microvascular problems like retinopathy, nephropathy, and neuropathy, management has traditionally concentrated on reaching glycemic targets. However, recent studies have shown that diabetes plays a major role in the development of mental health issues, liver dysfunction, macrovascular disease, and even some types of cancer.[3,4] As a result, the 2025 ADA Standards of Care emphasize the significance of all-encompassing management approaches that go beyond glycemia to encompass weight control, cardiometabolic health, psychological well-being, and health equity.[3]

Personalized care pathways are incorporating lifestyle frameworks, digital health technologies, and pharmaceutical advancements. Reducing treatment burden is the goal of once-weekly basal insulins, dual incretin therapies, and early sodium-glucose co-transporter-2 (SGLT-2) inhibitor use.[3,5] Self-management is changing as a result of telemedicine platforms, hybrid closed-loop insulin delivery, and continuous glucose monitoring (CGM).[3,4] At the same time, the guidelines emphasize social determinants of health, recognizing that inequalities in affordability and access continue to be major obstacles to global advancement.[1,4]

GLYCEMIC TARGETS

The recommended glycated hemoglobin (HbA1c) target is <7% for most nonpregnant adults to reduce the risk of microvascular complications,

TABLE 2: Individualization of glycemic targets.

Individual profile	*Target and rationale*
Young, newly diagnosed, low comorbidity	• *HbA1c:* ≤6.5% • Long-term prevention of complications
Middle-aged with ASCVD or CKD	• *HbA1c:* <7% • Balance of safety and protection from complications
Elderly, frail, multiple comorbidities	• *HbA1c:* <7.5–8% • Avoid hypoglycemia, preserve quality of life
Additional parameters	
Time in range (TIR)	>70%
Time above range (TAR)	<25%
Time below range (TBR)/ hypoglycemia	<4%

(ASCVD: atherosclerotic cardiovascular disease; CKD: chronic kidney disease; HbA1c: glycated hemoglobin)

while a stricter target of ≤6.5% may be considered in younger individuals with a shorter duration of diabetes, no significant comorbidities, and low risk of hypoglycemia. A more relaxed target of <7.5–8% is appropriate for older adults, those with long-standing diabetes, advanced complications, or significant comorbidities, where treatment risks outweigh benefits. Fasting plasma glucose targets are generally set at 80–130 mg/dL, and postprandial levels at <180 mg/dL **(Table 2)**.

DIABETES EPIDEMIOLOGY AND DISEASE BURDEN

Type 2 diabetes mellitus-related mortality has increased by more than 200% since 1990, according to recent global analyses. This sharp increase indicates a serious public health concern. This rise is concerningly becoming more noticeable among younger adult populations, a trend that is mostly attributable to fast urbanization and sedentary lifestyles.[6] The burden of T2DM is disproportionately felt by underprivileged groups, where socioeconomic stressors, poor food environments, and restricted access to healthcare all combine to increase prevalence and adverse consequences. These differences exacerbate the cycles of chronic illness and increase health disparities, highlighting the critical need for equity-focused interventions.[6]

Diabetes raises the risk of cardiovascular disease, causes progressive renal impairment, and deteriorates the nervous system, among other complications. With more hospital stays, longer-term treatment requirements, and a lower quality of life, these complications place a tremendous clinical, financial, and personal burden on patients as well as strain healthcare systems around the globe.[6]

Recent developments, such as artificial intelligence (AI) and CGM, are transforming diabetes care in order to address these epidemiologic and clinical issues. Real-time glucose insights are provided by CGM, and personalized glycemic management is made possible by AI-driven analytics, which enhances results and lowers the risk of complications. Additionally, cutting-edge techniques like transcutaneous auricular vagus nerve stimulation (taVNS), when combined with AI and CGM systems, hold promise for improving blood glucose regulation and comorbidity management through a customized, flexible approach.[7]

LIMITATIONS OF TRADITIONAL DIABETES METRICS: MOVING BEYOND GLYCATED HEMOGLOBIN

Despite being the gold standard for determining average glycemic control over a period of 2–3 months, HbA1c has a number of significant drawbacks:

- Fails to record transient glycemic changes that are clinically significant but obscured by the average HbA1c value, such as postprandial glucose spikes or nocturnal hypoglycemic episodes.[8,9]
- Glycemic variability is the term used to describe the intra- and interday fluctuations in blood sugar that lead to oxidative stress, endothelial dysfunction, and an elevated risk of micro- and macrovascular complications.[8,9]
- Nonglycemic variables that may affect HbA1c readings include changes in red blood cell lifespan brought on by anemia, hemoglobinopathies, renal disease, or recent blood loss.[8,9]

CONTINUOUS GLUCOSE MONITORING AND DIGITAL TECHNOLOGIES

Continuous Glucose Monitoring and Digital Ecosystems

By providing real-time, dynamic insights into glucose patterns, CGM has revolutionized diabetes care and greatly improved patient well-being and management:

- *Improved glycemic control:* CGM systems allow patients and healthcare professionals to quickly identify patterns, which reduces hypoglycemia episodes and improves glucose stability overall. Better time in range (TIR) and fewer glycemic excursions are correlated with these real-time metrics.[7]
- *Synergy with insulin delivery systems:* CGM makes hybrid closed-loop systems—often referred to as "artificial pancreas"—possible when combined with insulin pumps. By simulating the physiological insulin response, these systems automate insulin delivery based on glucose feedback, significantly raising TIR and reducing the risk of hypoglycemia.[7]
- *Emerging noninvasive and implantable technologies:* New developments include promising noninvasive tools that do away with the need for finger-stick sampling, which improves user comfort and adherence, and implantable sensors that provide long-term glucose monitoring without frequent skin pricks.[7]

- *Smartphone-enabled self-management:* Smartphone apps are becoming more and more integrated with CGM devices, enabling users to share data with healthcare providers, log meals and exercise, set alerts, and visualize trends. Patients are empowered, active self-management is encouraged, and dynamic patient–clinician collaboration is encouraged.[7]
- *Part of a broader digital ecosystem:* Nowadays, CGM is a single node in networks of digital health frameworks. Mobile apps, cloud-based platforms, and AI-driven analytics combine to form a clever ecosystem that provides tailored feedback, improving adherence, permitting lifestyle changes, and maximizing long-term results.[7]

The usefulness of CGM in the treatment of diabetes is becoming more and more clear. Regardless of the CGM modality or funding source, a 2024 meta-analysis of 28 randomized controlled trials (RCTs) showed that the use of CGM significantly improved HbA1c reduction, increased time-in-range, and decreased time above range.[10] CGM also improved glycemic outcomes, such as HbA1c, TIR, and TAR, in adults with T2DM.[11] However, open-label study designs and a lack of adequate complication data were mentioned. Building on this, a 2025 systematic review also emphasized how CGM helps individuals with T2DM improve their quality of life, reduce hypoglycemia, and improve glycemic control[12] **(Table 3)**.

TABLE 3: CGM and digital ecosystems.

Technology/innovation	*Impact/benefits*
CGM	Improves glycemic control, time-in-range, reduces hypoglycemia
Hybrid closed-loop systems	Simulates physiological insulin response, synergistic with CGM
Noninvasive/ implantable CGM	Enhanced comfort/ adherence, long-term monitoring
Smartphone and application integration	Data-sharing, trend visualization, alerts, active management
Digital health ecosystem	Integration of apps, cloud, AI for tailored feedback and improved outcomes

(AI: artificial intelligence; CGM: continuous glucose monitoring)

DIGITAL INNOVATIONS IN PATIENT EDUCATION AND SUPPORT

Through improving patient engagement, personalizing support, and encouraging peer-driven learning, digital health technologies are revolutionizing diabetes education and self-management:

- *Gamification and behavioral nudges:* Gamification techniques—points, badges, and motivational cues—are incorporated into mobile apps like mySugr to promote adherence to medication schedules, glucose monitoring, and lifestyle changes. These characteristics encourage behavior change and reinforce consistent self-management by transforming mundane tasks into interesting challenges.[7]
- *Integrated data platforms for lifestyle adjustment:* In addition to gamification, mobile platforms compile health data from multiple sources, such as patient-reported outcomes, dietary logs, wearables, and CGM. Through this integration, patients and physicians can reduce cardiovascular and metabolic risks by implementing real-time lifestyle changes, customizing interventions, and dynamically monitoring trends.[7,13]
- *Peer-led education and online communities:* Community-based engagement is becoming more and more important in digital ecosystems, as social networks and

platforms facilitate the sharing of knowledge between patients. In order to maintain behavior change in real-world situations, peer-led education, shared experiences, and emotional support are all fostered by online forums and digital hubs. These peer groups improve long-term treatment plan adherence, foster accountability, and lessen feelings of loneliness.[7,14]

- *Toward personalized digital education:* AI-driven adaptive education platforms, which customize instructional materials to each patient's unique profile, literacy level, and behavioral patterns, are another promising development in recent years. These developments complement the larger framework of personalized diabetes care by moving beyond generic educational materials to precision education.[13]

The substantial influence of digital health technologies on the treatment of diabetes is demonstrated by recent data. A 2022 systematic review highlighted the clinical advantages of digital self-management by showing that diabetes-specific mobile health apps and digital tools successfully decreased HbA1c across type 1 diabetes mellitus (T1DM), T2DM, and prediabetes.[15] To elaborate, a 2025 narrative review of 86 studies found that telemedicine, mobile applications, automated insulin delivery, and CGM significantly enhanced glycemic control and assisted in the management of complications associated with diabetes.[16] Similarly, digital health interventions in T2DM home-based care improved body mass index and blood glucose levels, according to a 2025 meta-analysis.[17]

ARTIFICIAL INTELLIGENCE: TRANSFORMING DIABETES CARE

- *AI-driven predictive models for risk and complication:* With over 80% accuracy in predicting the onset of the disease, its complications, and the response to treatment across a variety of patient populations, AI and machine learning (ML) are transforming predictive modeling in diabetes. These systems provide actionable insights that were previously unavailable through conventional statistical methods by analyzing complex multimodal datasets from wearable sensors, genomics, imaging, and electronic health records (EHRs).[18]
- *ML and deep learning approaches:* Strong predictive performance is shown for diabetes onset, cardiovascular and renal complications, and progression risk by algorithms like random forests, convolutional neural networks (CNNs), and long short-term memory (LSTM) networks. Clinicians can prioritize patients who would benefit most from intensive preventive interventions by using these models to generate early risk alerts by learning hidden temporal and spatial data patterns.[18]
- *Personalized risk stratification:* In order to accurately detect glycemic variability and other metabolic trends, recent frameworks combine wearable sensor data (such as activity trackers and CGM) with AI-driven analytics. This supports individualized management plans by enabling dynamic treatment adjustments and customized complication risk profiles.[7]
- *Patient-centered predictive ecosystems:* In order to facilitate real-time alerts and feedback loops between patients and clinicians, digital ecosystems are increasingly integrating predictive AI tools into telehealth services and mobile platforms. By improving patient involvement, adherence, and collaborative decision-making, these innovations facilitate the transition from reactive to proactive healthcare.[14]

In a variety of clinical settings, AI is becoming a potent instrument for improving diabetes care. Although there are still obstacles to clinical implementation, a 2025 systematic review on gestational diabetes found that AI models, in particular ML techniques, have great potential to improve prediction, screening, and management.[19] Similar to this, a 2025 review of ML models in diabetic kidney disease found that while these tools can enhance risk prediction, there are still issues because of variable methodological quality and a lack of external validation.[20] In support of personalized medicine and early intervention strategies, a 2024 review emphasized the increasing role of AI in predicting individual risk for T2DM and associated complications.[21]

Integration of Artificial Intelligence into Comprehensive Diabetes Ecosystems

Interoperability between CGM, insulin pumps, wearable technology, and smartphones is necessary for seamless diabetes management. The siloed nature of current device ecosystems restricts data integration and personalization. Semantic exchange of glucose, activity, sleep, and medication data is made possible by emerging standards like IEEE P1752 and FHIR (Fast Healthcare Interoperability Resources). By guaranteeing consistent data structures, these frameworks promote AI-driven personalization, improve clinical integration, and ease multicenter research. Interoperability is a crucial requirement for scaling digital and AI-enabled diabetes care.[7]

Concerns about algorithmic bias, privacy, and social equity are particular to AI-driven care. The risk of demographic disparities is decreased by federated learning and adversarial debiasing, and policy development prioritizes patient data protection and fair access to digital therapies, particularly for LMIC groups. Investments in infrastructure and digital literacy programs are required to optimize the benefits for all communities.[7] A key component of improving results is patient involvement. Adherence and glycemic control are greatly enhanced by digital self-management through interactive apps, voice assistants, and gamification when combined with AI analysis. Community-based initiatives that use aggregated data, customized educational materials, and peer mentoring empower people and contribute to the development of dynamic feedback cycles for technological improvement.[14]

Artificial intelligence and digital integration in diabetes care present both opportunities and challenges, according to recent reviews. A 2024 systematic review described developments in AI for diabetes prediction, emphasizing datasets, algorithms, and assessment techniques while stressing the significance of bias minimization and ethical implementation.[22] Similar to this, a 2025 systematic review discussed how AI can improve diabetes management, diagnosis, and prevention. It noted better results but also emphasized important concerns like infrastructure requirements, privacy, and equity.[23] These viewpoints were supported by a different 2025 review that emphasized the need for interoperability and standardized frameworks to guarantee the smooth integration of wearable technology, insulin pumps, and CGM into digital diabetes care.[16]

PHARMACOLOGICAL INNOVATION

Diabetes pharmacotherapy has changed significantly, now addressing weight control, heart protection, and metabolic health in addition to lowering blood sugar.

- *Glucagon-like peptide 1 receptor agonists (GLP-1 RAs):* In many cases of T2DM, especially in those with obesity or preexisting cardiovascular disease, GLP-1 RAs are now regarded as first-line therapy.[3,4] Agents such as semaglutide have demonstrated significant reductions in major adverse cardiovascular events, while also promoting weight loss of up to 15% in some trials.[5] In recognition of the wide-ranging metabolic advantages, the

American Diabetes Association (ADA) 2025 guidelines extend their use to people with metabolic dysfunction-associated steatotic liver disease (MASLD).[3]

- *Dual incretin therapies [glucose-dependent insulinotropic polypeptide (GIP)/GLP-1 RAs)]:* A paradigm shift has been brought about by tirzepatide, the first dual GIP/GLP-1 RA. With mean weight reductions of over 20% in certain populations, clinical trials like SURMOUNT and SURPASS have shown greater efficacy than GLP-1 RAs alone.[4] The medication's potential to improve liver histology and heart failure outcomes in MASLD extends beyond diabetes.[5]
- *SGLT-2 inhibitors:* Once thought of as adjunctive glucose-lowering agents, SGLT-2 inhibitors are now given priority early in the course of treatment.[3,4] They decrease cardiovascular mortality, decrease heart failure hospitalization, and offer strong renal protection.[24] Their systemic impact is highlighted by the fact that their benefits are extended to nondiabetic populations with heart failure and chronic kidney disease.[24]
- *Emerging therapies*: Once-weekly basal insulins, which are part of the 2025 pipeline, are intended to lessen the treatment burden related to daily injections.[3] Although there are still issues with bioavailability, oral insulin formulations are being studied.[25] Additional experimental agents include fibroblast growth factor analogues for metabolic disease and thyroid hormone receptor-β agonists, such as resmetirom, which target liver fat and fibrosis.[3]
- *Individualized therapy:* Treatment choices are influenced by a number of factors, including patient preference, cultural background, comorbidities, cost, and hypoglycemia risk.[3] Single-pill, fixed-dose combination regimens are becoming more structured to maximize results while reducing complexity, although polypharmacy is still a challenge.[4]

Large RCTs and meta-analyses continue to be the main sources of evidence in pharmacological innovation. GLP-1 RAs and dual GIP/GLP-1 agonists have been shown in recent meta-analyses to be superior in terms of weight loss and cardiovascular protection.[5] Similarly, SGLT-2 inhibitors have been shown in meta-analyses between 2023 and 2025 to consistently show significant reductions in cardiovascular and renal risk, thereby confirming their role as a crucial therapeutic class in the management of diabetes **(Table 4)**.

TABLE 4: Diabetes management.

Drug class/insulin type	*Mechanism of action*	*Advantages*	*Common side effects*	*Typical uses*
Biguanides	Decreases hepatic glucose production, improves insulin sensitivity	Weight neutral, low risk of hypoglycemia, inexpensive	GI upset, lactic acidosis (rare)	First-line drug for T2DM
Sulfonylureas	Stimulates pancreatic beta cells to secrete insulin	Rapid action, effective glucose lowering, low cost	Hypoglycemia, weight gain	Add-on therapy when metformin inadequate, cost-sensitive settings
Meglitinides	Stimulates rapid, short insulin release from pancreas	Short-acting, useful for postprandial glucose control	Hypoglycemia, weight gain, frequent dosing	Alternative to sulfonylureas for postmeal glucose spikes

Contd...

Contd...

Drug class/insulin type	*Mechanism of action*	*Advantages*	*Common side effects*	*Typical uses*
Thiazolidinediones (TZDs)	Improves insulin sensitivity in muscle and fat, reduces hepatic glucose output	Durable effect, improves insulin resistance, low hypoglycemia risk	Weight gain, edema, heart failure (HF) risk, bone fractures	Selected cases with marked insulin resistance (younger/obese patients)
DPP-4 inhibitors	Prevents breakdown of incretin hormones, increases insulin release post-meals	Weight neutral, low risk of hypoglycemia, well tolerated	Nasopharyngitis, headache, joint pain	Commonly used as add-on to metformin, safe in elderly
SGLT-2 inhibitors	Increases glucose excretion in urine by blocking renal glucose reabsorption	Weight loss, BP reduction, cardiovascular and renal benefits	Genital infections, urinary tract infections, dehydration, ketoacidosis (rare)	Preferred add-on in patients with ASCVD, HF, CKD; urban centers
Alpha-glucosidase inhibitors	Delays carbohydrate digestion and absorption in the gut	Targets postprandial hyperglycemia, low systemic effects	Flatulence, diarrhea, abdominal bloating	Adjunct for postprandial hyperglycemia
GLP-1 receptor agonists (GLP-1 RA)	Mimics incretin hormones, enhances insulin secretion, suppresses glucagon, slows gastric-emptying	Potent HbA1c reduction, weight loss, CV and renal benefits	GI intolerance (nausea, vomiting), rare pancreatitis, injectable route (except oral semaglutide)	Add-on in overweight/obese patients; CV/renal risk; high-cost limits widespread use
Dual incretin agonists (tirzepatide)	Dual action on GLP-1 and GIP receptors; enhances insulin secretion, reduces appetite, promotes weight loss	Superior glucose lowering, marked weight loss, CV/metabolic benefits	GI side effects, nausea, potential cost issues, injectable	Emerging option in India; strong efficacy for obese/poorly controlled T2DM
Rapid-acting insulin	Onset 10–20 minutes, peak 1–3 hours; controls postmeal spikes (e.g., Lispro, Aspart)	Mimics physiological insulin response, flexible dosing	Hypoglycemia, weight gain if overdosed	Used before/during meals to manage postprandial hyperglycemia
Short-acting insulin	Onset 30–60 minutes, peak 2–4 hours; short-term prandial control (e.g., Regular insulin)	Low cost, reliable prandial control	Hypoglycemia, weight gain	Used in hospital/ICU or as part of premix regimens
Intermediate-acting insulin	Onset 2–4 hours, peak 6–12 hours; basal coverage (e.g., NPH)	Once/twice daily dosing, inexpensive option for basal needs	Nocturnal hypoglycemia, weight gain	Affordable basal insulin in resource-limited settings

Contd...

Contd...

Drug class/insulin type	*Mechanism of action*	*Advantages*	*Common side effects*	*Typical uses*
Long-acting insulin	Onset 1–2 hours, minimal peak, duration ~24 hours; steady basal insulin (e.g., glargine, detemir, degludec)	Stable basal control, reduced hypoglycemia risk, convenient	Hypoglycemia (less than NPH), injection site reactions	Standard basal insulin for long-term therapy
Premixed insulin	Premixed ratios of short/intermediate insulin; covers both basal and meals (e.g., Mixtard, Humalog Mix)	Convenient dosing, widely used in India, covers basal + bolus	Hypoglycemia risk, weight gain	Commonly prescribed in India for convenience and affordability

(ASCVD: atherosclerotic cardiovascular disease; CKD: chronic kidney disease; CV: cardiovascular; DPP-4: dipeptidyl peptidase 4; GI: gastrointestinal; GIP: glucose-dependent insulinotropic polypeptide; GLP-1: glucagon-like peptide 1; HbA1c: glycated hemoglobin; ICU: intensive care unit; NPH: neutral protamine Hagedorn; SGLT-2: sodium–glucose co-transporter 2; T2DM: type 2 diabetes mellitus)

FUTURE HORIZONS

The treatment of diabetes is about to undergo revolutionary breakthroughs rather than merely incremental innovation.

- *Persistent gaps:* The inclusion of high-risk and underserved populations (such as children, older adults, and pregnant women), accurate diagnostics, and worldwide access to cutting-edge care and technologies are among the main areas lacking.[26]
- *Implementation challenges:* Infrastructure, education, and disparities often make new therapies (such as digital health tools and automated insulin delivery) expensive, complicated, and limited in their practical application, particularly in LMIC nations.[27]
- *Therapy-specific barriers:* Although stem cell and gene therapies are progressing, their practical widespread adoption is limited by issues with safety, scalability, and immunological rejection.[26]
- *Technology gaps:* In order to be accessible to all populations, next-generation technology (automated insulin delivery, AI, and digital twins) must better support a variety of daily routines, automate responses (meals, exercise), and protect patient privacy.[26]
- *Equity and access*: Global treatment disparities are still growing, and concerted efforts are needed to increase the accessibility, affordability, and digital literacy of cutting-edge therapies for disadvantaged populations.[27]

CONCLUSION

Harmonizing clinical innovation with systems-level commitment to affordability, accessibility, and ongoing education will be essential to making meaningful progress as diabetes prevalence and complexity continue to rise. With interdisciplinary cooperation and consistent international investment, the goal for 2025 and beyond is a future in which all people with diabetes receive comprehensive, efficient, and equitable care.

REFERENCES

1. International Diabetes Federation. IDF Diabetes Atlas, 11th edition. Brussels: International Diabetes Federation; 2025.
2. Deshpande PR, Jadhav S. Economic Burden of Type 2 Diabetes Mellitus in India with

Bibliometic and Quality Analysis of Studies: A Systematic Review. Med J Dr. DY Patil Vidyapeeth. 2025;18(3):412-30.
3. American Diabetes Association Professional Practice Committee. Summary of Revisions: Standards of Care in Diabetes-2025. Diabetes Care. 2025;48(1 Suppl 1):S6-S13.
4. ADA Newsroom. (2024). American Diabetes Association Releases Standards of Care in Diabetes—2025. [online] Available from https://diabetes.org/newsroom/press-releases/american-diabetes-association-releases-standards-care-diabetes-2025 [Last accessed March 2026].
5. Jastreboff AM, Aronne LJ, Ahmad NN, Wharton S, Connery L, Alves B, et al. Tirzepatide once weekly for the treatment of obesity. N Engl J Med. 2022;387(3):205-16.
6. American Diabetes Association Professional Practice Committee. 2. Diagnosis and Classification of Diabetes: Standards of Care in Diabetes-2025. Diabetes Care. 2025;48(1 Suppl 1):S27-S49.
7. Zhang K, Qi Y, Wang W, Tian X, Wang J, Xu L, et al. Future horizons in diabetes: integrating AI and personalized care. Front Endocrinol (Lausanne). 2025;16:1583227.
8. Huang JH, Lin YK, Lee TW, Liu HW, Chien YM, Hsueh YC, et al. Correlation between short- and mid-term hemoglobin A1c and glycemic control determined by continuous glucose monitoring. Diabetol Metab Syndr. 2021;13(1):94.
9. Chehregosha H, Khamseh ME, Malek M, Hosseinpanah F, Ismail-Beigi F. A view beyond HbA1c: role of continuous glucose monitoring. Diabetes Ther. 2019;10(3):853-63.
10. Tan YY, Suan E, Koh GC, Suhairi SB, Tyagi S. Effectiveness of continuous glucose monitoring in patient management of Type 2 Diabetes Mellitus: an umbrella review of systematic reviews from 2011 to 2024. Arch Public Health. 2024;82(1):1-23.
11. Jancev M, Vissers TA, Visseren FL, van Bon AC, Serné EH, DeVries JH, et al. Continuous glucose monitoring in adults with type 2 diabetes: a systematic review and meta-analysis. Diabetologia. 2024;67(5):798-810.
12. Barchiesi MA, Calabrese A, Costa R, Di Pillo F, D'Uffizi A, Tiburzi L, et al. Continuous glucose monitoring in type 2 diabetes: a systematic review of barriers and opportunities for care improvement. Int J Qual Health Care. 2025;37(3):mzaf046.
13. Sabari VD, Brindha GR, Veeraragavan PD, Sathya A, Thiruvengadam M. Personalized lifestyle recommendations for improved diabetes management leveraging machine learning. Biomed Signal Process Control. 2025;108:107983.
14. González-Rivas JP, Seyedi SA, Mechanick JI. Artificial intelligence enabled lifestyle medicine in diabetes care: A narrative review. Am J Lifestyle Med. 2025;15598276251359185.
15. Stevens S, Gallagher S, Andrews T, Ashall-Payne L, Humphreys L, Leigh S. The effectiveness of digital health technologies for patients with diabetes mellitus: a systematic review. Front Clin Diabetes Healthc. 2022;3:936752.
16. Maida E, Caruso P, Bonavita S, Abbadessa G, Miele G, Longo M, et al. Digital Health in Diabetes Care: A Narrative Review from Monitoring to the Management of Systemic and Neurologic Complications. J Clin Med. 2025;14(12):4240.
17. Xiao Y, Wang Z, Zhang L, Xie N, Chen F, Song Z, et al. Effectiveness of digital diabetes management technology on blood glucose in patients with type 2 diabetes at home: Systematic review and meta-analysis. J Med Internet Res. 2025;27:e66441.
18. Adetunji O, Evah PT. Developing personalized diabetes management plans using artificial intelligence and machine learning. World J Adv Res Rev. 2025;27(2):605-24.
19. AlSaad R, Elhenidy A, Tabassum A, Odeh N, AboArqoub E, Odeh A, et al. Artificial Intelligence in Gestational Diabetes Care: A Systematic Review. J Diabetes Sci Technol. 2025;19322968251355967.
20. Li Y, Jin N, Zhan Q, Huang Y, Sun A, Yin F, et al. Machine learning-based risk predictive models for diabetic kidney disease in type 2 diabetes mellitus patients: A systematic review and meta-analysis. Front Endocrinol (Lausanne). 2025;16:1495306.
21. Wang SC, Nickel G, Venkatesh KP, Raza MM, Kvedar JC. AI-based diabetes care: Risk prediction models and implementation concerns. NPJ Digit Med. 2024;7(1):36.
22. Khokhar PB, Gravino C, Palomba F. Advances in artificial intelligence for diabetes prediction: insights from a systematic literature review. Artif Intell Med. 2025;103132.

23. Khalifa M, Albadawy M. Artificial intelligence for diabetes: Enhancing prevention, diagnosis, and effective management. Comput Methods Programs Biomed Update. 2024;5:100141.
24. Zinman B, Wanner C, Lachin JM, Fitchett D, Bluhmki E, Hantel S, et al.; EMPA-REG OUTCOME Investigators. Empagliflozin, cardiovascular outcomes, and mortality in type 2 diabetes. N Engl J Med. 2015;373:2117-28.
25. Eckhardt J. (2025). Emerging Breakthroughs in Diabetes Treatment: A New Era of Hope. [online] Available from https://www.forbes.com/sites/juergeneckhardt/2025/03/18/emerging-breakthroughs-in-diabetes-treatment-a-new-era-of-hope/ [Last accessed March 2026].
26. Jacobs PG, Levy CJ, Brown SA, Riddell MC, Cinar A, Boughton CK, et al. Research Gaps, Challenges, and Opportunities in Automated Insulin Delivery Systems. J Diabetes Sci Technol. 2025;19(4):937-49.
27. Iacobucci G. Diabetes: Global treatment gap is widening, study finds. BMJ. 2024;387:q2515.

Index

Page numbers followed by *f* refer to figure, *fc* refer to flowchart, and *t* refer to table.

C

D

E

F

I

J

K

L

M

N

O

P

Q

R

S